YOUR PERSONALITY PRESCRIPTION

YOUR PERSONALITY PRESCRIPTION

OPTIMAL HEALTH THROUGH PERSONALITY PROFILING

Roberta Schwartz Wennik, M.S., R.D.

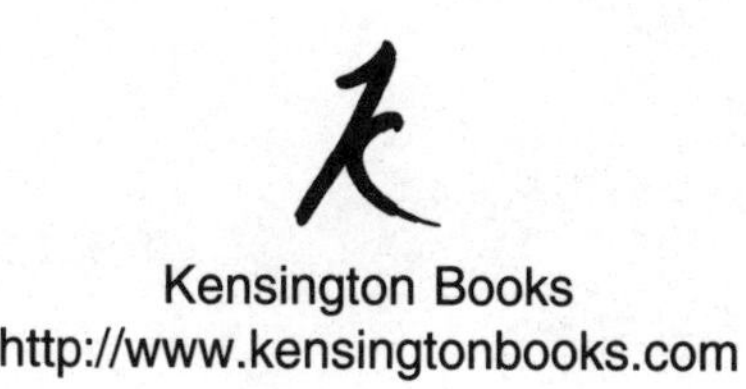

Kensington Books
http://www.kensingtonbooks.com

The names of people in this book have been changed to protect their privacy and anonymity. Myers-Briggs Type Indicator® and MBTI® are registered trademarks of Consulting Psychologists Press, Inc.

This book is intended for informational purposes, not as a substitute for the medical advice of a physician. Because nutritional needs vary from individual to individual based on age, gender, height, weight, and health status, it may be beneficial for you to consult a registered dietitian. The author and publisher disclaim any liability arising directly or indirectly from the use of this book.

KENSINGTON BOOKS are published by

Kensington Publishing Corp.
850 Third Avenue
New York, NY 10022

ISBN 1-57566-401-1

First Printing: April, 1999
10 9 8 7 6 5 4 3 2 1

Printed in the United States of America

To Larry—my husband, friend, and everlasting love
For all your help, support, and encouragement

and

To Debbie, Shari, and Muffy—who make my life complete

Acknowledgments

Not until you have written a book do you realize how many people contribute to the process and make it what it is. My appreciation to all who were involved reaches far beyond the words on this page.

I am very fortunate to have had Tracy Bernstein as my editor. She has the perfect *personality prescription* for the job, having brought to it not only insight and guidance but an eye for detail that added immeasurably to the book. *Your Personality Prescription* became richer because her ISTJ personality type saw things from a different perspective than my ENFJ viewpoint. Her good-natured attitude made working with her a delight. Thank you, Tracy! Best of all, I now have a new friend with whom I share something special—the delivery of our two "babies": my book and her daughter.

I also want to express heartfelt thanks to Judith Riven, my literary agent, who made it possible to work with Tracy and Kensington Publishing. Because of her belief in this book, it is now a reality.

Many other people deserve my thanks—my clients, who proved personality profiling *does* work in changing your habits; my friends, who helped pretest the Personality Profile Questionnaire and provided valuable input; and my colleagues, who encouraged me with this book because they could see the value of it for their own practices.

Contents

Introduction

This is the book for you if you:

1. Didn't lose weight on that last diet you tried
2. Did lose weight but gained it back
3. Weren't able to stick to the exercise program you started
4. Never could get yourself started on an exercise program
5. Let stressful situations in your life get to you and couldn't relax, no matter how hard you tried
6. Have habits you want to change but haven't yet found the right method *to* change

I'm sure you could add to the list. I want to say up front: *You* have not failed. The approach you've taken has failed you!

Let me repeat that: **You have not failed. The approach you've taken has failed you!** Keep that in mind as we search for what *is* the right way for you.

When you see people changing their habits successfully, you probably assume that they are stronger than you—that they have the willpower and determination you lack. They seem to exude confidence. What they've got that you don't is the *right approach,* one that fits them like comfortable shoes. You, too, can have that confidence, if you read on.

Many people embark on a journey of losing weight and improving their lifestyle habits, but few of them arrive at their destination. As people get older and "wider," they longingly remember how good they used to look and how well their clothes used to fit. They jokingly allude to some unknown phenomenon in their closet that is shrinking their clothes. They know all too well, when huffing and puffing up a flight of stairs, how out-of-shape they have become. When their friends nickname them "Spud" because of the couch potato they have become, they think about dusting off the athletic club membership card they haven't used since they joined the year before.

Maybe you're saying to yourself, "You wouldn't believe how many times I have tried to lose weight and change my habits. If there was a new diet on the market, I was on it. If there was a new miracle food, I ate it. If there was a new piece of exercise equipment, I bought it. While I experienced some success with everything I tried, before I knew it, I was back where I started." Then there are some people who cannot even claim any level of success. "Put a donut in front of me and I'm a goner (and so is the donut!)." "I would get the latest book on how to relax, but then get stressed out because I never got around to reading it!" Sound familiar?

As a nutrition consultant, I hear similar stories from many of my clients. They fervently want to change their habits so they can lose weight and improve their health. They know that their bad habits are leading them down a road of self-destruction. When they look at themselves in the mirror, they assess their character in terms of their weight and berate themselves for "letting themselves go" like that. Of course, not looking good in their clothes is minor in comparison to what carrying around excess weight can do to their health. If they don't already have high cholesterol, high blood pressure, or blood sugars that are out of control, being overweight can lead to these conditions—and then on to the development of diabetes, heart disease, high blood pressure, stroke, and a host of other problems.

Something's Wrong Here

When counseling my clients, I used to take a different approach than I do now. We would discuss their goals and what they wanted to achieve, and, after taking a medical and diet history, I would develop an eating and exercise plan for them. They would also get a weekly assignment to help them incorporate the new knowledge they were receiving. At the end of two to three months, my clients were normally well on their way to achieving their goals. They would continue with me for some months after they had reached their goal to make sure they could maintain what they had accomplished. After that, it was time for them to go it on their own.

When some of my clients were back on my doorstep nine months to a year later, I found it puzzling and disconcerting. They shared with me how good they had been at first, practicing everything they had learned. But slowly they found themselves falling back into their old habits. I felt bad for them and wondered what had gone wrong. Why were *these* people having problems when my other clients were maintaining their new lifestyle habits?

I questioned what had gone wrong. Did the *approach* I had taken with these clients fail them in some way? Or did they fail themselves? While under my care, they fully participated in the process and achieved their goals. One would assume, then, that the approach itself was beneficial. But something was happening when they were on their own. What was it?

Nor was this scenario something that was happening only to my clients. When we look at the track record of the weight-loss industry as a whole, the rate of relapse is staggering. The easy excuse is to blame the individuals, and conclude that they are simply weak-willed. However, you have to ask yourself why anyone would go through all the effort to achieve a health goal (such as losing weight or lowering blood cholesterol), and then, once the goal is reached, let it slip away. I realized that something deeper must be causing the problem.

When my returning clients and I tried to analyze what had gone wrong, a common theme began to appear: It seemed they had looked at the goals they set as *end points.* Once the goal was achieved, they felt they could give up the method they had used to get there. This often felt like a great relief because, in order to reach their goals, they had relied on sheer willpower—with all its connotations of self-denial and strict self-control. Not wanting to let me down or embarrass themselves, they did what it took to reach their goal and get that proverbial gold star—and then collapsed!

Willpower takes a diligence most of us cannot maintain. It's a short-term Band-Aid® that can eventually backfire, sending people retreating to their old habits with a vengeance. If *you* have tried using willpower, you know the feeling of sacrificing, of giving something up, but missing it all the more. Finally, under the strain of being on your guard every moment and worrying that you will return to your old ways, you inevitably do. Using willpower often results in your sabotaging your good work.

Reminding myself that not all my clients were reverting to their old ways, I had to ask: What was working for some of them—enabling them to maintain their new approach to eating, exercise, and stress-reduction—that was *not* working for the others?

An Interesting Discovery

As luck would have it, about the same time some of my clients were returning to me, I was introduced to *psychological type.* It was developed by the Swiss psychologist, Carl Jung, and later elaborated by two women, Isabel Myers and her mother, Katharine Briggs, who had been studying Jung's theories for some time. What interested them was how we use our mind, our values, and our feelings in the everyday business of living. With so much information available for the taking and so many decisions to make every day, something within us must be guiding us in the process. They saw this guiding force as our personality, with its many facets coloring our lives and influencing our behaviors. In order to find out what those facets were, Myers and Briggs developed a questionnaire, the Myers-Briggs Type Indicator® (MBTI®). Using it, they were able to group people into sixteen different types according to their characteristics and values.

Psychological type, also referred to as personality type, has been used for a long time to help people discover appropriate career paths and improve their communications and relationships. To my knowledge, it has never been used to help people change their lifestyle habits and, in turn, to help them lose weight, lower their blood cholesterol, stabilize their blood sugars, reduce their risk of disease, increase their energy, and generally feel their best. With that in mind, I started to explore, from the perspective of psychological type, the reason some clients were returning.

It dawned on me that the health and weight-loss program I gave all of my clients worked for the successful ones simply because it *matched their personality*. They were able to comfortably make changes that were compatible with their personality and then maintain those changes. Those who had experienced relapse had failed because the program was not a good fit with their personalities.

In the course of helping an individual lose weight, lower blood cholesterol, stabilize blood glucose, or optimize wellness, health-care professionals tend to tailor the health program to that person's physical needs by adjusting calorie levels, teaching about appropriate food choices, and proposing some sort of exercise regimen that fits the individual's capability. However, the basic weekly approach or plan used to make the necessary changes is usually the same for everyone (for example, telling each person to keep a daily food and exercise diary). If your personality favors the approach, the chances are you will achieve your goals. If not, you're back to blaming yourself for being a failure.

Once I made personality profiling part of my practice, I realized that "one plan does not fit all." Due to our differing personality types, not everyone feels comfortable keeping food diaries, hanging pictures on the refrigerator of how they want to look when they have lost weight, keeping track of the number of fat grams they are eating, or scheduling an appointment with themselves each day to relax. Some people can't take that much structure, while others can. Some people need greater variety in their choices than others. Some people want to be shown the way, while others need to do it their own way.

What's the Right Plan?

If you were to do a survey of the people with a healthy lifestyle, you would find that they are not all doing the same thing. They don't all eat the same things or exercise the same way. To paraphrase the title of the Frank Sinatra song, "They do it their way." And their way utilizes their personality to make the choices that are right for them. Now you, too, can do it your way with the help of this book. There *is* a right approach for you. You will find out what your personality type is and how it has contributed to:

1. Eating for the wrong reasons
2. Eating too much and not the right foods
3. Avoiding exercise and opting for a sedentary lifestyle
4. Letting stress run your life instead of being in control

The exciting part comes when you learn how to use the different components of your personality type to make a healthy lifestyle a habit. Then losing that extra weight, maintaining the loss, having more energy, and literally feeling like a new person will come naturally.

This is an approach that will last you a lifetime. It isn't a quick fix; it's a permanent fix. That's because you will be discovering ways to eat, exercise, and relax that work with *your* personality type, *your* way of life, *your* needs. You were born with your personality type and it will be with you until you die. Therefore, it just makes good sense to make changes to your habits in a way that is compatible with your personality. Then those changes are yours for the rest of your life. You will say about your new lifestyle approach, just as did Cinderella when she tried on the glass slipper, that "It fits perfectly." (And don't forget, Cinderella lived happily ever after!)

PART I

YOU AND YOUR PERSONALITY

1

Know Where You're Headed and Why

This could be your first attempt or your hundredth attempt to improve your lifestyle habits, but I'm confident it will be your last. This time you are going to do it differently. Hopefully you really feel ready this time. While motivation gives you the *why* of embarking on the journey, commitment gives you the *staying power* to see your journey to its end. It's the fuel to reach your goal. Your personality is the *vehicle* you will use to find the best means to get there.

Appreciate that this journey you're about to start will take time. Change should be a gradual process. Overnight change is quickly followed by overnight relapse. It probably took you years to form the habits you have. Therefore you need to give yourself time to become accustomed to new ways of doing things. Think about the piano player who must first learn the notes on the piano, then practice scales, before moving on to playing concertos. The more the pianist practices, the more comfortable he or she feels with the instrument and the more adept at playing it. Eventually, little thought need be given to the mechanics of playing. That is the way habit changes take place.

Keep in mind that while the destination of your journey is important, the journey itself is every bit as important. I suppose I could tell you exactly what to do, step by step, to reach your destination (and there may be some of you who would be very content with that). However, how prepared will you be if something comes along that I never addressed? Using your personality to determine what works for you is in keeping with an ancient Chinese saying that goes:

Give a man a fish, and you feed him for a day.
Teach a man how to fish and you feed him for a lifetime.

As you learn to use your personality to make lifestyle habit changes, you will be feeding yourself for a lifetime. It should be an enjoyable and comfortable process. Otherwise, you're doomed from the start because you will have to rely on sheer willpower to get the job done.

You Must Be "Myth-taken"

Myth #1: All It Takes Is Willpower

Most people use methods to reach their goals that they would never consider using for a lifetime. They figure that they can discontinue them once they arrive at their destination. That's why they are amenable to using willpower, accepting that—for a short while—they will be denying themselves certain things and having to be in absolute control of themselves. The less people perceive themselves as being able to change, the more strongly they employ willpower.

Using willpower implies that we have to avoid "forbidden fruits"—which, by most people's definition, includes everything they like that isn't healthy. That would mean eliminating chocolate, ice cream, steak, butter, lazing around watching television, . . . (I'm sure you could add to the list!) The problem with this thinking is that it won't last a lifetime. I have to be honest with you. I'm not willing to give up chocolate for the rest of my life unless a doctor tells me I must.

You may mistakenly believe that those who are able to avoid these forbidden fruits are naturally strong-willed while you, who may succumb to them, are weak-willed. It could well be that they have already made the difficult behavior change and so appear strong. You may feel weak because you have tried to change some behaviors and have failed. Once you learn how to use your personality to make decisions, however, nothing need be forbidden unless your doctor has told you to eliminate certain foods from your diet or to avoid certain exercise. Barring such medical prohibitions, you can make constructive decisions based on what you've already eaten for the day, what will fit into your daily nutrient allowances, whether you plan to exercise to burn a few extra calories, and many other issues. When you do decide to have something, it definitely won't be because you were weak-willed. While I believe that nothing should be off-limits, I do believe that everything should be done within a defined context of your needs, which we will discuss in Part II.

One of the main disadvantages of using willpower is that, instead of responding to the needs of your body, you are implementing the dictates of some eating or exercise plan. Let's say you've read or were told that you should not snack between meals. Three meals a day should be more than sufficient food, so it says. Yet, you find that by midmorning your stomach is growling. Your body is sending you a message, but you will "show it who's boss" and use willpower to get you through. Maybe you manage not to eat anything, but you make up for it at lunchtime by stuffing yourself. With your body being such a smart machine, you really should take the time to listen to what it has to say. The conflict arises when your mind and emotions get involved in the process, so that you no longer react naturally to your bodily needs.

This book will help you find a way that works with your personality, so that the process of change is also the process of living. There is less likelihood of relapse when the way you change becomes a part of you, a natural and effortless approach.

It isn't willpower you need to employ in your pursuit of healthy habits. It's conscious awareness. It's keeping your eye on your target at all times. By constantly checking and rechecking your strategies and moves, making sure they are in line with your goal, you can reach your goal. Some people find that willpower makes them more conscious of what they are doing. Unfortunately, that usually lasts only until the rubber band of willpower stretches so tightly it breaks.

Myth #2: The Changes Will Never Last

I'm sure that many of you are asking yourself why this time should be any different than all your other attempts at making changes. There could be many reasons why your previous attempts failed. Maybe you weren't ready the last time you tried to change your unhealthy lifestyle habits. Think back and ask yourself whether you tried changing because you wanted it or someone else wanted it for you. The only change that is going to endure is one *you* really want.

Another reason you might think the change won't last is that previously you were attacking the symptoms of the problem, not the problem itself. For example, Stephanie had gained quite a bit of weight when she was going through an emotionally trying time with her boyfriend. She had turned to food for comfort. When she decided to lose the weight she had gained, not surprisingly, she failed. What needed fixing first was her relationship with her boyfriend.

Have you tried the "let's-do-this-quickly-and-get-it-over-with" approach? It rarely lasts. Little is learned in the process that you can use for the rest of your life. It could also be that the methods you have tried were not right for you. Just because they worked for someone else doesn't mean they will work for you.

The reason you'll have success this time is that you are going to determine what is right for you by using your personality. I'm not going to *tell* you what to do. Your personality is going to do that. The more control you have over your destiny, the more you'll enjoy the process of getting there.

Myth #3: You Can Give Up a Goal Once You've Achieved It

Many people who have set such goals as losing weight, lowering their blood cholesterol, or improving their energy level often believe that once they have achieved these goals, they can give them up. They figure they did what it took to accomplish the feat and now, thank goodness, they can get on with their lives. However, this type of thinking sets people up for gaining back the weight, increasing their cholesterol, and so on. Before too long, they are setting the same goals. Their problem is simply that they are setting the wrong goals and thinking short-term instead of considering how they can make this change last a lifetime.

Maybe You're Setting the Wrong Goals

Why do Americans insist on setting goals such as weight-loss, cholesterol reduction, and so forth? I'm not saying that being overweight, having high cholesterol, high blood pressure or any adverse health condition is a good thing or that, because you have these conditions, there is nothing you should do or can do about it. I'm just saying that these are the wrong goals, and that by setting them, people set themselves up to fail.

Think about why you bought this book. You must have some unhealthy lifestyle habits that you know are causing you problems and that need replacing. What do you think would happen if you set and achieved the goals of healthy eating, healthy fitness, healthy attitude, and healthy habits for life? I'll tell you. You would be able to lose weight, lower your cholesterol, control your blood sugar, decrease your risk for disease, have more energy, and feel better about yourself, along with a host of other healthy conditions. Your weight, your blood cholesterol, your energy level, and so on just become measurements of how well you're succeeding with your new habits and how your body has responded to the changes. They are no longer end points.

These healthy habits are like a wheel (see Figure 1), because there is no beginning or end to them. You need to have all these habits working for you all the time. Some of them you may already have. However, only when all the spokes of the wheel (all the healthy habits) are present can the wheel of life turn smoothly.

What's Your Incentive for Changing?

Everyone has their own reasons for changing, but too often they involve short-range thinking—"I have to get my cholesterol down by the time of my company physical," "I bet my friend that I could cut out desserts for a month." The outcome of this kind

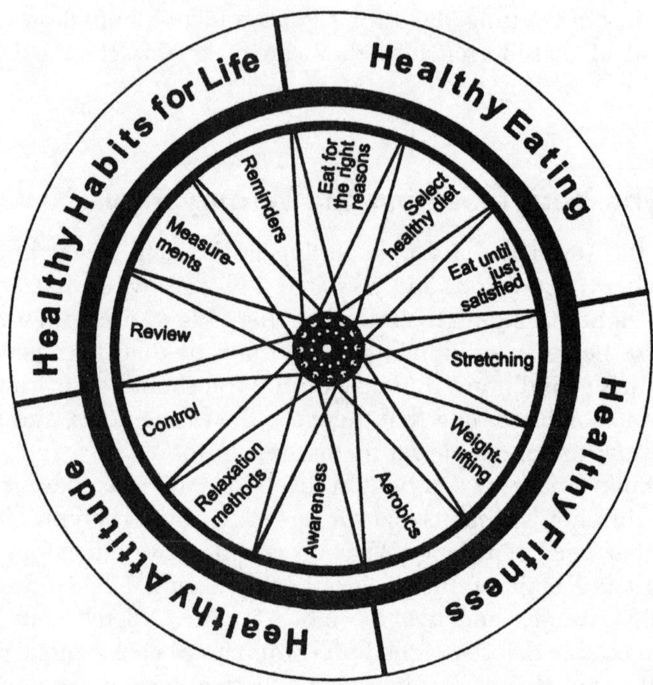

Figure 1. The Wheel of Healthy Habits

of thinking is that once you have achieved the results, whatever efforts you used to get there no longer seem necessary. Take the example of Lucy, mother of the bride. Lucy wanted to lose weight so she would look good at her daughter's wedding. On the day of the wedding, everyone was congratulating her on the great job she had done. (They should only know the methods she used, from diet pills to fasting to grapefruit five times a day!) However, six months later, Lucy had regained all the weight she had lost and then some. You see, once the wedding was over, so was the reason for her losing weight. Lucy was missing what I call a *life vision.*

A *life vision* is the *why,* or purpose, behind your efforts, what you see for yourself regarding your health that will last you a lifetime. It is measured in the amount of drive and motivation you have to see it happen. It is the eternal carrot in front of you that constantly pulls you forward toward something far bigger than individual goals or healthy habits.

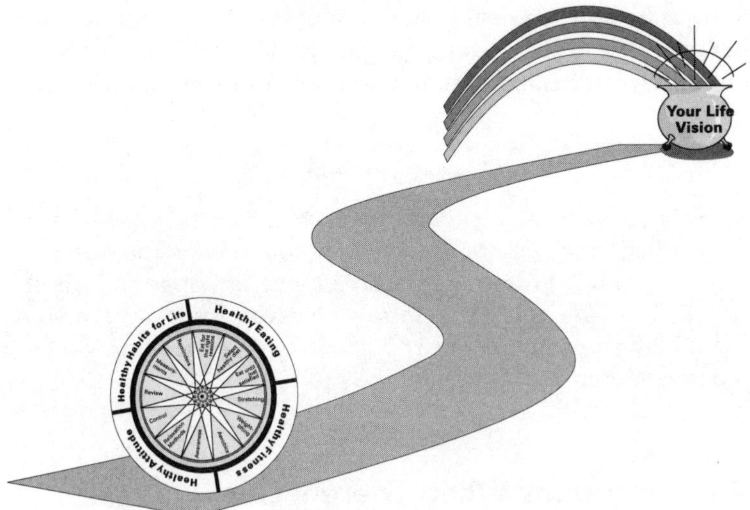

Figure 2. The Road to Optimum Health

If you were to say that your vision is to lose weight, I would ask you "Why? What is your reason for losing weight?" You might say, "To fit into my clothes," and I would tell you that that isn't a strong enough reason to last you a lifetime. (You can always get a larger size. Besides, the baggy look is in!) If you were to say that your vision is to lower your cholesterol to a normal level, I would again ask you "Why?" You might say, "To avoid a heart attack." With that comment, you are getting closer to making a vision statement, but not quite. I could again ask you "Why do you want to avoid a heart attack?"

As long as you can ask the question "Why?" in answer to a stated health goal, you have not come up with a *life vision.* I'm hoping that you will come to the same conclusion or vision as I have for you: to improve the quality of your life and potentially extend the quantity or length of your life. That's what I see as the pot of gold at the end of the rainbow. That should have enough pulling power to get you to change and to maintain that change. When you have a complete Wheel of Healthy Habits headed toward a *life vision,* you are literally whirring along. (See Figure 2.)

A *life vision* is for the long term and needs to be the guiding force for the rest of your life. What if Lucy had set as her vision to be as healthy as possible so that she would be around to enjoy her grandchildren? Losing weight would have been only one objective or measurement among many to reach that vision.

Take a Moment . . .

Think about what you want your *life vision* to be. Make it something that will continually draw you forward through the coming years. Write it down on a piece of paper and put it away in a safe place (not so safe that you forget where you put it)! Every so often you should look at it to see how you're doing in your pursuit of your vision.

What Happens When There's One Missing Piece

Let's look a little more closely at Figure 1, The Wheel of Healthy Habits, which will serve as your basis for setting goals. There are four major parts to it: healthy eating, healthy fitness, healthy attitude, and healthy habits for life. Within each of these categories are the lifestyle habits we will be working on throughout the remainder of the book. To achieve **Healthy Eating,** you need to learn about food selection, eating for the right reasons, and knowing when enough is enough. **Healthy Fitness** includes three major habits of exercise: stretching for flexibility; weight-training to increase the ratio between muscle and fat; and aerobics for endurance. **Healthy Attitude** involves being aware of and understanding how stress can negatively affect you; finding effective ways to relax; and learning to control the situation before it becomes stressful. Lastly, **Healthy Habits for Life** means learning how to maintain these healthy habits and prevent relapse by continually monitoring, reviewing, and reminding yourself of your *life vision.* Being able to achieve and maintain your *life vision* amounts to maintaining your new healthy lifestyle habits.

Every category and every habit within a category is very valuable in reaching a *life vision.* If there is just one part missing, you will not see the same level of results. Some people don't enjoy exercising and can't imagine themselves becoming an exerciser.

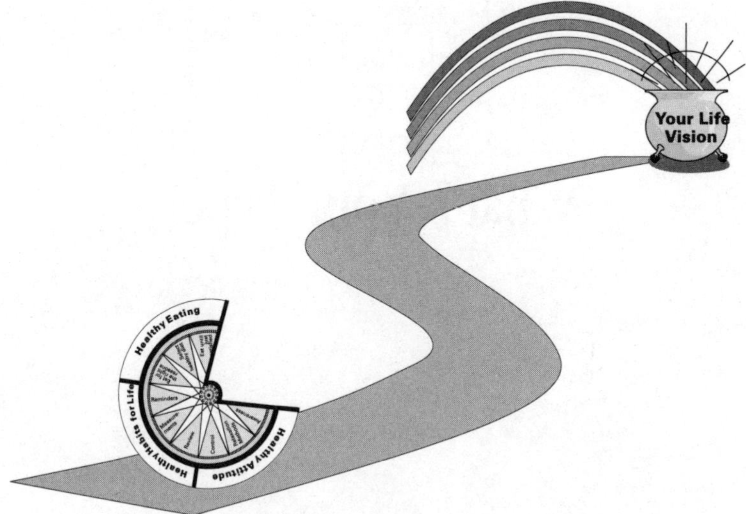

Figure 3. Whirr, Thump, Whirr, Thump . . .

They figure that they can just eat healthfully, do a little relaxation, and that will do it. Yet good nutrition and stress management without exercise is like driving around on an old stage-coach wheel with part of its rim missing. The ride won't be very smooth, and it's questionable whether the destination can be reached without there being a breakdown. That's what we see in Figure 3. Instead of your life whirring along, your journey sounds more like ''Whirr, **thump,** whirr, **thump**.'' The greater the number of missing healthy habits, the more thumping than whirring you will experience. The results will show up in your physical condition, and there will be less likelihood of your arriving at your *life vision.* Appreciate the fact that the amount of thumping is up to you. You determine how much effort you are willing to expend.

2

What's Your Type?

While we would all like to boast that we are unique, we need only look around us to see that there are others who think and act just like us. Of course, there are some people who are not at all like us. What makes us the same or different? According to Carl Gustav Jung, a Swiss psychiatrist, it's our personalities. We may feel most comfortable with people who are similar to us, but we are often attracted to those who are different because they have characteristics we wish we had. What we learn from those differences can contribute to our own growth.

In 1921 Jung published his theory of personality preferences he called *psychological type.* He believed that our personalities predict our behavior. For example, if you tend to nurture others, Jung would view your acts of kindness not as a random behavior but as a product of your personality. Knowing your personality, he could predict what you would do. He proposed that the differences in people's behavior stemmed from their different personality preferences. Once he established what these preferences were, he was able to create a personality classification system that allowed him to group people into various personality types.

The system took into account how you prefer to deal with life, make decisions, and act on those decisions, as well as what influences your decision-making process. It could be as simple a decision as, "Should I sleep for another fifteen minutes?" or as complicated as, "Should I accept that job offer?" Your personality type can predict and affect what decisions and actions you take. The fact that not all personality types come up with the same response makes for a more colorful and varied kaleidoscope of life.

Jung's theory moved from the clinical office into the public arena, when it became popularized by two American women, Katharine Cook Briggs and her daughter Isabel Briggs Myers. Neither Briggs nor Myers were psychologists, but during World War II they realized that many people who had been forced into the war effort were doing jobs for which they were unsuited. Through rigorous observation and documentation, they set out to create a way of measuring the differences among people to determine how better to use their skills and abilities. The result was the Myers-Briggs Type Indicator® (MBTI®). It captured the essence of Jung's theory and shaped it into a tool that could be used for many different purposes. Over the years, countless people have been tested, most often in connection with determining their career aptitudes. Marriage counselors have often used the MBTI® to help partners deal with interpersonal issues. In businesses the MBTI® has been used for team building and improving communications. New applications for the MBTI® continue to be found—among them, the ones you'll discover in this book.

It's Yours for Keeps

You are born with your personality preferences and, as you mature, they slowly express themselves. The older you get, the more fully your personality becomes evident to yourself and others. There's no question that your environment influences how your preferences are expressed, but it doesn't change what is innately yours.

Keep in mind that there are no good or bad personality types. Identifying your type is not meant to put you into a rigid box or assign you a scarlet letter as a means of explaining who you are and why you behave as you do. The human personality is too complex for that. While you are much more than type can explain, type gives you a basic understanding of why you and others behave in certain ways. *Your Personality Prescription* presents an exciting new application of the work of Jung, Myers, and Briggs. It shows you how your personality may have promoted some of your unhealthy habits and how you can use your personality to change those habits.

The Basic Four Categories

Jung came up with three categories of preferences for personality typing, to which Briggs and Myers added a fourth. Each category is essential to your total personality and how you function in life. How they combine determines your type. The four categories involve:

1. What stimulates you
2. What is significant for you to know
3. How you make decisions
4. The way you handle life

Before I go into any detail about the categories, I want you to answer the Personality Profile Questionnaire (PPQ), in Figures 4 and 5, to identify your type. When you take the PPQ, do it in a comfortable place where you won't have any interruptions. You will see that on each line there are a pair of words or phrases. Select the word or phrase from each pair that seems to best apply to you. Don't think too deeply about each set of words. Your first impression or feeling about the words will be more representative of you than the answer you might come up with if you analyzed what they mean. Consider your response in terms of what is generally true or natural for you, not situational, connected with work, or how you would like to be. Don't take the PPQ right after you have had an argument or been in a deep discussion of some matter, because that will also influence your responses. Note the category type to help you put the terms into a particular context. Place a checkmark in the box in front of that word. When you have finished a particular category, add up the checkmarks in each column and write the total in the box.

Category: **What Stimulates You**

E		I
❑ group	*or*	❑ one-on-one
❑ introduce others or self	*or*	❑ get introduced
❑ talkative	*or*	❑ quiet
❑ energized by group	*or*	❑ energy drained by group
❑ self-revealing	*or*	❑ private
❑ always have fun at parties	*or*	❑ sometimes bored at parties
❑ speak, then think	*or*	❑ think, then speak
❑ participate	*or*	❑ watch
❑ being in the spotlight	*or*	❑ being in the background
❑ outgoing	*or*	❑ reserved
❑ broad friendships	*or*	❑ deep friendships
☐ *Total*		☐ *Total*

Category: **What's Significant to You**

S		N
❑ rely on my senses	*or*	❑ rely on my instincts
❑ discover	*or*	❑ create
❑ practical	*or*	❑ imaginative
❑ verbatim	*or*	❑ representation
❑ familiar	*or*	❑ unfamiliar
❑ routine	*or*	❑ novelty
❑ actual	*or*	❑ theoretical
❑ conventional	*or*	❑ innovative
❑ facts	*or*	❑ ideas and theories
❑ want details	*or*	❑ want the big picture
❑ what is	*or*	❑ what might be
☐ *Total*		☐ *Total*

Figure 4. Personality Profile Questionnaire.

By the way, if you have taken the MBTI® before and can remember your type, skip the PPQ. However, if you decide to take the PPQ anyway and get a different result from the MBTI®, read the descriptions of preferences and type that follow to see which assessment results are more accurate.

Category: **How You Make Decisions**

T		F
❑ head	*or*	❑ heart
❑ accepted standards	*or*	❑ personal values
❑ analyze	*or*	❑ sympathize
❑ objective	*or*	❑ subjective
❑ fair	*or*	❑ compassionate
❑ faultfinding	*or*	❑ uncritical
❑ impersonal	*or*	❑ personal
❑ truthful	*or*	❑ tactful
❑ argue	*or*	❑ harmony
❑ impact on situation	*or*	❑ impact on people
❑ logic over sentiment	*or*	❑ sentiment over logic
☐ *Total*		☐ *Total*

Category: **The Way You Handle Life**

J		P
❑ decisive	*or*	❑ inquiring
❑ punctual	*or*	❑ leisurely
❑ controlled	*or*	❑ impulsive
❑ firm	*or*	❑ flexible
❑ making lists appeals to me	*or*	❑ don't like making lists
❑ early starting	*or*	❑ last minute catch-up
❑ goal-oriented	*or*	❑ process-oriented
❑ structured	*or*	❑ unstructured
❑ rapid closure	*or*	❑ keeping options open
❑ orderly	*or*	❑ easygoing
❑ arranged	*or*	❑ spontaneous
☐ *Total*		☐ *Total*

Figure 5. Personality Profile Questionnaire, continued.

What Your Results Mean

I intentionally kept you in the dark about what the letters at the head of the columns in the PPQ stood for. I didn't want you to be biased by their names. Now I'll tell you. They are preference alternatives or opposite ways of dealing with a particular category, as you can see in Table 1.

TABLE 1. Preference Alternatives

Category	Preference Alternatives
What stimulates you	Extraversion (E) or Introversion (I)
What's significant to you	Sensing (S) or iNtuiting (N)
How you make decisions	Thinking (T) or Feeling (F)
Way you handle life	Judging (J) or Perceiving (P)

Note: You may be wondering why the letter *N* is the shorthand way of writing "iNtuiting." Since Jung had already assigned the letter *I* to "Introversion," he had to come up with another letter. Throughout this book, the word will be written as "iNtuiting" rather than the conventional way.

Jung, Myers, and Briggs appreciated that we all possess all the preferences. But since it is hard to be both extraverting and introverting at the same time, we generally prefer to do one rather than the other in most situations. The same holds true for sensing and iNtuiting, thinking and feeling, or judging and perceiving.

Think of the duality of preferences in terms of the hand you normally use to write. Are you left-handed or right-handed? If you said "right-handed," it only means that you have a *preference* for writing with your right hand. However, if you were to break your right arm, you would struggle and eventually succeed at writing with your left hand, even though it would take some effort and concentration on your part. Depending on how long you had to practice writing with your left hand, you might get very proficient at it. Once your right arm was healthy again, you would most likely go back to writing with your right hand, but still be capable of writing with your left hand.

Personality preferences work the same way. Within any one category, there is a preferred way of acting and behaving most of the time. Yet if you were to practice using the other preference within that category, you might find yourself becoming more comfortable with it. You might even start to appreciate its value. That's what you will be learning to do to change your habits.

To give you a general idea of the differences between the preferences, let me share with you how each might experience the Grand Canyon. The *Sensing* preference would notice the size

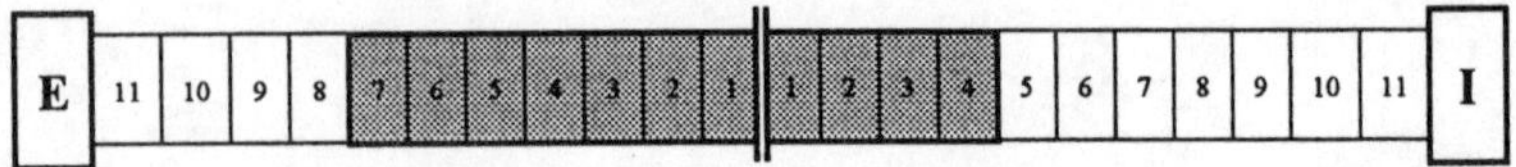

Figure 6. Example of Charted PPQ Results

and depth of the Grand Canyon, the maze the river has created, the color of the rock, the fact that this looks exactly like a photograph seen in a *National Geographic* magazine. Contrast that to the *iNtuiting* preference, which would marvel at how nature could create such a wonder. The *Thinking* preference would look at the scene and consider the scientific and geological principals that would govern such a creation. The *Feeling* preference, in comparison, would be overwhelmed by the grandeur and beauty of the scene.

Charting the PPQ Results

Transfer the totals for each of the columns on the PPQ onto the bar graphs provided in Figure 7, counting off the number of squares equal to your totals. For example, if your total for *E* (Extraversion) was 7 and your total for *I* (Introversion) was 4, your results would look like the graph in Figure 6.

Shading the boxes makes it easier to see what side of the center line you favor. The individual in this example had a somewhat clearer preference for Extraversion than Introversion. When you see your results graphed like this, it becomes clearer how much more you favor one preference over another. It also shows you that you do have the opposite preference at your disposal if you need to call it into action. It is a very rare individual who is totally one way or the other. If it happens, it is probably because you are responding to the word pairs from a situational perspective.

The letter of the preference with the higher total within a category becomes part of your type name. In the example in Figure 6 that shows "Extraversion" having a higher total than "Introversion," the test taker would include the letter *E* in his or her type name.

Now fill in the following blanks with your preference letters, listing them in the order that the categories appear above:

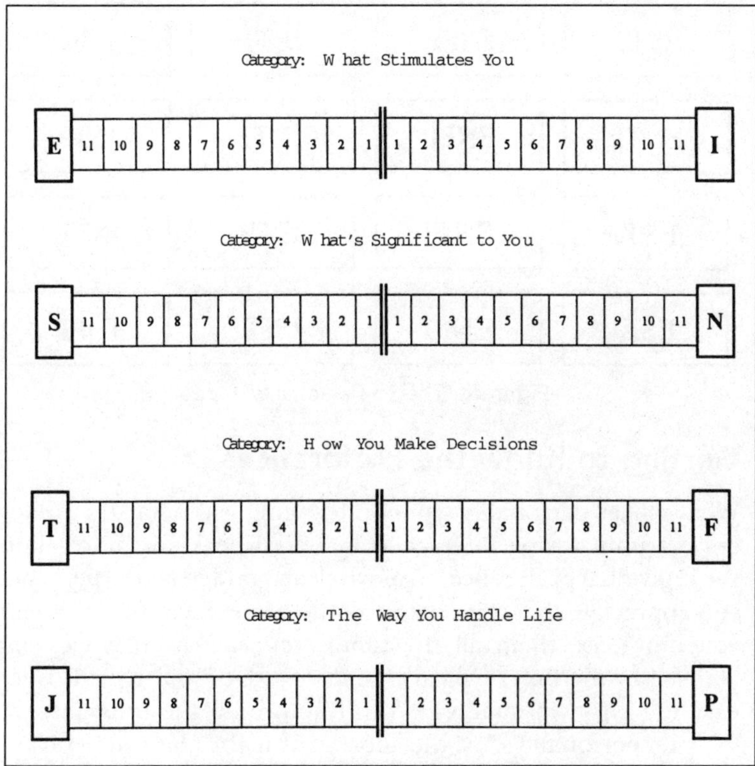

Figure 7. Charting Your PPQ Results

My type is ___ ___ ___ ___.

Note: If you want a more in-depth assessment of your personality type, locate a qualified MBTI® practitioner in your area or contact Consulting Psychologists Press, Inc., 3803 East Bayshore Road, Palo Alto, CA 94303 (1-800-624-1765).

The 16 Personality Types

As Figure 8 illustrates, there are 16 combinations of preferences that give us the following types:

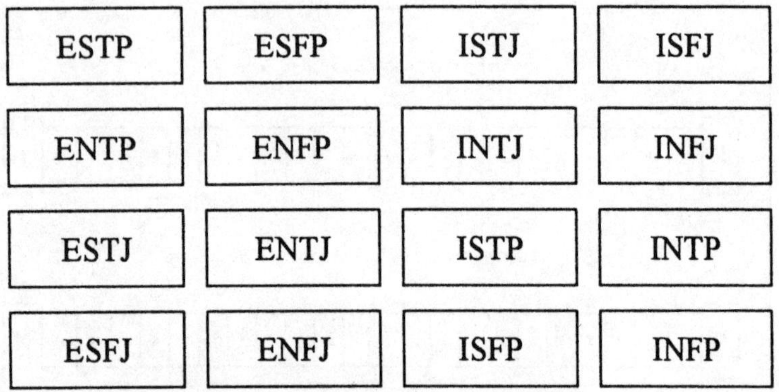

Figure 8. The 16 Personality Types

Getting to Know the Preferences

What makes personality typing interesting is the way the preferences within a type interact. It is helpful to know more about the individual preferences to more clearly understand type. When you appreciate that you possess all the preferences (even though you don't use them all the time), you can avoid typecasting yourself by the stereotypical characteristics of your type. It is too easy to say, "I'm an ENTP" and ignore all the other aspects of your personality. Yet the more you learn about the various preferences (not just the ones in your type name), and how to use them in your daily life, the easier it will be to change your habits. All the preferences are equally valuable.

As you read the following descriptions, you may find aspects of each preference that seem to describe you. However, within each category, one preference will feel like the better fit overall. Also, as you read about the Sensing, iNtuiting, Thinking, and Feeling preferences, you will probably find one that stands out as most like you. That's because the discussion about these preferences describes how that preference acts when it dominates your type. The dominant preference is the one you most naturally turn to make decisions, help you out in various situations, and guide you. (In Chapter 5 you'll learn what is your dominant preference.)

You will be meeting some of my clients throughout the book. Some of them came to me for various health problems. Others wanted to have a nutrition makeover, being concerned that their diet was inadequate. A good number of my clients wanted to lose weight. Some wanted to improve their athletic performance and realized that nutrition was an important component. No matter what reason people came to see me, they inevitably had some unhealthy habits they wanted to change. As you read about these people, you may find some you relate to more than others because they remind you of yourself. In some ways it is comforting to know you are not alone in having certain unhealthy lifestyle habits. It is also uplifting to see that others with the same personality type as you have changed their behaviors. If they can do it, so can you.

Category 1—What Stimulates You

The Extravert and the Introvert

Their Source of Energy

Extraverts focus their attention on—and derive their energy from—people, things, and events. Their concern is how they relate to the outside world, and they often respond to its demands or requirements at the expense of their own needs. If you questioned them about it, they would say that it's their pleasure to help, and they'll get around to their own needs later. The Extraverts who are in balance learn to integrate their own needs with taking care of the people and things outside themselves that are important to them.

Extraverts can be the life of the party. You probably know people who seem to become more lively in a crowd. They're the ones at a party who have to be practically shoved out the door by the host if anyone is to get any sleep that night. Give them a chance to talk and they'll never give up the stage. From the Introvert's point of view, Extraverts are too loud and tend to talk too fast. They control the airwaves by repeating themselves.

Their body language can be just as excitable. They use dramatic arm motions and facial expressions to give full impact to what they are saying. Extraverts don't like too much silence. If you're an Extravert, you can probably recall how you felt on a first date when the Introvert you were with seemed too quiet. Someone had to fill the void, and so you found yourself rambling on about who knows what.

Being with others actually charges the batteries of Extraverts. You can appreciate that when you see them in a conversation with someone. They're like a top that is wound tightly and then let loose. If you look at their address book, you'd wonder how they have the time to have so many friendships. However, they tend to have broad friendships with many people rather than deep friendships with just a few.

Introverts are just the opposite, looking within themselves for their energy. Their attention is on how something relates to them. Their focus is inward, responding to personal needs. The immature Introvert is self-centered, whereas mature Introverts look within to see how they can best serve the outer world. It is a matter of integrating their own priorities with the demands of other people, things, or events. They appreciate that participating in the outside world is the best way to fulfill their own priorities. They tend to concentrate their attention on their own ideas, thoughts, observations, and musings. They are very content to be by themselves because it gives them time to ponder.

You'll also recognize the Introverts at a party. They aren't necessarily the wallflowers. However, they prefer to be with just one or two other people. More than that becomes overwhelming. They'll be leaving the party hours before it's over, feeling drained from the experience. To recharge their batteries, they need to get away by themselves. Deep friendships with just a few people are more important to Introverts than being able to boast about the number or variety of people they know.

How They Think

It's interesting how Extraverts think. The more they talk, the clearer become their thoughts. A lively or intense discussion about a subject is much more enjoyable to them than spending too much time in deep, individual thought. Their thoughts tend to skim the surface of subjects rather than delve deeply into any one topic.

Introverts' conversation is often more subdued than Extraverts'. It's not that they aren't paying attention to the group. Just don't expect them to contribute much right at that moment. They need time to process what is going on before responding. For them, it's easier to formulate ideas when they are alone. Then they will mentally rehearse how they plan to present those ideas to others and what the potential responses will be. This two-way conversation in their mind gives them a greater sense of security when they finally vocalize their thoughts.

Getting to Know Them

It is easier to "read" Extraverts than Introverts. With so much of their energy being projected outward, the Extraverts are constantly revealing their personalities. Besides, they are more than happy to share personal information with others. They are open and ready to engage in conversation. It doesn't matter whether they are standing in line at the grocery store or attending a seminar. There's always something to talk about. They also can be distracted more easily. Better to have a face-to-face encounter with them than to write them letters.

Introverts are more cautious about what they share about themselves. If they appear standoffish, don't take it personally. They don't mean to offend you. If they do carry on a conversation, they like to go into depth about certain subjects. When they're talking, try not to interrupt. Since they gave you concentrated time to state your thoughts, they would appreciate the same in return. Compared to Extraverts, Introverts are much happier getting something in writing because it gives them time to absorb what was written and evaluate its meaning.

Getting the Job Done

Variety is the Extravert's middle name. Without it, he or she will be bored and quickly lose interest. Extraverts can charge right in and get the job done without a second's thought. Their philosophy is, "Do it first, *then* think about it—maybe." They figure they can always come back and fix it later. They believe in group effort. The Extravert's byword is *action,* and the best place for that is in the outside world, where its results can be seen.

Introverts have an easier time staying focused and on task if—provided they can work on just one or two things at a time. It's best not to interrupt Introverts at work. They get very frustrated when they lose their concentration. They prefer to think about what needs doing, follow through if action is required, and then evaluate the results. The Introvert's byword is *reflection,* and the best place for that is in the inside world of the mind.

An interesting note: The dictionary definition of *extravert* is someone who is gregarious or unreserved. That isn't always true of Extraverts—except in comparison with Introverts.

The dictionary definition of *introvert* is someone who is shy. That isn't always true of Introverts, but because they tend to keep to themselves, they may appear so.

Greta, the Extravert

As Greta put it, "I've had it with myself. I never feel in control of what I eat, and my eating habits are atrocious." I had Greta take the Personality Profile Questionnaire (PPQ) to find out her personality type. One aspect of her personality turned out to be Extraversion. As I shared the characteristics of an Extravert with her and we started to analyze why Greta was feeling out of control about what she ate, it became clear how her personality was involved.

Greta's strong preference for Extraversion had her accepting every luncheon date, every dinner invitation, and every latté break request, even if she wasn't hungry. She couldn't resist any opportunity to get an "energy fix" from being with a group of people. But it seemed that the amount she ate went up in direct proportion to the number of people at the event. She would start out calm and in control of her food choices. She would be careful about the quantity she was eating, promising to keep an eye on herself. However, before she knew it, she would be swept away by the energy of the group and, totally forgetting her good intentions, would be eating everything on her plate and ordering something else. Buffets were a complete disaster for her.

David, the Introvert

About six months before coming to see me, David signed up with a weight-loss clinic hoping to lose 35 pounds. The consultant at the center explained to him that he would receive a half-hour one-on-one counseling session each week. On the day of his visit, he would also be required to attend a 45-minute group session. At these sessions he would be given various weight-loss tips (about eating out, snacks, and so on) and have the opportunity to share any challenges he was currently facing in his struggle to lose weight.

David dropped out of the program after just two weeks—and felt like a failure for doing so. He went back to struggling on his own, not really quite sure how to lose weight (other than by the extreme measure of not eating!). That's when a friend of his recommended that he give me a call. During our first session, he answered the PPQ I gave him. We found out that part of his personality type was Introversion.

When I explained to him that he wasn't a failure for dropping out, he looked at me quizzically. How could that be? He hadn't finished the program, nor had he lost the 35 pounds he had set as his goal. David told me that the one major problem he had with the weight-loss center was having to publicly share his personal struggles with the group. The group leader kept trying to draw him out. Obviously, she tried one too many times for David's comfort level, making him decide this approach to weight loss wasn't for him. Had she realized that David was—in Jungian terms—an Introvert, she would have allowed him to sit and absorb what he needed and, if he felt it appropriate, to ask for support. David needed to go home and process what had happened that day. By internalizing the information, he could then see how to apply it in his own life. Being asked to speak out on something that he hadn't had the opportunity to process made him feel very uncomfortable.

Category 2—What's Significant to You

The Sensor and the iNtuitive

Their Source of Information

For Sensors, "What you see is what you get." If they can't see it, smell it, taste it, touch it, or hear it, it probably doesn't exist. That's why firsthand experiences are important to them. It's their main way of learning new things. For them, "Seeing is believing." iNtuitives would rather trust their hunches than rely solely on their senses because they believe that intuition reveals more than the senses can. Both preferences can be involved with immediate experiences. Sensors use their five senses for a direct experience of the world, while iNtuitives use their "sixth" sense to capture an experience's essence—that deeper something that goes beyond mere reality.

Their Focus

To the Sensor, "what is"—the present, the here-and-now—is much more important and relevant than the iNtuitive's "what will be." The iNtuitive is wondering how the Sensor can be so *now*-focused when the possibilities for the future are so endless. In their imagination, iNtuitives can always see how much better life will be "one of these days."

To make a job worthwhile, Sensors need to see tangible results. iNtuitives, with their forward-looking philosophy, don't need those tangible results to make their efforts valuable. They believe with their intuition and gut-feel that whatever their efforts, there will eventually be some reward. In a crap game, they are the ones willing to "bet on the come."

You could say that many Sensors are pleasure seekers because they know how to enjoy the moment. iNtuitives are willing to put off immediate pleasure, believing that what they could possibly have in the future will be even better. They keep hoping that one day they'll find ultimate pleasure.

What's Important to Them

Being in the present, Sensors have a need for facts. Sergeant Joe Friday on the television show *Dragnet* summed it up best for the Sensor when he said, "We need the facts, Ma'am, just the facts." Sensors also want exact details. Whether being given information or providing it, they want it as precise as possible. Their weight isn't "about 150 pounds." It is "152½ pounds." They believe that what is inferred is not as reliable as what is explicitly stated. It annoys Sensors when the real meaning of an action or statement is left to the imagination.

By contrast iNtuitives would say, "What difference do facts make if you have an overall picture of things?" For the iNtuitive, the details are just boring and just get in the way of seeing the bigger picture and its meaning. The bigger picture requires that there be an acceptance of generalizations and approximations, especially since things could change tomorrow anyway. To an iNtuitive, what's important are the connections and the way things relate to each other.

Applying Information

Once they know the facts, Sensors need a practical application for them. Going to a cooking class to learn how to make a meal worthy of a five-star restaurant would be totally impractical for the Sensor with two toddlers and a "meat and potatoes" spouse. She probably wouldn't even sign up for a class teaching such new skills in the first place—she'd rather rely on the skills she has. The only thing she'd like about a cooking class would be the clear, step-by-step fashion in which cooking methods were taught. Sensors learn best when given information in a sequential order.

For the iNtuitive, the same class would have a totally different impact. The class would just serve as a springboard for her to exercise her creative juices. The adventure of learning new skills would be half the fun of the class. She could even see the possibility of converting her "meat and potatoes" spouse to a gourmet. As for the toddlers, she'd consider it a good thing to expose them to the unusual, since from the iNtuitive's point of view, that's what makes life interesting. The likelihood of the iNtuitive preparing the meal according to the step-by-step instructions provided would be pretty slim. iNtuitives prefer to be more random, jumping past prescribed steps when they can see other connections or ways of doing the job. They will probably even change the recipe as they go along, imagining how it could be improved.

Solving Problems

When there is a problem to solve, Sensors try to find a standard solution for it. It's even better when they've had previous experience with the problem so they can use the same approach to fix it. They already have the concrete data and can now just apply it. Their approach is to look at the specific parts to the problem and figure out how they actually interact. You can understand why they make great mechanics. Sensors tend to be very good at work that requires precision.

That type of job wouldn't work for iNtuitives, who look at patterns and relationships when trying to solve a problem. They are best when using their strength in creating designs. The more abstract the problem, the more they enjoy the challenge. They make great scientists because of their anticipation of what could be. The author Jules Verne must have been an iNtuitive, considering the foresight he had in such books as *The Time Machine* and *20,000 Leagues Under The Sea.* iNtuitives are fascinated by the possibilities.

A major difference between Sensors and iNtuitives is their attitude toward problems. The Sensor's philosophy is, "If it isn't broken, don't fix it." The iNtuitive would rather break it and find a better way to make it. Sensors prefer to get on with life as it is, enjoying what is there, while iNtuitives want to improve on life as it is.

Susie, the Sensor

Susie came to me with a mild case of bulimia. It scared her when she got out of control. As a Sensor, she gave no thought to what this condition could do to her in the future; bulimia seemed to satisfy her needs at the moment.

(Remember that Sensors are here-and-now people.) Susie made sure her refrigerator and pantry were always well stocked. At the same time Susie was seeing me for nutritional advice, she was getting psychological counseling. The two types of care helped her break the habit.

Megan, the iNtuitive

Megan could best be called a daydreamer. If you asked her what life would be like in five years, she'd give you a complete rundown. She would describe the house she'd be living in, the type of job she would have, the number and type of pets she would own. With iNtuition as part of her personality type, she could create a picture of the future in her mind.

That picture included a slim Megan. When she came to see me, she was 20 pounds overweight. She wanted to lose weight because her class reunion was coming up the following year and she didn't want to embarrass herself in front of her old classmates. Two images of the reunion danced in her mind—one of a trim Megan surrounded by old friends asking how she had been able to maintain her high school weight, and another of an overweight Megan, wanting to hide behind the palm plant for fear of what her old friends would think.

One would expect that an iNtuitive like Megan would be able to see where her present actions are leading since iNtuitives are so good at envisioning possibilities. Yet because the changes they need to make have to be made in the present, their challenge is to stay in the here-and-now to effect those changes. When Megan had an extra helping of food, her line would be "Come Monday, I'll start my diet." She reminded me of Scarlett O'Hara in the movie *Gone With the Wind*, when she says "Tomorrow is another day." She and Megan both avoid facing up to problems when they occur.

Category 3—How You Make Decisions

The Thinker and the Feeler

Their Basis for Making a Decision

Thinkers make logical decisions. They analyze information, subjecting it to impersonal considerations using accepted standards and rules. While others may see them as lacking sympathy, they see themselves as being objective. To them there is no other way of being fair to either a cause or other people.

Feelers, on the other hand, worry about the effect their decisions will have on other people and themselves. Therefore, their basis for decision making is a personal, subjective value system. That system will reflect what they like or don't like, their values, and their personal reactions. They seem to have a natural gift for understanding and empathizing with others.

What's Important to Them

For Thinkers, being right is more important than being liked. Feelers believe in just the opposite. They need to be liked. While Feelers are showing compassion, Thinkers are showing reasonableness. While Feelers are tactfully trying to see the positive points about someone, Thinkers are being truthful, often quick to criticize and find flaws. While Feelers are seeking harmony, Thinkers are looking for clarity, even if someone's feelings are at stake.

Seeing It from Both Sides

Feelers tend to view strong Thinkers as cold and calculating—too hard, too tough, too lacking in heart. Thinkers see strong Feelers as "bleeding hearts"—too soft, too "touchy-feely," too likely to take things personally. What both need to appreciate is that at different times and places, each of these preferences can excel and shine. Thinkers do well in business when analyzing strategic plans. Feelers do well in business when doing performance reviews. Thinkers do well in the home when setting up a budget. Feelers do well in the home when the kids get into an argument and need help settling it.

Communication Styles

Thinkers will be more than glad to talk with you as long as you keep it brief and concise. State your case, citing the pros and cons of the alternatives you are presenting. The more logical, scientific, and fact-based the information, the more credible you'll be. Don't be surprised when Thinkers tell you exactly what they think about what you've said. The adage that ''You can catch more flies with honey than with vinegar'' doesn't apply to Thinkers. They figure they can convince others by presenting logical reasons.

On the other hand, Feelers tend to drizzle honey over everything they touch. They would never think of hurting someone's feelings. Share an idea or thought with them, and they'll show great appreciation for it and bestow that same appreciation on the giver. They convince others with what they believe is ''meaningful'' information.

An interesting note: The data show that the Thinking and Feeling preferences are gender-related. About two-thirds of males are Thinkers, and about the same proportion of females are Feelers. It could be the roles that men and women have historically played. It also could be due to their upbringing. Girls are expected to play at human relations with dolls, while boys are given action-oriented toys like erector sets and toy guns.

With that said, don't think that Thinkers have no emotions and Feelers can't analyze. It's just not their first mode of action.

Bob, the Thinker

Bob became a client of mine when his doctor referred him to me for nutritional counseling to help him reduce his cholesterol and weight. It made a great impression on Bob when his doctors presented him with his ''numbers.'' His cholesterol of 235 mg/dl (milligrams per deciliter) was more than 35 mg/dl too high. His weight of 215 pounds was 50 pounds greater than what is considered healthy for his height. His blood pressure, 140/90, was in the hypertensive range. These were elements he could deal with—hard facts that could be measured against accepted standards. His doctor didn't sugarcoat the news, but leveled with Bob about his chances of suffering a heart attack. Bob's doctor laid out a strategy with him. Bob would come to me for nutritional advice, sign up at the health club with a personal trainer to establish an exercise program, and attend a stress-reduction class offered at the local hospital outpatient department.

It wasn't hard for Bob to adopt the plan. It was logical and made sense. How else was he going to improve his chances of avoiding a heart attack like the one his dad had suffered? Bob became almost fanatical in his attempts to change his habits. He figured people would just have to understand when he turned down their dinner invitations or wouldn't accept the cake they gave him for his birthday. The right thing to do was to get his "numbers" where they belonged.

Jennifer, the Feeler

Jennifer was at the end of her radiation and chemotherapy treatments for breast cancer when she started coming to me. Months earlier, when she had been diagnosed with the disease, she had started reading everything she could about it. One point that kept being underlined was that there were things she had control over that could decrease her risk of the breast cancer returning. Her genetic predisposition for breast cancer was out of her hands; her lifestyle habits she could control.

Because of her strong Feeling preference, when she heard the diagnosis from her doctor, her first concern was for her family. She was the mother of two toddlers. The idea of not successfully curing this disease was unthinkable to her. The picture of her toddlers without a mother was unacceptable. Jennifer assumed that she was going to have to cook separate meals for herself since she didn't want to deprive her children of the foods they liked. When I told her that a cancer-prevention diet was a healthy diet suitable for her whole family, it pleased her that food wouldn't be a divisive issue.

Category 4—The Way You Handle Life

The Judger and the Perceiver

Taking Action

Judgers speak with a sense of authority and want to see others conform to the standards they espouse. There are rules that need to be followed. They are not afraid to give people advice, whether they want it or not. Since they don't tolerate uncertainty very well, they make sure they do their homework to get the information they think necessary to make a decision. However, in their haste to have the matter settled and out of the way, that research may not be as complete as it could be. They might even ignore new facts that could cloud the issue once the decision has been made. Their approach to decision making is quite methodical: (1) they collect the information (but don't spend too much time doing it); (2) they narrow down the possibilities; (3) they select from those possibilities; (4) they make the decision (one they rarely second-guess). Judgers are great at goal setting.

For Perceivers, the more possibilities there are the better. If one doesn't work, they can try another. It keeps them from being tied down to just one right answer. Who knows for sure that it is *the* right answer, without seeking new information and testing it? Besides, exploring the unknown can be so much more fun than just following the tried-and-true way. Don't be surprised when, after Perceivers have made a decision, they question it, sometimes fretting that maybe they've made the wrong decision. That's why they have a hard time setting goals. They're continually trying to determine *if* they should set goals and, if so, what they should be. On the surface, Perceivers appear to be procrastinators. However, it's often more a matter of being reluctant to commit to just one approach and thus close off other options.

You would think that as long as it takes them to finally make a decision, they would be quite sure of it. However, they're still thinking that maybe they didn't collect enough information and didn't spend enough time considering it. They can agonize as much over a $5 purchase as over a $500 purchase.

Keeping a Date

You can always recognize Judgers. They're the ones who carry a calendar with them wherever they go. It may be a small version of the one they have at home or work. However, they wouldn't think of being unprepared in case someone asked them to lunch, a meeting, or a movie. You can be sure that when they get back to work or home they'll update their main calendar. You can also be sure that they will be on time for anything that they have set up. Schedules make life more settled for the Judgers. They know exactly what they are doing morning, noon, and night. No surprises for them. Of course, there will be days when things don't go quite as planned—then you have a frazzled Judger.

Perceivers are the just the opposite. They probably don't even keep a calendar, much less write on it if they do. Once they commit to a date, they feel boxed in by it. Just as the Judgers can't handle too little structure, Perceivers can't handle too much of it. They really prefer to leave themselves open for last-minute options. While Judgers are schedule-type people, Perceivers are spontaneous-type people; for them, adapting to an exciting new plan is less a problem than a pleasure.

Endings Versus Beginnings

Judgers are pleased when a project gets underway, but not half as pleased as when the project is completed. They have a persistence that keeps them going. However, they like to see things get done quickly. Finishing something brings closure and allows them to move on to the next project. Completing the project on time makes it all the better. Last-minute stresses don't sit well. Planning each step of the project and keeping to the timetable helps, too. Judgers need to have a sense of control over whatever they do. Leaving anything to chance is terribly uncomfortable for them.

Perceivers love to start projects, but are less concerned about getting them done. It's the experience they're after, figuring that what they haven't tried yet is going to be exciting. Their open-ended attitude allows the project to change course many times before the end. For Perceivers, variety is what makes life interesting. A project that looks as if it won't be done on time is not a problem. The last-minute pressure energizes Perceivers and spurs them on to completion. To them, the process along the way is what really counts anyway.

Order Versus Chaos

Judgers thrive on order. Making plans allows them to know exactly what is expected of them and others. They are the list makers. There are to-do lists, lists of where everything is located in their homes, lists of errands with exactly what, where, and in what order they are to be done. Once completed, a line can be drawn through the item. What a marvelous sense of closure that is for Judgers. At work, they are the ones with all their files organized, labeled, and put away where they belong. At home, their shoes are all in labeled boxes to make finding the right pair quick and easy. They may even have them organized according to color and type. To Judgers, it just makes sense to have such orderliness. Why waste time trying to find something because you didn't put it back where it belongs?

Perceivers, on the other hand, tend to be more flexible, not wanting to commit to the rigidity that the Judger's orderliness requires. It doesn't make any sense to Perceivers to make lists, since they aren't going to stick to them anyway. Lists and plans are just too stifling. It doesn't bother Perceivers to have things scattered about at work and at home. Being neat is not high on their lifestyle list of to-dos, though they wouldn't mind a *little* order in their lives (just not too much!). They almost always seem to find what they need. It may take a little longer than if a Judger were looking for something he or she put away. However, from the Perceivers' perspective, since they didn't waste as much time with the labeling and organizing in the beginning, they can make up for it by searching a little longer. If they're really lucky, someone will come along to interrupt their search and they can put off finding whatever it was until later. What's really important in life is being able to be spontaneous.

Words like *should* and *ought* underlie Judgers' own actions and their expectations of others. They need a basis upon which to run their lives (and often the lives of others). They live by structure, organization, and rules. You know you're having a conversation with a Judger when it sounds as if they prepared it with an outline. One point leads to the next, until they reach the conclusion. They also believe that work comes first. Once completed, then it's time to play (if there is any time left).

Words like *could be, maybe,* and *perhaps* underlie Perceivers' own actions and their expectations of others. They are flexible, adaptable, and tolerant. Their lives need to be unstructured, leaving room for change and opportunity. Their philosophy is to let life happen. Anything new that comes along could be a pleasurable experience. They avoid commitment as long as possible. Perceivers try to combine play with their work whenever possible. It helps take the structure and rigidity out of the job. Conversations with Perceivers are sometimes hard to follow. They may start on one topic and before you know it, whatever they were talking about triggers another thought, which takes them down another road of topics. They often do end up back where they started, but not always. Then they may have to run through their conversation backward to know what it was that they were originally trying to share.

An interesting note: Keep in mind that being a Judger doesn't mean you are judgmental, though you might be. Being a Perceiver doesn't mean you are perceptive, though you might be.

Henry, the Judger

Henry was referred to me when he was diagnosed as having diabetes. Fortunately, Henry's diabetes could be controlled with pills, an improved diet, and exercise. He had a few extra pounds around his middle he said he certainly wouldn't miss. From a nutritionist's point of view, helping a Judger make changes is a real pleasure. Once the Judger buys into the plan, he or she will become very methodical about carrying it out. When we decided that Henry should eat three meals and three snacks during the day, his comment was, "Just give me a schedule or time sheet and a list of foods, and I'll do fine. I'm ready to get started."

Millie, the Perceiver

Millie was upset that her husband, Henry, had been diagnosed with diabetes. However, she realized his personality type would have an easy time sticking to a diabetic meal plan. Had she been the one diagnosed with it, she wondered what success she would have. The idea of having to stick to a rigid plan, eating at specific times, was completely foreign to her. If her friends asked her at the last minute to join them for coffee, she would go. The more spontaneous the occasion, the better. Millie always answered when opportunity knocked.

Because she loved Henry and wanted to spend many more years together, she was determined to do what she could for him. When I impressed upon her that the plan for Henry was a healthy approach to eating that would benefit her as well, she became an eager learner for them both.

Consistent Results

Do you think the results of your PPQ are consistent with the descriptions you just read? I want you to be sure that you have identified the type that fits you best, since much of the rest of the book is based on it. The section Putting It All Together that begins on page 45 provides a description of each of the types. When you read about your type, you may find what seem to be a few inconsistencies. There are several possible reasons for this:

- You may have answered according to how you would *like* to be or feel you *should* be.
- How you were feeling emotionally at the time influenced your answers.
- You answered with a particular situation in mind.

TABLE 2. **Percentage Estimates for the Different Preferences**

Personality Type	Percentage of Population	Personality Type	Percentage of Population
Extraversion	75%	Introversion	25%
Sensing	75%	iNtuiting	25%
Thinking (female)	35%	Feeling (female)	65%
Thinking (male)	60%	Feeling (male)	40%
Judging	55%	Perceiving	45%

You can either retake the PPQ or select the preferences from the descriptions that seem most like you. Put the letters of the preferences together to give you your type name.

People-Watching

It's interesting how, once you get involved with personality profiling, you start looking at people differently. You wonder what their type is and try to understand them based on it. It would be so helpful if we knew everyone else's type. There would probably be fewer misunderstandings. We'd allow for people's differences because we would now recognize what they are. The differences would be our gain once we learn to appreciate them.

Looking at the distribution of preferences within the general population, we can understand why we have the differences we do. We are seeing and living life from a different perspective. Isabel Myers's percentage estimates for the different preferences are given in Table 2.

One note of caution: Though you would expect that two people of the same type would act in the same manner, it rarely works that way. Jane and Joe are both ESTPs working at a fund-raising event. As you watch them, you notice that Joe is getting much more pumped up by the crowd than Jane. His speech is faster and louder, while Jane's conversational tone seems more subdued. You might think that Jane is actually an ISTP, not an ESTP. That's because your assessment of their type is based on comparing the two. The situation can dictate the way people use their type. While Joe may be more flamboyant at this fund-raising event, Jane might outshine Joe if they were at a class reunion, for example.

I hope you start watching people, trying to figure out what their type is—especially the people who seem to have the healthy habits. Ask yourself what they seem to be doing that you're not. Talk with these people if you can and get a firsthand account. What's in their personality type that is working for them in such a positive way?

By the way, for those who are curious, I am an ENFJ. I suppose you could say I am a nurturer and teacher, which is probably why I got into the nutrition field in the first place. It seemed like an area where I could make a difference in people's lives. And I do hope that this book can make a difference for you.

Putting It All Together

The brief descriptions you'll find below will help you become more familiar with your type—and that of others. The general attributes, assets, and challenges of each type, as well as what causes stress for each type are listed. (Please note: The challenges listed for your type tend to be what other types pick up on, though for you, they may be blindspots.) Keep in mind that these descriptions reveal the basic tendencies and values associated with the type, not necessarily developed skills. You may find some points in each category that fit you perfectly and others that aren't quite as accurate. That's only logical, considering that each of us is unique, even if we do share certain attributes, assets, and challenges with others of our personality type.

If You're an ESTP

ATTRIBUTES

Present-oriented
Playful
Outgoing
Risk taker
Jump in before knowing what's involved

Enjoy life to the fullest
High-energy
Pleasure seeker
Prefer strong sensations (for example, spicy foods)
Easygoing
Adventurous
Tolerant
Spontaneous
Results-oriented
Action-oriented
Enjoy hands-on experiences
Practical
Prefer to deal with facts and details as opposed to ideas and theories
Dislike rules because they are too restrictive
Believe closure isn't important since it's the process that's meaningful
Take what you see at face value

ASSETS

Realistic
Adaptable
Resilient
Troubleshooting
Keen observer
Quick to size up a situation without allowing personal feelings to interfere
Able to foresee consequences of an immediate situation, especially as it pertains to you
Calm and efficient in a crisis
Open-minded
Flexible
Expedient
Able to improvise
Negotiator
Logical in regard to the way things are
Detail-oriented
Good at sales or jobs using your hands
Problem solver

CHALLENGES

Excessive pleasure seeking
Impulsive
Easily distracted
Poor follow-through once project gets going
Become easily bored without variety
Getting buried by details and missing the big picture
Short-sighted
Difficulty with situations that require intellectual pursuits rather than physical action
Desire for instant gratification
Overextending yourself
Not being organized
Being blunt and curt with people

STRESSORS

Deadlines
Too many commitments
Boring or mundane tasks
Being told "you have to"
Rules and regulations
Too much alone time
When results aren't immediate or tangible
Too much preplanning
Too much theory without some practical application

If You're an ESFP

ATTRIBUTES

Present-oriented
Considerate
Enjoy life to the fullest
Pleasure seeker
Sociable
Outgoing
Playful
Practical
Tolerant
Action-oriented
Spontaneous
Enjoy hands-on experiences
Prefer strong sensations (for example, spicy food)
Dislike rules because they're too restrictive
Risk-taker
Jump in before looking and knowing what's involved
Want reward or praise immediately
Believe closure isn't important since it's the process that's meaningful
Prefer to deal with facts and details as opposed to ideas and theories
Strong need for harmony
Take things at face value without looking for reasons or motives
Results-oriented

ASSETS

Realistic
Keen observer
Detail-oriented
Practical
Good in a crisis
Expedient
Adaptable
Ability to improvise
Work well with others
Aim for harmony
Considerate
Empathetic
Open-minded
Flexible

Resilient
Troubleshooting
Good at jobs involving people or using your hands

CHALLENGES

Excessive pleasure seeking
Become easily bored without variety
Getting buried by details and missing the big picture
Not good at long-range planning
Shortsighted
Little consequential thinking
Poor follow-through once project gets going
Impulsive
Tendency toward instant gratification
Impulsiveness causes decisions to be based on what feels good, not what is logical
Finding theories and concepts confusing
Easily distracted
Not being organized
Overextending yourself
Sensitive to criticism

STRESSORS

Deadlines
Too many commitments
Too much alone time
Lack of variety
Results that aren't immediate or tangible
Too much theory without some practical application
Not being appreciated for what you do
Being told "you have to"
Trying to please everyone
Personal conflicts
Too much preplanning
Long-range goal setting

If You're an ISTJ

ATTRIBUTES

Selective attention
Excited by the impression an object gives rather than by the object itself
Results-oriented
Need tangible results from your efforts
Practical
Not a risk-taker
Traditionalist

Good memory for facts, details, and impressions
Quiet
Reserved
Conservative
Reflective
Objective
Analytical
Cautious
Work well independently
Believe actions speak louder than words
Present-oriented
Rely on tried-and-true methods rather than experimenting
Conformist
Follow rules and established ways of doing things
Strong work ethic—work before play
Rely on previous experiences for decision making
Enjoy hands-on experiences
Need to be in control
Prioritize projects based on what is most logical
Rarely show your emotions
Unwilling to take chances

ASSETS

Strong sense of responsibility and duty
Realistic
Ability to organize and provide structure
Commitment both to job and family
Hardworking
Logical
Precise, accurate, and thorough
Good at follow-through
Persistent
Ability to solve practical problems
Efficient
Draw on previous experiences and stored knowledge
Appear calm during a crisis, even if anxious inside
Ability to schedule and plan
Dependable
Synthesis thinking
Able to foresee consequences of an immediate situation, especially as it pertains to others and the environment

CHALLENGES

Being too rigid and inflexible
Making decisions so quickly as to overlook important information
Becoming overly systematic
Difficulty in adapting
Not delegating enough

Impatience
Being too critical of others
Difficulty in working on more than one thing at a time
Fear of future unknowns
Missing the big picture
Not a long-range planner
May blame others for your problems
Not generous with compliments or praise
Being stubborn
Dogmatic under stress
Getting locked into routine approaches even if not effective
Ignoring the feeling side of a situation, inadvertently hurting people
Too many "oughts" and "shoulds"
Once a decision is made, you rarely change it
Doing someone else's job to be sure it's done and done right

STRESSORS

Working with people who are slow and don't contribute
Messy room or desk
Too many projects to do at one time
Not having enough alone time
Being put in the position of having to finish a task at the last minute
Having to deal with ideas rather than facts
Group brainstorming
Not being appreciated
Being thrown off schedule because of others
Having to deal with people's emotions
Having to do something unconventionally
Working on a project that has no obvious purpose

If You're an ISFJ

ATTRIBUTES

Selective attention
Excited by the impression an object gives rather than by the object itself
Need tangible and immediate results from your efforts
Not a risk-taker
Conservative
Traditionalist
Conformist

Good memory for facts, details, and impressions, especially of things and people with personal meaning
Quiet
Reserved
Work well independently
Reflective
Results-oriented
Believe actions speak louder than words
Present-oriented
Rely on tried-and-true methods rather than experimenting
Practical
Follow rules and established ways of doing things
Considerate
Helpful and caring
Empathetic
Desire harmony
Make decisions based on values
Loyal
Prioritize projects based on what is most dear
Strong work ethic—work before play
Enjoy hands-on experiences
Need to be in control
Rely on previous experiences for decision making
Unwilling to take chances

ASSETS

Strong sense of responsibility and duty
Ability to organize and provide structure
Commitment
Draw on previous experiences and stored knowledge
Ability to schedule and plan
Dependable
Supportive of others
Tactful
Value harmony
Precise, accurate, and thorough
Good at follow-through
Persistent
Hardworking
Use efforts to produce immediate, tangible, and practical results
Efficient
Realistic
Good organizer, especially of people

CHALLENGES

Getting locked into routine approaches even if they are not effective
Difficulty in adapting
Not a long-range planner
Being stubborn
Having difficulty saying "no," leading to overwork

Being too rigid and inflexible
Making decisions so quickly as to overlook important information
Impatience
Fear of future unknowns
Missing the big picture
Failure to use logic to solve problems and make decisions
Becoming overly systematic
Difficulty in working on more than one thing at a time

STRESSORS

Messy room or desk
Too many projects to do at one time
Not having enough alone time
Interruptions
Being put in the position of having to finish a task at the last minute
Having to deal with ideas rather than facts
Group brainstorming
Confrontation or conflict
Having to do something unconventionally
Working on a project that has no obvious purpose
Having an opinion based on your personal value system challenged

If You're an ENTP

ATTRIBUTES

Creative
Able to improvise
Rarely accept the way things are
Entrepreneurial
Ambitious
Future-driven
Adventurous
Risk-taker
High-energy
Playful
Competitive
Perfectionist
Find the process more fascinating than the end result
Work must include a play element
Intellectually curious
Action-oriented
Need for novelty and variety
Enjoy a good challenge
Need proof to change your mind
Objective
Analytical

Spontaneous
Flexible
Unstructured
Tend to do things at the last minute
Prefer to get essence of situation without distraction of facts and details
Tolerant
Don't like to be boxed in by rules

ASSETS

Logical analysis of creative ideas to determine if feasible
Innovative problem solving of real-life problems
Good debater and communicator
Synthesis thinking
Resourceful
Open-minded
Long-range planning
Seeing the big picture
Seeing the possibilities
Group brainstorming
Insightful

CHALLENGES

Losing interest when creative process over
Difficulty translating ideas into reality because it requires more patience, structure, and follow-through than is comfortable
Being easily sidetracked
Lacking attention to detail
Overlooking facts by being too future-oriented
Critical, especially of self, because of unrealistically high standards
Easily bored
Overly competitive
Living too much in the future so you may miss what the present has to offer
Changing course before reaping benefits from the present one
Becoming overextended
Overcautious in stressful situation
Stubborn at times
Focusing on your body and any of its shortcomings when under stress

STRESSORS

Deadlines
Too many commitments
Not knowing the "why" behind a matter

Not getting feedback
Routine
Being forced to do something in a prescribed way
Having to live by rules
Too much structure
Too much outside stimuli when trying to think
Seeing no connection between your actions and the future
Having to work alone on a project
Working with people you don't respect or feel are incompetent

If You're an ENFP

ATTRIBUTES

Creative
Able to improvise
Curious
Entrepreneurial
Future-driven
High-energy
Charismatic
Competitive
Rarely accept the way things are
Idealistic
Spontaneous
Flexible
Adventurous
Risk-taker
Enjoy challenges
Unstructured
Dislike details and rules
Need for novelty and variety
Not singularly focused
Tolerant
Interested in harmony
Know how to persuasively enlist help of others to fulfill your personal agenda
Treat people favorably so you will be liked and well received
Tend to do things at the last minute using a burst of energy to get the job done
Find the process more fascinating than the end result
Work must include a play element
Looking for personal purpose in life
Persevering
Commitment to personal values

ASSETS

Creating ideas to benefit others and the environment
Innovative problem solving
Seeing the big picture as it relates to others and things
Long-range planning
Seeing the possibilities
Resourceful
Adaptable
Insight into other people's needs and potential
Good debater, communicator, and motivator

CHALLENGES

Lack of patience
Being easily sidetracked
Can't deal with routine
Easily bored
Losing interest when creative process is over
Changing course before reaping benefits from the present one
Lacking attention to detail
Living too much in the future so you miss what the present has to offer
Poor follow-through
Becoming overextended
Difficulty in making decisions if presented with too many alternatives
Focusing on your body and any of its shortcomings when under stress

STRESSORS

Routine or anything done repetitively
Too much paperwork that seems unnecessary
Strict schedules
Deadlines
Being alone too much
Being over-committed
Being forced to do something in a prescribed way
Confrontation
Not being appreciated
Working with people who lack vision
Not getting feedback
Having to spend time on a cause that is not personally meaningful
Difficulty in saying "no" to new experiences, resulting in overload

If You're an INTJ

ATTRIBUTES

Perfectionist
High achiever
Independent
Like to be in control
Confident
Rarely accept the way things are
Need proof to change your mind
Logical and analytical
Objective
Ignore rules if they don't make sense
Need for closure
Future-oriented
Enjoy challenges
Need for novelty
Decisive
Reflective
Reserved
Persevering
Intellectually curious
Creative
Insightful

ASSETS

Long-range planning
Problem solving
Consequential thinking
Strategic planning
Seeing the big picture
Sharing insights clearly
Being tough when necessary
Appearing calm in a crisis
Good at prioritizing and organizing
Original thinking
Individual brainstorming
Synthesis thinking

CHALLENGES

Supercritical of others and self because of unrealistically high standards
Too demanding
May hurt people's feelings unknowingly
Inflexible
Too independent to seek others' help
Speak with such unquestioning decisiveness and authority as to make others feel inferior
May appear arrogant
Controlling
Might not attempt something you think you can't succeed at

Under stress, will overindulge, overeat, become overstimulated
Impatience
Scant with praise
Making decisions so quickly that important information or input from others is overlooked or not requested
Living so much in the future as to miss what the present has to offer
Difficulty in adapting
If project not considered personally important, you give sparingly of your time

STRESSORS

Unfinished projects
Corporate culture
Disorganization
Routine
Not being appreciated
Having to follow what you think are useless rules
Work that has no evident purpose
Not knowing "why"
Too many things going on at once
Not sticking to schedule
Messy room or desk
No time to reflect
Lack of control in a situation
Incompetent people
Having to deal with people's emotions

If You're an INFJ

ATTRIBUTES

Idealistic
Looking for life's purpose
Searching for meaning
Prefer to get essence of situation without distraction of facts and details
Need for closure
Future-oriented
Creative
Decisive
Empathetic
Accepting of people
Interested in harmony
Want your deeds and contributions to serve as evidence of who you are
Keep feelings to yourself
Believe it isn't nice to criticize
Insightful
Independent

Reserved
Nurturing
Warm, considerate, and compassionate
Reflective
Need for novelty
Rarely accept the way things are
Dreamer

ASSETS

Good at solving people problems
Insight into other people's needs and potential
Encourage harmony within a group
Being a motivator
Seeing value in each individual
Long-range planning
Can see the big picture as it relates to self and ideas
Group brainstorming
Organized
Loyal
Persuasive

CHALLENGES

Overcautious in stressful situations
Bottling up feelings until they become so overwhelming that you blow up
Making sacrifices in the name of harmony
Overlooking facts by being too future-oriented
Often making decisions too quickly
Under stress, will overindulge, overeat, become overstimulated
Setting unrealistically high standards for self and others
Sometimes inflexible
Coming up with ideas but never putting them into action

STRESSORS

Unfinished projects
Having to finish a task at the last minute
Disorganization
Routine
Work that has no evident purpose
Not sticking to the schedule
Too many things going on at once
No time to reflect
Competition
Confrontation
Not being appreciated

If You're an ESTJ

ATTRIBUTES

Analytical
Objective
Traditionalist
Conservative
Live by rules, standards, and established ways of doing things
Conformist
Rely on previous experiences for decision making
Need to be in control
Outspoken
Strong work ethic—work before play
Schedule all aspects of life, from work to play
Like action and variety
Excited by the impression an object gives rather than by the object itself
Cautious
Not a risk-taker
Practical
Need tangible results from your efforts
Present-oriented
Rely on tried-and-true methods rather than experimenting
Prioritize projects based on what is most logical
Unwilling to take chances

ASSETS

Use efforts to produce immediate, tangible, and practical results
Logical
Realistic
Good at prioritizing, scheduling, and planning
Efficient at organizing, especially of facts
Attention to administrative details
Efficient
Dependable
Hardworking
Conscientious
Persistent
Strong sense of responsibility and duty
Good at follow-through
Synthesis thinking
Commitment
Able to see consequences of the immediate situation, especially as it pertains to others and the environment
Leadership skills

CHALLENGES

- Getting locked into routine approaches even if they're not effective
- Inflexible
- Making decisions so quickly as to overlook important information
- Impatience
- Not a long-range planner
- Missing the big picture
- Ignoring the feeling side of a situation, inadvertently hurting people
- Being too critical of others
- May blame others for your problems
- Difficulty in adapting
- Dogmatic under stress
- Failure to delegate enough
- Too many "oughts" and "shoulds"
- Difficulty in working on more than one thing at a time
- Becoming overly systematic
- Once your mind is made up, it is hard to change it

STRESSORS

- Not being appreciated
- Having to deal with people's emotions
- Working with people who are slow and don't contribute
- Having to work alone on a project
- Having to do something unconventionally
- Messy room or desk
- Having to deal with ideas rather than facts
- Not sticking to schedule
- Put in the position of having to finish a task at the last minute

If You're an ENTJ

ATTRIBUTES

- Analytical and logical
- Objective
- Live by rules and standards
- Like to be in control
- Assertive
- Outspoken
- Future-oriented
- High-energy
- Need for closure
- Decisive
- Insightful
- Need for novelty and variety

Good communicator and leader
Perfectionist
Persevering
Ambitious
Strong drive and ego
Rarely accept things as they are, since you believe everything can be improved
Need proof to change your mind—especially logical proof
Enjoy a good challenge
Competitive
Intellectually curious

ASSETS

Organization problem solver
Leadership skills
Logical
Good at prioritizing and organizing
Good at long-range planning
Can foresee problems
Group brainstorming
Creative
Synthesis and hypothetical thinking
Strategic planning
Seeing the big picture
Being tough when necessary
Appear calm in a crisis
Hardworking
Enjoy challenges
Productive
Decisive

CHALLENGES

Making decisions so quickly that important information or input from others is overlooked or not even sought
Impatience
Difficulty in adapting
If you don't consider a project personally important (or once the creative part is completed) you give sparingly of your time and effort so you can head off to a new project
Scant with praise
Inflexible
Controlling
Intimidating
Might not attempt something you think you can't succeed at
Too demanding
Being stubborn and overpowering
Overly competitive
Under stress, will overindulge, overeat, become overstimulated

Supercritical, often without concern for hurting people's feelings
Setting unrealistically high standards for yourself and others
Living so much in the future as to miss what the present has to offer

STRESSORS

Not being appreciated
Not getting feedback
Having to deal with people's emotions
Having to work alone on a project
Messy room or desk
Routine
Others keeping you from sticking to a schedule
Unfinished projects
Disorganization
Having to follow what you think are useless rules
Work that has no evident purpose
Lack of control in a situation
Indecisive or incompetent people
Inefficiency
Not knowing "why"
Corporate culture
Step-by-step instructions

If You're an ISTP

ATTRIBUTES

Present-oriented
Action-oriented
Adventurous
Spontaneous
Risk-taker
Impulsive
Jump in before looking and knowing what's involved
Enjoy hands-on experiences
Pleasure seeker
Quiet and reserved
Independent
Practical
Prefer strong sensations (for example, spicy food)
Dislike rules because they're too restrictive
Closure not important since it's the process that's meaningful
Prefer to deal with facts and details
Tolerant
Analytical
Love the outdoors

ASSETS

Realistic
Keen observer
Good in a crisis
Troubleshooting
Able to improvise
Expedient
Open-minded
Solving immediate problems
Efficient
Able to foresee consequences of an immediate situation, especially as pertains to you
Logical
Flexible
Good at sales and jobs using your hands
Adaptable
Resilient
Curiosity about how things work

CHALLENGES

Excessive pleasure seeking
Easily distracted
Getting buried by details and missing the big picture
Tendency toward instant gratification
Not organized
Overextending yourself
Often taking the first available, easy-to-follow approach that may not be adequate for the task
Shortsighted
Not good at long-range planning
Poor follow-through once project gets going
Reactive rather than proactive
Overlooking emotional needs of people because of logical and analytical focus

STRESSORS

Deadlines
Too many commitments
When results aren't immediate
Too much newness
Being told too much theory without some practical relevance
Being told "you have to"
Too much preplanning
Working without tangible or practical results

If You're an INTP

ATTRIBUTES

Reflective
Quiet
Reserved
Independent
Tolerant
Spontaneous
Flexible
Future-driven
Entrepreneurial
Rarely accept the way things are
Enjoy a good challenge
Ambitious
Perfectionist
Adventurous
Risk-taker
Unstructured
Objective
Prefer novelty
Dislike rules and routine
Tend to do things at the last minute
Find the process more fascinating than the end result
Prefer that work include a play element
Intellectually curious
Need proof to change your mind
Prefer to get essence of situation without distraction of facts and details
Your solutions to problems may not be practical

ASSETS

Open-minded
Logical analysis of creative ideas to determine if feasible
Innovative problem solving of real-life problems
Synthesis thinking
Long-range planning
Seeing the big picture and the possibilities
Curious
Resourceful
Being prepared
Insightful
Good at coming up with theories for what exists
Creative
Able to improvise

CHALLENGES

Losing interest when creative process is over or inspiration diminishes
Can be easily sidetracked
Lacking attention to detail
Critical, especially of self
Appear indecisive
Easily bored
Challenging the rules
Living so much in the future as to miss what the present has to offer
Dealing with people problems
Changing courses before reaping benefits from the present course
Poor follow-through
Becoming overextended
Overcautious in stressful situations
Stubborn at times

STRESSORS

Deadlines
Not getting feedback
Incompetent people
Too much structure
Having to live by rules that seem useless
Being forced to do something in a prescribed way
Too much stimuli when trying to think
Not knowing "why"
No time to reflect

If You're an ESFJ

ATTRIBUTES

Selective attention
Excited by the impression an object gives rather than by the object itself
Live by rules and standards if you believe in them
Rely on previous experiences for decision making
Traditionalist
Present-oriented
Need tangible results from your efforts
Practical
Not a risk-taker
Considerate
Helpful and caring
Value harmony
Going along with the group
Cooperative

Rely on tried-and-true methods rather than experimenting
Decisions based on values consistent with tradition and accepted standards
Failure to use logic to solve problems and make decisions
Strong work ethic—work before play
Good memory for facts, details, and impressions, especially of things and people with personal meaning
Prioritize projects based on what is most dear
Want variety
Conservative
Conformist
Enjoy hands-on experiences
Cautious
Want to be in control
Outspoken

ASSETS

Use efforts to produce immediate, tangible and practical results
Realistic
Good at prioritizing, scheduling, planning, and organizing
Dependable
Precise, accurate, and thorough
Good at follow-through
Hardworking
Conscientious
Persistent
Focus on people's needs and desires
Supportive of others
Tactful
Good people organizer
Strong sense of responsibility and duty
Committed
Efficient

CHALLENGES

Getting locked into routine approaches, even when they're not effective
Being too rigid and inflexible
Becoming overly systematic
Becoming overworked because of difficulty in saying "no"
Difficulty in adapting
Not a long-range planner

Making decisions so quickly as to overlook important information
Impatience
Unwilling to take chances
Fear of future unknowns
Missing the big picture
Being stubborn
Inflexible
Difficulty in working on more than one thing at a time
Taking failure personally
In attempt to help and please others, you may overlook your own needs

STRESSORS

Having to work alone on a project
Feeling you are not needed
Having to do something unconventionally
Messy room or desk
Being given too many projects to do at one time
Being put in the position of having to finish a task at the last minute
Having to deal with ideas rather than facts
Confrontation or conflict
Not sticking to a schedule
Too many new challenges
Not being appreciated
Competition in which someone has to lose
Rules that don't appear fair or nice

If You're an ENFJ

ATTRIBUTES

Idealistic
Looking for life's purpose
Rarely accept the way things are
Prefer to get essence of situation without distraction of facts and details
Need for closure
High achiever
Future-oriented
Creative
Warm and considerate
Accepting of people
Nurturing
Charismatic
Want to please even if at the expense of yourself
Interested in harmony
Enjoy doing for others
Persevering
Sensitive to criticism
Want to be accepted

Decisive
Assertive
Enjoy a challenge
Need for novelty and variety
Leadership skills
Empathetic
Compassionate
Want your deeds and contributions to serve as evidence of who you are
Act according to personal values
Reflective
No hidden agendas
Assume it is your responsibility to make events fun and entertaining

ASSETS

Solving people problems
Long-range planning
Group brainstorming
Coming up with a variety of solutions
Organized
Seeing the big picture as it relates to self and ideas
Being a motivator, helping to bring out the potential in others
Seeing value in each individual
Generous with praise
Search for meaning
Loyal
Good communicator, mediator, and facilitator
Persuasive
Encourage harmony and cooperation within a group
Insight into people's needs and their potential
Search for meaning
Bettering others' lives

CHALLENGES

Overcautious in stressful situations
Once creative part of project is completed, give sparingly of your time and effort so you can head off to new project
Setting unrealistically high standards for yourself and others
May make decisions too quickly
Avoiding conflict instead of confronting a problem
Making sacrifices in the name of harmony
Easily hurt
If something goes wrong, worrying if you are at fault
Failure taken personally

Overlooking facts by being too future-oriented
Under stress, will overindulge, overeat, become overstimulated
Sometimes overlooking the logical consequences of your actions

STRESSORS

Unfinished projects
Corporate culture
Disorganization
Too much routine
Work that has no evident purpose
Not being appreciated
Having to spend time on a cause that is not personally meaningful
People being critical
Competition
Confrontation

If You're an ISFP

ATTRIBUTES

Present-oriented
Action-oriented
Enjoy hands-on experiences
Pleasure seeker
Playful
Adventurous
Risk-taker
Independent
Practical
Quiet and reserved
Spontaneous
Tolerant
Accepting of others and things as they are
Considerate
Prefer strong sensations (for example, spicy food)
Dislike rules because they're too restrictive
Impulsive
Jump in before looking and knowing what's involved
Want reward or praise immediately
Closure not important since it's the process that's meaningful
Prefer to deal with facts and details
Commitment to inner circle of family and friends
Prefer to blend in with crowd

ASSETS

Realistic
Keen observer
Troubleshooting
Able to improvise
Expedient
Good in a crisis
Work well with others
Cooperative
Empathetic
Aim for harmony
Open-minded
Flexible
Good at jobs involving people or using your hands
Adaptable
Resilient

CHALLENGES

Excessive pleasure seeking
Getting buried by details and missing the big picture
Not good at long-range planning, especially goal setting
Little preparation
Poor follow-through once project gets going
Tendency toward instant gratification
Impulsiveness causes decisions to be based on what feels good, not what is logical
Finding theories and concepts confusing
Short-sighted
Little consequential thinking
Easily distracted
Not organized
Overextending yourself
Don't reveal the true you

STRESSORS

Deadlines
Too many commitments
Too many new things at one time
Results that aren't tangible or immediate
Being told too much theory without some practical relevance
When not appreciated for what you do
Being told "you have to"
Trying to please everyone
Personal conflicts
Too much preplanning

If You're an INFP

ATTRIBUTES

Creative
Able to improvise
Future-driven
Rarely accept the way things are
Curious
Challenge the rules
Idealistic
Reflective
Spontaneous
Flexible
Adventurous
Risk-taker
Unstructured
Prefer novelty
Enjoy challenges
Dislike details and structure
Independent
Self-directed
Reserved
Tend to do things at the last minute
Find the process more fascinating than the end result
Prefer that work include a play element
Empathetic
Look for personal purpose in life
Commitment to personal values

ASSETS

Creating ideas to benefit others and the environment
Innovative problem solving
Long-range planning
Seeing the big picture as it relates to others and things
Insight into people's needs and their potential
Being a motivator
Seeing the possibilities
Resourceful
Adaptable

CHALLENGES

Lack of patience
Losing interest when creative process is over
Being easily sidetracked
Lacking attention to detail
Poor follow-through
Becoming overextended
Easily bored
Living so much in the future as to miss what the present has to offer
Changing course before reaping benefits from the present one

Unrealistic expectations of what you can accomplish

Taking personally the failure to accomplish something

STRESSORS

Routine or anything done repetitively

Overcommitting yourself

Having to spend time on a cause that is not personally meaningful

Being forced to do something in a prescribed way

Confrontation

Not being appreciated

Working with people who lack vision

Too much paperwork that seems unnecessary

Strict schedules

Not getting feedback

Competition

No time to reflect

Too many things going on at once

Too structured an environment

Rules and regulations that stifle creativity

3

Killer Habits

What's the first thing you think of when I say the word *habit?* Most people respond with: "I have plenty of them, and a lot of them aren't healthy." Those who need to lose weight might add: "Just look at me. These extra pounds I carry around are the result of those habits." According to the *Random House Dictionary,* the definition of *habit* is:

> **1.** A customary practice or use. **2.** An acquired behavior pattern regularly followed until it has become almost involuntary.

The day you were born, you had no habits. You were a clean slate upon which you started writing down or acquiring certain behavior patterns. As a toddler, you might have learned that when you pounded the table with your cup, you could get your mother's attention. The first time you did it, it was an unplanned event. Getting the results you wanted was reinforcing. After trying it a few more times and getting the same reaction from your mother, you were rapidly making this behavior a habit (that is, unless your mother nipped that habit in the bud!).

All habits come about in a similar way. You do something, see the results and experience the way it makes you feel, and then determine whether it's worth repeating the behavior. The first time you took a hot pot off the stove without a potholder and burned your hand, you knew immediately that it wasn't a behavior you wanted to make a habit. Generally speaking, having habits can be beneficial. Habits allow you to act in certain ways without having to constantly think about your actions. Take tying your shoelaces, for example. When you were first shown how to tie your laces, you probably felt all thumbs. Eventually, though, with enough practice, you could easily tie your laces. I'm sure you no longer think about what you actually do when you tie them, because it's become a habit.

Just to prove my point, why don't you try something that you may find very frustrating. Give someone a step-by-step description of tying shoelaces as you are doing it. You'll find that you've become all thumbs again. That's because tying your shoelaces has become "almost involuntary," as the definition states. By describing the process in detail, you're forcing the process into conscious awareness, something you don't normally do with habits.

Here's another task that can be equally frustrating. Fold your arms across your chest. Note which arm is on top. Now unfold your arms, then fold them again, except this time, put the other arm on top. Does it feel strange to you? Can you even do it? That's because crossing your arms in a certain way has become a habit—fortunately one that won't cause you any harm.

Because many of our habits get us into trouble, we tend to apply a negative connotation to the word. For many people, the words *bad* and *habit* seem to go together naturally. Yet, a habit only becomes bad when the result of the habit causes problems. The habit of eating a candy bar for a snack every afternoon is a bad habit when it adds to your weight and takes the place of something healthier. The habit of parking as close to the mall as possible so you don't have to walk too far is a bad habit when you have little other physical activity in your life. On the other hand, the habit of eating a nutritious breakfast each day is a good habit because it gives you the necessary fuel to perform at your best throughout the day. The habit of buckling up your seat belt in the car is a good habit because it reduces your risk of serious injury in an accident.

It's curious that people who know better still allow bad habits to persist. The reasons they give may have a plausible ring to them, but still keep them on the road to destruction. They find that their habits bring them pleasure both physiologically ("I love the taste of chocolate") and psychologically ("I deserve this little treat"). They rely on those habits to get through times when there is little stimulation ("I'm so bored; tossing popcorn into my mouth will at least keep me busy") or too much stimulation ("I'm so stressed out, maybe a bowl of ice cream will make me feel better"). Then there is the influence of others ("If you're going to have dessert, I'll join you") or environmental influences ("With that big plate of cookies just sitting there, I couldn't resist").

A Time for Reckoning

Before I share with you the **Top Ten List of Unhealthy Habits** and the **Top Ten List of Excuses** for those habits, I'd like you to create your own lists. Take a piece of paper and draw two columns. Make the heading of the first column, "Habits I'd Like to Change and Their Consequences." Make the heading of the second column, "Excuses for These Habits." In the first column write the unhealthy habits you want to change, immediately followed by what you think are the potential consequences of those unhealthy habits. Then list what excuse or excuses you are using to continue this habit. Here's how Joann started her list, for example:

Habits I'd Like to Change and Their Consequences	Excuses for These Habits
Eating a bowl of ice cream every night before I go to bed.—*It's probably the cause of my gaining five pounds in the last month.*	My husband makes me feel guilty for not joining him when he wants a bowl of ice cream.

Now let's see how your list compares with the **Top Ten List of Unhealthy Habits** that my clients helped me create. As in the tradition of David Letterman, the night-time talk show host, I have listed them in reverse order, saving the best for last.

Top Ten List of Unhealthy Habits

10. Over-committing yourself.
9. Not taking time for yourself.
8. Eating too much of the not-so-healthy foods without balancing them out with healthy foods.
7. Not living in the present moment.
6. Eating for all the wrong reasons: (a) because you associate it with an activity (e.g., eating popcorn at the movies); (b) because you're depressed, bored, lonely, frustrated; (c) because you're trying to avoid a job; (d) because it's there; (e) because your friends are having something, so you decide to as well.
5. Setting unrealistic goals for yourself and seeing yourself as a failure when you fall short of them.
4. Smoking or drinking excessively.
3. Overeating or eating when not hungry.
2. Leading a sedentary lifestyle, not exercising, or being physically inactive.
1. Making excuses for all of the above.

The worst habit of all is making excuses for having a bad habit. Whenever you provide an excuse, you are trying to justify something you know in your heart isn't really justifiable. Realize that making excuses doesn't change the habit and, when you take the time to think about the excuse, it reinforces your feeling of failing to do something about the habit. In addition, excuses won't protect you against disease, illness, a shorter life span, or becoming overweight.

We need to air those excuses now so we can begin to release their grip on us. If we don't have any excuses to hide behind, we are more likely to face up to the challenge of changing our unacceptable habits. Here's the **Top Ten List of Excuses** people give for not changing their habits. Did your list have some different ones? (If you didn't make a list, it's just one example of your personality at work. I do hope that, at the very least, you thought about some of your unacceptable habits and the excuses you make for them. Later, we'll find out more about the personality types that enjoy the structure of writing things down and those that do not.)

Top Ten List of Excuses

10. "I've got so many changes to make. It just seems too overwhelming."
9. "It's too much work and too inconvenient for me to exercise and prepare healthy meals."
8. "It will cost too much."
7. "It's hard for me to picture how things will be different when I change my habits."
6. "I don't know how or what to change. One day I read about a nutrition study that supports eating one way, only to have it contradicted the next day. It's too confusing."
5. "I'm under too much stress to put my mind to changing right now."
4. "At this point, it's force of habit with me, and I don't know whether I can change."
3. "I have no willpower or self-control."
2. "I don't want to give up my favorite foods or deprive my family of theirs."
1. "I don't have the time."

The list of bad habits and excuses could go on and on. What's distressing is that people may be digging themselves into an early grave with their habits and excuses. What you eat and how much you exercise, whether you let stress get to you, whether you smoke, and how much you drink—all are factors that impact your future health. Along with genetic components in heart disease, stroke, hypertension, cancer, and diabetes, it's now known that lifestyle habits can greatly influence our chance of developing these diseases. Lifestyle habits also contribute to our becoming overweight, a condition that can hasten the onset of these same diseases.

It would probably help for you to become a little more familiar with these serious diseases and what habits you might have that raise your risk for them. We'll be looking at heart disease, cancer, and diabetes, the three major diseases in the United States.

Cardiovascular Disease

Did you know that heart attacks amount to the single-biggest killer in the United States? (Stroke is the third-biggest killer.) The statistics from the American Heart Association are even more chilling. They tell us that about every 33 seconds someone in this country dies from some form of cardiovascular disease (CVD), which includes heart disease, stroke, and hypertension (high blood pressure). Every 20 seconds an American suffers a heart attack, and about every minute someone dies from one. Every 3.4 minutes someone dies of a stroke. One in four Americans has high blood pressure.

Heart Disease

The heart is a muscle. It is surrounded by arteries that supply it with oxygen and nourishment. The health of those arteries influences the health of your heart. If they become narrower, there will be a reduction in blood flow. That means that less oxygen and fewer nutrients can get to the heart.

When your blood cholesterol level is high, there's a greater chance of damage to your arteries. Cholesterol, along with other materials, damages the walls of the arteries by invading them and forming what is known as *plaque.* As more and more plaque forms, the walls thicken and start to bulge, inward, making the passageway of the artery narrower. Sadly, plaque can begin to develop at a fairly early age.

Picture two garden hoses, one with a diameter half as large as the other. Now turn on the faucet to each hose, keeping the water pressure the same for both. The flow in the narrower hose will be slower. Apply that image to the arteries leading to your heart. Less oxygen and fewer nutrients get to your heart when the diameter of the arteries is narrowed by the formation of plaque. (See Figure 9.)

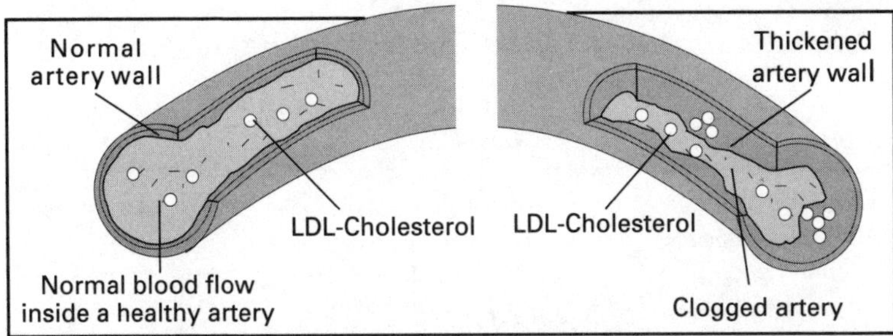

Figure 9. Healthy and Clogged Arteries

Now imagine that a pebble has gotten into your hose and totally blocks the flow of water. That's what happens when a blood clot occurs in an artery. Almost no blood gets to the heart muscle at that point, and some of the heart muscle dies. Whether the heart can continue to beat will be determined by how severe the blockage is and how much of the heart muscle has died.

When was the last time you had your blood cholesterol level checked? The next time you do, keep the following desirable numbers in mind:

- Your **Total Cholesterol (TC)** should be less than 200 mg/dl.
- You want your **LDL-Cholesterol** to be less than 130 mg/dl. (LDL is considered the "bad" cholesterol because it's what clogs your arteries.)
- Your **HDL-Cholesterol** should be 30–80 mg/dl if you're a woman, and 30–70 mg/dl if you're a man. (HDL is considered the "good" cholesterol because it acts like a street cleaner, picking up and getting rid of excess LDL-cholesterol that wants to clog your arteries.)

One other very important number is the **Ratio of TC to HDL-Cholesterol** (TC ÷ HDL, written as TC:HDL). It should be less than 3.5. You might be okay with a high total cholesterol as long as you have a high HDL-cholesterol level to go with it. The more HDL you have, the more LDL-cholesterol can be swept up. Therefore, the smaller the TC:HDL ratio, the lower is your risk for CVD. (See Table 3.)

TABLE 3. **Blood Cholesterol Values**

Blood Cholesterol	Desirable Level	Borderline Level	High Level
LDL-Cholesterol	< 130 mg/dl	130–159 mg/dl	≥ 160 mg/dl
HDL-Cholesterol			
Female	30–80 mg/dl		
Male	30–70 mg/dl		
Total Cholesterol (TC)	< 200 mg/dl	201–239 mg/dl	≥ 240 mg/dl
TC:HDL-Cholesterol Ratio	< 3.5		

mg/dl = milligram per deciliter

Stroke

Stroke is similar to heart disease except that the arteries affected by a stroke are in the brain. Complete blockage of an artery there starves the brain of blood and oxygen, causing permanent damage. (A temporary interruption of blood flow may not cause permanent damage.) Stroke can affect speech, the ability to move (when one side of the body is affected, it means the opposite side of the brain was injured), and the ability to accomplish everyday tasks like getting dressed.

Hypertension

High blood pressure is often listed on death certificates as a cause of death. That's because it contributes to heart attacks, strokes, heart failure, and kidney damage. Hypertension can sneak up on you without any symptoms, so it's a good idea to have your blood pressure checked every year or so. When you do, you will be given two numbers. The first will be the larger of the two, and is called the *systolic* pressure. It represents the pressure in your blood vessels as your heart contracts. The second, or smaller, number is your *diastolic* pressure, the pressure as your heart relaxes between beats.

Your blood pressure tends to vary slightly, depending on what you're doing. It rises when you're exercising or are excited. It drops when you're asleep or sitting quietly. These changes are normal. According to the National Heart, Lung, and Blood Institute, a reading of 120/80 is normal for most people. When it gets above 140/90, hypertension has set in.

Your heart pumps blood through large blood vessels called arteries, which are elastic and flexible when healthy. As the heart pumps blood, an artery stretches to accommodate the influx of fluid. The artery contracts when the heart muscle relaxes. Under normal conditions, this stretching and contracting can occur 60 to 80 times a minute. The health of your arteries—that is, how elastic and open they are—is one determinant of how much pressure the heart must exert to push the blood through. The less elastic and more narrowed the artery, the higher the blood pressure. Again, think about it in terms of your garden hose. When you have the nozzle wide open, the water flows freely with little pressure. However, if you partially close the nozzle, the water pressure builds up.

Hardening of the arteries, *arteriosclerosis,* occurs with age, often starting with some damage to the lining of the arteries. However, the process speeds up when you have high blood pressure, which only adds insult to injury. Your risk for stroke and heart disease becomes that much higher.

Most people think that to avoid high blood pressure, they should eliminate salt from their diet. Research shows that unless you are salt-sensitive, decreasing your intake to abnormally low levels won't be of much help. The American Heart Association's recommendation for salt intake is 2400 mg, or about one teaspoon of salt per day. Keep in mind that that means salt from all sources, both naturally occurring and what you add to foods. Diets that are low in potassium, calcium, and magnesium may also play a part in causing hypertension.

The most important thing you can do when you have high blood pressure is lose weight. Even as little as a 10 percent change in your weight can affect your pressure.

Who Gets CVD?

What are the chances that you'll get cardiovascular disease? There are risk factors involving your lifestyle habits that you can do something about, and there are other factors over which you have no control. First, let's look at what might be genetically working against you.

Family If someone in your family has had the disease, your risk is higher.

Gender Men are more prone to heart disease than premenopausal women. However, older women lose their gender advantage. This is because menopause lowers their levels of estrogen, a hormone that has a protective effect against heart disease.

Age Our chance of getting CVD increases as we age. The highest rate of CVD in men occurs when they're between 50 and 60 years old. In women, that increased incidence doesn't occur until they're between 60 and 70 years old. If a woman is on estrogen-replacement therapy after menopause, her risk level goes down even as she ages. There is much we can do in our younger years to try to prevent CVD. Changing our habits should be high on the list.

Race Black males have a 50 percent higher rate of CVD than white males, and black females suffer 69 percent more deaths from CVD than white females.

Even though there is nothing you can do about the genetic factors, let's not forget all the habits you do have control over that pave the road to CVD: smoking, eating a high-fat diet, living a sedentary lifestyle, being overweight, allowing stressful situations to get to you. It's up to you whether you want to do something about them.

Did you know:

A person with a body weight that is 20 percent or more above a healthy weight runs a much greater risk of CVD than a person of normal weight.

Do You Have Any of These CVD Killer Habits?

Cigarette smoking

Cigarette smoking ranks extremely high among the habits that increase your risk of developing heart disease. The smoke contains what are known as *free radicals.* (We're not talking about the rebels during the Free Speech movement in the late 1960s!) Chemically, these free radicals are molecules that are missing an electron, and they will do most anything to find one. The easiest way is to be a thief and steal the electron from another molecule.

As the chemicals from smoking travel through your bloodstream, they find easy prey in the LDL-cholesterol. When the free radicals found in the smoke take an electron away from the LDL-cholesterol, they *oxidize* the LDL-cholesterol, making *it* a free radical looking for an electron. As the LDL enters the blood vessel walls, it goes after electrons there and damages the tissues. The body rushes to repair the damage, surrounding that area with fatty streaks and cholesterol, where eventually plaque forms *within* the lining of the arteries. Many people have incorrectly thought that cholesterol clogs arteries by collecting *along* the lining of the artery cavity, somewhat like sludge in a drainpipe. Now we know differently.

An Overdose of Fat and Cholesterol

The type and amount of fat, along with how much cholesterol you eat, to a large extent determines your blood cholesterol level. Too much total fat, saturated fat, and dietary cholesterol lead to a high blood cholesterol. Some of the fat and cholesterol from your food goes directly to your fat cells. The rest goes to your liver to be repackaged as LDL-cholesterol, HDL-cholesterol, and other forms of cholesterol. The more saturated fat you eat, the greater number of LDL-cholesterol packets made by the liver. That means there is more of the "bad" cholesterol traveling around in your bloodstream to cause problems.

What you choose to eat can have a strong influence on your cholesterol level, and in turn, on your risk for CVD. Because the liver is capable of making cholesterol, you don't need to include *any* cholesterol in your diet. However, with most Americans relying on a meat-based diet, it's unlikely that that will happen. (Cholesterol is found only in animal proteins.) The meat-based diet also means a high saturated-fat diet. The American Heart Association recommends that fats contribute less than 30 percent of our total calories and saturated fats less than 10 percent. Later in the book you'll find out more about creating a diet based on these numbers.

Before we go any further, I want to clear up one misunderstanding many people have. When I talk about the "good" cholesterol (HDL-cholesterol) and the "bad" cholesterol (LDL-cholesterol), I'm referring to the type of cholesterol the body makes. There is only one type of cholesterol in food, and it is neither good nor bad. What is harmful is giving your body too much of it, along with too much fat—especially saturated fat.

That brings me to my next point: How much fat are you eating each day? In addition to the *type* of fat, the *amount* is an important consideration. The more fat you eat, the more cholesterol packets your body is going to make to transport it through the bloodstream. And the more packets there are, the higher will be your total blood cholesterol. Fat is also a very concentrated form of calories. Too much fat means too many calories, which, in turn, can lead to weight gain, one of the risk factors for CVD.

The higher your blood cholesterol level without a correspondingly high HDL-cholesterol level, the more plaque can build up in your artery walls. When you eat too much fat, cholesterol, and calories, you are literally feeding the plaque (and filling out your waistline!). Don't get me wrong. I'm not saying you have to give up your favorite foods. As you will see later in the book, all foods are legal (unless your doctor has told you certain foods must be eliminated from your diet).

In most cases, a high-fat diet also means a low-fiber, low fruit, and vegetable diet. That's too bad, since fiber can help lower your cholesterol. Also, there appear to be natural chemicals in vegetables and fruit that protect your heart. More about that later.

A Sedentary Lifestyle

Regularly eating too many calories and leading a sedentary life is definitely going to show up on the bathroom scale. It also will wreak havoc on your body's health. Each morning, as you step on the "truth-sayer," you pray that the numbers won't keep climbing, but they defy you anyway. Even worse is the way you feel. Whether you're feeling sluggish because of the extra weight or because you're out of condition, the bottom line is that you aren't operating at your best. Lack of exercise could be the problem.

There are so many benefits to exercising. Just a few of the most important ones are these:

1. Exercise promotes the production of the good cholesterol, HDL.
2. When you exercise, you build muscle. Muscle burns calories and fat doesn't.
3. Exercise strengthens your heart muscle. The stronger your heart muscle, the less work it has to do to pump the blood around your system.
4. Exercise helps relieve stress. If you like to be outside when you exercise, it gets you a little closer to nature. Noticing the new growth on the trees, the colors of the flowers, the feel of the wind and the sound of the birds tends to take your mind off your problems.

Cancer

Cancer is the second leading cause of death in the United States. According to the American Cancer Society, one out of every four deaths in the United States is from cancer. That amounts to more than fifteen hundred people dying from cancer every day. Lung cancer heads the list, followed by cancer of the breast, uterus, cervix, and ovary in women, and cancer of the prostate in men. But cancer can affect almost any part of the body; nine percent of new diagnoses of cancer involve the colon and rectum, for example.

There's nothing we can do about the unavoidable risk factors of heredity, age, and gender. When a member of your family has had cancer, your chances of getting it are greater. And the older you get, the more your risk increases, partly because a cancer that may have started years before finally grows large enough to be detected. Gender is also a factor because our hormones can play a role in promoting cancer of the breasts, ovaries, uterus, and prostate.

Yet there are many avoidable risk factors—smoking, poor nutrition, sunbathing, exposure to X rays, lack of exercise, and becoming overweight—that you can do something about. The apple- versus pear-shaped woman who carries her weight around her middle has a higher risk of uterine cancer. It may even increase her chances of breast cancer after menopause. It is thought that the fat from the abdominal area causes levels of estrogen to rise. Increased estrogen is associated with an increased risk for breast and uterine cancer. Leaner women make less estrogen, and, in turn, tend to have lower rates of cancer of the female organs. Even though estrogen has a protective effect against heart disease, it is better to have a doctor monitor your level of estrogen and supplement it as necessary, knowing your family history for heart disease and breast cancer, than to be overweight and increase your risk for these cancers. Men could be facing a similar scenario with prostate cancer. That rubber tire around their middle contributes fat that is converted into excess testosterone, which in turn affects the condition of the prostate.

What Is Cancer?

Cancer starts out as a single cell that multiplies at an abnormally rapid rate. It becomes a problem when it invades healthy tissue and destroys it. Where in the body this takes place and how much damage it causes, depends upon what type of cell became cancerous and how it spread through the body. No one knows for sure what causes a cell to go haywire and become cancerous. However, it is known that repeated contact with cancer-causing agents, or *carcinogens,* seems coincident with the development of cancer.

Carcinogens can be found almost everywhere—in our air, water, and food. Cigarette smoke contains high levels of them. The body is a pretty amazing machine, able to fend off carcinogens by deactivating them and eliminating them from the body. However, a carcinogen may occasionally become activated, enter

TABLE 4. Promotors and Inhibitors of Cancer

Promotors	Inhibitors
Cigarettes, cigars, pipes	Vegetables
High-fat foods	Fruit
Sex hormones	Fiber
Sunlight	Low-fat foods
Alcohol	Exercise
X rays	Sunscreen
Excess salt-cured, smoked, or charcoal-broiled foods	

a cell, and attach itself to the cell's DNA, the blueprint for making similar cells. Even then, the body has a chance of destroying the cancer cell by cutting it off from the DNA before the cell duplicates itself. If the cell divides into two cells before the DNA has a chance to be repaired, the cells with the cancerous DNA continue to duplicate. The availability of *promotors* and *inhibitors* determines how fast the cancer cells grow. Inhibitors include vitamins, minerals, antioxidants, and fiber found in vegetables, fruits, and grains. Fat is an especially potent promotor, as are sex hormones. (See Table 4.)

The seriousness of cancer is heightened when it isn't detected before it starts to spread in the body. Then it is much more difficult to treat and cure. There are symptoms that are associated with cancer, but they are not sure signs of cancer. For example, a sore, cut, or bruise that is taking too long to heal could be cancerous. If you become constipated or have diarrhea or if you are urinating too often or not often enough and these symptoms last for more than several days, it's worth seeing your doctor. It could simply be a change in your eating or living patterns or a current physical or emotional stress, but it's best to know for sure. Women who notice a lump in their breast during self-examination should see a doctor. Difficulty in swallowing or a persistent cough could also be due to cancer. Again, it should be checked. Appreciate that the sooner cancer is diagnosed, the less invasive the treatment will be and the greater the chance of a cure.

Diagnostic Tests

The more we learn about cancer, the more diagnostic procedures are being developed. There are X ray and nuclear scans as well as blood tests that can be done. Mammography (a breast X ray) is a very important tool for diagnosing breast cancer. The American Cancer Society recommends that women over 40 years old have a mammogram once a year. An annual pap smear is also a good idea. It takes but a moment during a pelvic exam for a health care professional to take a swab of cells from the cervix for examination under a microscope. The American Cancer Society recommends that men over 50 years old have a PSA (prostate specific antigen) blood test each year as a screening approach for prostate tumors. A rectal and colon exam should also be part of your annual physical checkup.

Do You Have Any of These Cancer-Risk Habits?

Smoking

There are little hairlike bodies called *cilia* in your lungs that act like brooms to sweep out particles, germs, and dirt. Smoking a cigarette makes the cilia sluggish, and the more smoking you do, the higher your risk of actually destroying the cilia. Without them, you take away one of your body's first lines of defense against infection and environmental hazards such as air pollution.

Did You Know:

Just one cigarette can

- Increase your heart rate
- Increase your blood pressure
- Affect the blood flow and air in your lungs

Every time you inhale the smoke from a cigarette, you introduce several very damaging substances: nicotine, tar, and carbon monoxide. Nicotine makes blood vessels constrict, impeding the flow of blood and the delivery of nourishment and oxygen around your body. (Smoking also forces your heart to pump harder, which, as we saw with cardiovascular disease, increases your chances for hypertension, heart disease, and stroke.) The tar in cigarette smoke is very hard on the delicate tissue of the lungs. As the particles in the tar cool in the lungs, they form a brown, sticky sludge over the cilia. You're asking a lot of the cilia to even function under these conditions, let alone stand up to this exposure to harmful gases. Have you ever heard of someone committing suicide through carbon monoxide poisoning by attaching a hose from their car's tailpipe into their car's interior? Smoking is not that different. It robs your red blood cells of oxygen and replaces it with the carbon monoxide from the cigarette smoke. Is this just a slower death? No wonder someone who smokes excessively becomes easily winded when having to do anything physical.

Smoking cigars and pipes also increase the risk of cancer. However, it's more likely that cigars and pipes will cause cancer of the mouth, tongue, and throat than cancer of the lung. If you are one of those who think they can avoid cancer by chewing tobacco, think again. Cancer of the mouth is very common among tobacco chewers.

What about the poor nonsmoker who is subjected to secondhand tobacco smoke? The smoke contains over 4000 chemicals, many of them known poisons. It's not only the smoke exhaled by the smoker that is damaging, but also the smoke rising from the burning tobacco of the cigarette. Some studies have found that there is more tar, nicotine, and carbon monoxide in the smoke from the burning tobacco than there is in the smoke exhaled by the smoker.

I've spent a great deal of time on cigarette smoking because I believe it's imperative that we give up this damaging and destructive habit. It is a major risk factor in too many of our country's most serious health problems.

Poor Food Choices and Cancer-Causing Preparations

There is much about what you eat and how you prepare your food that affects your chances of getting cancer. Eating a **high-**

fat, low-fiber diet is just asking for trouble. As noted earlier, fat is a concentrated form of calories, and we all know where too many calories end up (everywhere you don't want the fat—the hips, the behind, the stomach). Also, the types of fat you eat can be a problem. A diet too high in polyunsaturated fats (which are found in large quantity in vegetable oils) is more cancer-promoting than one that relies on monounsaturated fats (found in such fats as olive and canola oil).

Without enough fiber, you lack the bulk in the intestine to trap potential carcinogens and carry them out of your body. Without fiber, the passage of waste through the intestines slows down because the muscles of the intestine have nothing against which to exert pressure.

Your mother was right when she said, "Eat your vegetables." However, it seems that too few people have taken that instruction to heart. Few of us eat the recommended daily requirement of three to five servings of vegetables and two to three servings of fruit, along with six to eleven servings of bread, grains, and pasta. This **lack of vegetables, fruits, and grains** in the diet is also causing a lack of the necessary fiber, vitamins, minerals, and antioxidants.

Have you ever thought about what makes a hot dog red and why, when you cook it, the color remains the same? It's because of the **nitrates and nitrites** it contains. Ham, bologna, salami, sausage, jerky, and corned beef also contain nitrates and nitrites, which, when combined with protein, form powerful carcinogens called *nitrosamines.* Frying cured meats at high temperatures can also form nitrosamines. If meat processors add some ascorbic acid (vitamin C), sodium ascorbate, and sodium erythrobate in the curing process, some nitrosamine formation can be prevented. If you plan to eat cured meat, reading the label can help you find the products that contain these beneficial additives. However, moderation should be the key here.

When the warm weather comes, people head outside to **barbecue.** The irresistible smell of grilled meat, fat searing in the fire, is very inviting, but unfortunately, the National Academy of Sciences' Committee on Diet, Nutrition, and Cancer found that there is a link between the way we prepare our foods and the incidence of cancer. This is how it works: When the fat drips from the meat onto the charcoal, it forms a carcinogenic substance that then rises in the smoke, depositing that carcinogen onto the surface of the meat.

The heat of the charcoal alone can convert proteins in the meat into substances that damage the DNA in your cells. It could be the trigger for initiating or promoting cancer. (By the way, it doesn't matter whether you are cooking over real charcoal, stones, gas, or electric burners.) I don't want you to feel that you have to give up barbecuing. Just make it a once-in-awhile cooking process.

Broiling meat is not as much of a problem. The heat source is above the meat, so the fat doesn't drip onto it, and thus doesn't create smoke filled with carcinogens.

Lastly, if you drink **alcohol,** try to do so in moderation. Even though alcohol in moderation has been found to be somewhat protective of the heart, excessive consumption can cause liver cancer. Mix that alcohol with cigarette smoking, and you increase your odds of developing cancer of the mouth, esophagus, and larynx. Besides, alcohol is low in most nutrients and high in calories.

Sun-Worshipping

Why is it that we think people with a tan look healthy, when in reality they are at a far greater risk of getting skin cancer because they've exposed themselves to the ultraviolet radiation from the sun? If you have a fair complexion, you are at an even greater risk of developing skin cancer than someone with darker skin. And avoiding this danger is so easy. Sunscreen and protective clothing not only defend your skin against ultraviolet radiation but keep you from getting prematurely wrinkled.

A Sedentary Lifestyle

About 10 percent of the cancer deaths in 1997 were from colon cancer. Studies have shown that people with a sedentary lifestyle have a higher risk of colon cancer. It may be that exercise helps to speed waste through the intestine, reducing the amount of time cancer causing substances are in contact with the lining of the large intestine. Exercise also helps you keep your weight within a healthy range. And don't forget that being overweight is a risk factor for many cancers, not just colon cancer.

Diabetes

According to the American Diabetes Association, there are sixteen million people in the United States with diabetes. Unfortunately, only half of them know it. Diabetes is the fourth-leading cause of death in the United States. Complications of diabetes include blindness, kidney disease, heart disease, stroke, and nerve disease that could lead to amputation of the lower limbs. Each year, 12,000 to 24,000 people lose their sight because of diabetes. Some 10–21 percent of people with diabetes will develop kidney disease. People with diabetes are 2–4 times more likely to experience heart disease or a stroke and 15–40 times more likely to require the amputation of a leg than those who don't have diabetes.

There are two forms of diabetes. Type I (formerly known as IDDM or Insulin-Dependent Diabetes Mellitus) most often occurs in children and young adults. It is due to an autoimmune disease that causes the body to produce little or no insulin, which is necessary for the metabolism of glucose (sugar). These people must give themselves daily insulin injections to survive. Type II (formerly known as NIDDM or Non-Insulin-Dependent Diabetes Mellitus), on the other hand, results from the inability of the body either to make enough insulin or properly use what it makes. Often all that is required is a healthier diet, weight loss, and exercise. Occasionally medication is recommended. This type of diabetes is much more prevalent, accounting for 90–95 percent of all cases.

If you experience frequent urination, unusual thirst, or extreme hunger, you may have diabetes. Frequent infections, blurred vision, tingling/numbness in the hands or feet, fatigue or irritability can also point to diabetes. You should consult your physician and be sure to get a fasting blood glucose test, which measures the amount of glucose in your bloodstream in the

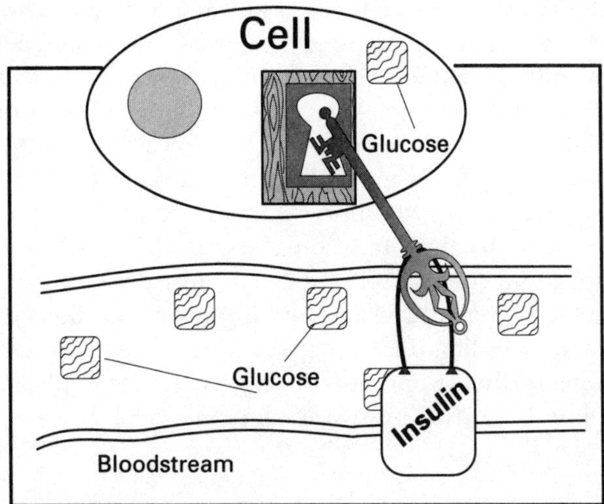

Figure 10. Getting Glucose into the Cell

morning before you have eaten anything. A value of ≥ 126 mg/dl confirmed by a repeat test on a different day indicates you have diabetes. A value of 110 mg/dl on the same kind of test is considered the upper limit for a normal blood glucose. Don't be tempted to self-diagnose by using the finger-prick test that people with diabetes use for monitoring their blood glucose level. It's not reliable enough. You need to have a fasting blood glucose test evaluated by a laboratory.

Insulin is necessary to move glucose from the bloodstream into the cells. When you have a fasting blood glucose of ≥ 126 mg/dl, it means that something isn't working right in your body. It could be that your pancreas is not producing enough insulin for the job. It also could mean that your body has become *insulin-resistant*—i.e., the cells have become less receptive to insulin. Somewhat as in a lock-and-key mechanism, insulin is the key to opening the lock on the cell's door to let the glucose in. When the cells don't respond to the insulin present in the bloodstream, there's no way to move the glucose into the cells. So it remains in the bloodstream, where it raises your blood sugar level. (See Figure 10.)

That may not sound all that bad, but many things are being

adversely affected. The cells are beginning to starve. They need the glucose for energy. The brain is a glucose junkie and performs poorly without it. When there is no glucose available because of insulin resistance, the requirements of the cells and brain are partially satisfied by the body breaking down fat. Now you may be thinking that this is a real benefit in losing weight. It isn't. The fat must be converted into what are known as *ketones* before it can be used by the brain and the cells. Too many ketones running around your bloodstream can cause confusion and nausea. The high blood glucose inflicts havoc on your body in many other ways, including damaging your arteries and nerves, which leads to heart disease and also to serious nerve complications in your feet and hands, digestive system, and eyes.

Who Gets Diabetes?

Genetics can play a part in getting diabetes. Also, it appears that certain racial and ethnic groups have a higher risk of becoming diabetic—in particular, African-Americans, Hispanics, and Native Americans. Type II diabetes risk increases in people over 45 years old. Yet there are many risk factors for Type II diabetes that can be controlled. Being overweight and not exercising regularly are two of them. When you are overweight, you set yourself up for insulin resistance. Losing weight causes the cells to become more receptive to insulin.

Do You Have Either of These Diabetes-Risk Habits?

Poor Food Choices

Most people want to point to the eating of too much sugar as the cause of diabetes. While excess sugar can aggravate diabetes, it does not cause it. However, too much sugar does add up to too many calories, and too many calories add on the pounds, which does contribute to the development of diabetes. The same is true of too much fat in the diet. I can't stress enough the harmful effect of being overweight. Low-fiber diets are also a problem. The more fiber in the diet, the better your glucose control. That's because the fiber helps slow the entrance of glucose into the bloodstream. The slower the rate, the less likelihood of a rapid rise in blood glucose. Without the rapid rise, your pancreas does not need to produce as much insulin.

The Sedentary Lifestyle

Leading a sedentary lifestyle is just as much a risk factor for diabetes as it is for cardiovascular disease. The major problem is that you don't burn enough calories. The law of balance says that to maintain your weight, the number of calories you consume must be the same as the number of calories that you burn. If you want to lose weight, you have to tilt the balance so that you are eating fewer calories and/or burning more.

Did You Notice?

Did you notice the killer habits that were common among the various diseases:

- Cigarette smoking
- Poor food choices—high-fat, high-sugar, high-calorie, low-fiber foods
- Sedentary lifestyle

You could add "Stress" to that list, as well, because stress leads people to smoke, eat poorly, and never seem to get around to exercising. Now you should have a good idea of what habits you need to work on.

I hope that what I've just shared with you about cardiovascular disease, cancer, and diabetes has helped motivate you to change your habits. Don't forget about your *life vision.* Whether your motivation to change your habits is to lose weight and look better or lose weight and feel better, succeeding in your quest will also take you a long way in protecting yourself against these diseases. Considering that the life expectancy at birth is 76.1 years (based on 1996 data), you have many good years left. Why not do what it takes now to make the best of those years?

Remember, the ability to change your habits rests in your hands. When you find out how easy it is to do just that by using your personality, those unhealthy lifestyle habits can become ancient history!

4

Healthy Habits

To live longer, to live healthier. Who wouldn't jump at the chance? Researchers believe a 115-year life span is possible. There's one catch, though. For you even to have a shot at it, you have to be willing to get rid of your unhealthy lifestyle habits and establish healthy ones. The future is in your hands.

Life is far more than a roll of the dice and far more than the genes you were born with. Oh, sure, genetics has some influence on your risk for certain diseases. But we all have a chance at longevity and a good quality of life based on what we are willing to do for ourselves. We may not have control over our genes (at least, not yet), but what we do have control over can have some pretty powerful results.

- *Eat nutritiously,* and you supply your body with the nutrients necessary to maximize your physiological potential, perform at your optimum level, decrease your risk for many fatal diseases, and maintain a healthy body weight.
- *Exercise,* and you increase your muscle mass, decrease your body fat, improve your oxygen distribution, and increase your stamina and energy level.
- *Stop smoking,* and you avoid serious risk to your lungs and other vital organs, cells, and tissues and reduce your risk for cancer and heart disease.

- *Incorporate relaxation techniques* such as yoga, meditation, deep breathing, and visualizing, and you destress your life and eliminate its negative effects on your body.
- *Establish a support network,* whether it be with a group or an individual, and you can increase your general resistance to stress and disease by sharing ideas, assistance, camaraderie, and good will.

These are just a handful of lifestyle changes that can make major differences in how you feel and how long you live. It's amazing how, once you start to do good things for yourself, you will continue to do good things for yourself. It reinforces itself.

If you stop exercising, you'll miss it. Several days away from it and your body will feel like lead—stiff and unable to move. If you stop eating nutritiously, you'll miss it. Going back to a diet high in fat, high in sugar, high in calories, and low in fiber will not only take its toll on your alertness and energy level but increase the amount of indigestion you experience, and show up in the weight registered on your bathroom scale. If you stop taking time to relax, you'll miss it, too. You'll feel the return of depression, frustration, and moodiness in your daily life.

Creating a New Comfort Zone

Let's face it. Your habits are your comfort zone. They release you from having to make any decisions because they are habits. Your life is literally on autopilot. Yet you may not like the results of some of those habits. What I don't understand is how people can continue to do what they've always done and expect different results. Talk about wishing for miracles. If you want different results, you're going to have to do some things differently. That's why using your personality is so exciting. You get to try new ways of doing things, but only if they feel right for your personality. Then you can easily slip into a healthier comfort zone.

Watch healthy people. What are they doing? They seem so full of energy and "have it all together." They aren't free from stress, but they know how to handle it. They're faced with eating decisions every day but seem to lean toward the more nutritious foods without sacrificing some of their favorites or eating those favorites with guilt. Exercise is part of their lives. They do all of this willingly, enjoying how they look and feel. Be assured that, unless it felt comfortable to their personality, they wouldn't be doing it (unless they're martyrs!). They are in their comfort zone of good health.

Celebrity Role Models

A number of celebrities come to mind who seem to have used their personalities to be healthy and in their comfort zone. One is Jack Lalanne. He took the PPQ for me, revealing that he is an ESFJ. He is quite an amazing man, still going strong at 84 years old. I enjoyed talking with him, finding out about his past, his philosophy, and what's important to him in the field of fitness. In 1936 he opened the nation's first health club. In the 1940s and 1950s, he designed exercise machines that predated Nautilus fitness equipment. He has had his own show on television. He set out to prove to the world that there is a relationship between health, the food people eat, and the amount of exercise they get (a great use of his Sensing preference). At the age of 60, he challenged himself and succeeded in swimming the San Francisco Bay from Alcatraz Island to Fisherman's Wharf, handcuffed, shackled, and towing a 1000-pound boat. To top that feat, at the age of 70 he towed 70 boats carrying 70 passengers through Long Beach Harbor, again handcuffed and shackled. His judging preference provided the structure he needed to train and then accomplish such feats. Here is a man who takes his health seriously. He has a great mental outlook on life. He has always loved what he does, likes to share it with others, and is still sharing it (the Feeling preference displaying itself).

Actress Jane Fonda—very probably an INTJ—is another fitness guru of the 1980s and 1990s. At the age of 42 she opened the Jane Fonda Workout Studio in Beverly Hills. Since then she has become one of the world's leading health and fitness advocates, producing videos, audio programs, and books. Her iNtuiting preference would lead her to believe that no matter what your age, exercise and healthy eating can make a difference.

The Judging part of her type would provide the structure that underlies her exercise programs and her life. She has served as an inspiration for many Americans, making them believe that they, too, can be fit. At 60 years old, she is still going strong.

"Sweatin' to the Oldies" Richard Simmons knows how to both entertain and get people off the couch. Most likely an ESFP, Richard has had to fight a weight problem since childhood. With Sensing as his dominant preference, he ate whatever food he saw, believing (with his Feeling preference) that the food could comfort him and make him feel better about himself. Once he was able to lose weight, his ability to show others how to do it, too, provided his Extraversion a great avenue for hamming it up. Richard has probably learned to tap into his iNtuiting and Thinking preferences because, left to its own devices, the _S_P combination will go for instant gratification, whatever the consequences.

Then there is Oprah Winfrey, television personality and a likely ESFP. After many quick-get-it-off-me-now diets, most notably the Optifast® liquid diet weight loss plan, and many pounds lost and regained (showing her Perceiving preference in action), she met Bob Greene, a personal trainer. He shared with her the habits of healthy people (appealing to her Sensing preferences), and she became a believer and a follower, as told in their book, *Make the Connection.* I believe Bob serves as the Judging counterpart to Oprah's Perceiving, giving her the structure needed to change her ways. By using other aspects of her personality not previously tapped into, along with a personal commitment to change, Oprah has been able to lose weight and become more physically fit.

Jack, Jane, Richard, and Oprah are all in the public spotlight. They set a fine example of what we need to do to stay healthy. My clients, too, while not in the public spotlight, have used their personalities to become healthier people. Many of them will share with you how they did it. See if you can recognize their personalities at work.

The Healthy Habit of Healthy Eating

Jennifer, the ENFJ

Jennifer, one of my clients, is a great role model. She's also the envy of all her friends because she seems to have it all together, especially when it comes to the way she eats. She is almost textbook perfect—not too much fat in her diet, not too many calories, plenty of fiber. Her motto is variety, moderation, and balance. Her repertoire of foods has greatly expanded to include all sorts of cuisine (showing her iNtuiting preference). By being sensible, and not overdoing it, she gets to enjoy all kinds of foods. She is learning to become more flexible, allowing herself to eat foods without guilt. She now balances high-fat, high-calorie foods with lower-fat, lower-calorie foods.

It wasn't always like that for Jennifer, however. Her diet used to be based on what she felt others needed (Feeling preference). Being a mother, she wanted to make her kids happy. If they wanted to go to "the golden arches" for lunch, she ate there, too. If everyone wanted to get an ice cream cone, she wasn't one to say "no."

While Jennifer's genetic background was a major factor in her developing breast cancer (her mother had also had breast cancer), her eating habits contributed to the problem. Her diet was too high in fat and too low in fruits and vegetables. Once she was diagnosed, one of her first concerns was how her condition would affect her family and loved ones (again showing her Feeling preference). She worried that not taking care of herself would, in some way, let those she loved down. She underwent chemotherapy and radiation treatments and came to me to learn how to make the necessary changes in her diet (trying to tap into her Thinking and Sensing preferences). Annual mammograms and checkups give her the reassurance that her cancer has not come back. And with her new approach to eating, she is now feeling better than ever.

Bob, the ESTJ

A similar scenario is true of Bob. He started coming to me after he was told, during his annual physical, that his blood cholesterol level was 235 mg/dl, he was 50 pounds overweight, and his blood pressure was too high. If he wasn't careful, said his doctor, he would succumb to heart disease as his father had. Hearing the results of his physical was a wake-up call for Bob. Somehow there was no reality to his condition until he heard the numbers (Sensing and Thinking preferences). No one had to tell him that the donuts he ate on his coffee break or the hamburgers he had for lunch or the pasta with cream sauce he had for dinner weren't good for him. All that fat, especially the saturated fat variety, was helping to raise his blood cholesterol. He had read about it in the media but ignored it, not wanting to give up his favorite foods. He figured that if he did anything, it was going to be all or nothing. Remembering how his father had suffered, he decided it was time to change.

Rachel, the INFJ

Fortunately for Rachel, she is part of the "being-fit-is-in" generation and came to me to be sure she was on the right track. She, like many of her peers, is very concerned about what she eats. Eating from all of the food groups, with an emphasis on grains, vegetables, and fruits, just makes sense to her. Her choices tend toward the unusual, taking advantage of the cornucopia today's supermarkets have to offer. Sometimes she gets overzealous in her attempt to do her best nutritionally. Fearing that our food is depleted of essential nutrients because of the soil and environment in which they are grown (her iNtuiting and Feeling preferences at work), she often relies on supplements. With a little coaching and counseling, Rachel now realizes that, with a balanced diet, supplements aren't really necessary. She is still working on removing the concept of "good foods/bad foods" from her thinking (Feeling preference). It's hard for her to believe that there are no bad foods, just bad diets. Having grown up and heard the "good food"/"bad food" philosophy so often, it's difficult for Rachel to accept that "all foods can be legal."

Henry, the ENTJ and Millie, the ISFP

Henry and Millie are part of the "silver" generation. They came to me for nutritional counseling because Henry had recently been diagnosed with diabetes. They both grew up with the meat-and-potatoes approach to eating. But what they were hearing in the media and reading in books and magazines convinced them that they were not too old to make some improvements in their diet. They were looking forward to reaching their golden years together. (Henry's perfectionist _NT_ wants to do it right, and Millie's _S_P wants it to happen immediately. This is a fortunate combination since Millie's type can help get Henry's type to do something *now* that he might otherwise put off.)

Millie accompanied Henry to his appointments with me, since she would be the one doing the cooking. She also figured that what was good for him would probably be good for her (Feeling preference). They haven't given up meat entirely, but now it's more of a side dish than the main attraction on their plate. Where canned vegetables used to be the order of the day, they now enjoy eating more raw vegetables. (Who said you can't teach old dogs new tricks!)

The Healthy Habit of Exercise

Jennifer, the ENFJ

It pleased Jennifer that she had been able to improve her eating habits. However, she was a little more concerned about trying to improve her exercise habits. She always seemed to have some excuse why she couldn't fit exercise into her daily routine. Fortunately for her, her friend Lisa was looking for a walking partner. Jennifer was glad she didn't want a jogging partner; she didn't feel comfortable jogging.

She and Lisa set a schedule of walking together (Judging preference) early in the morning (so her husband could watch the kids before he had to leave for work). She had originally feared that she wouldn't be able to get up that early and did occasionally consider calling Lisa to make up some excuse. Luckily, her conscience never let her make the call because she didn't want to let her friend down (Feeling preference). After their walk, she would notice how great she felt, ready to face the day. Each week Jennifer was finding energy she never thought she had. The more energy she had, the more she got accomplished. (Of course, because Jennifer is an _NF_, it never seemed to be enough!)

Bob, the ESTJ

In years past Bob used to be more active, playing basketball and occasionally racquetball. But when he moved from New York to Seattle, he never seemed to have the time to find a local team to join. His job seemed to take up all his free time and involved many hours in front of a computer screen—which, of course, doesn't consume a lot of calories. Without any physical activity, Bob began his slow ascent to his overweight status. The results of his annual physical, along with feeling winded whenever he climbed a flight of stairs, made Bob realize it was time to get back to the "good old days."

On leaving his doctor's office, Bob went directly to the YMCA to sign up for basketball (Sensing and Judging preferences). The team at the Y met twice a week after work. Bob was glad the games were a scheduled event (Judging preference); as long as it appeared on his calendar, he would probably do it. Bob even recruited a small group from work to play together on weekends. When Bob visited his doctor for a follow-up checkup about a month later, his weight had started to go down, as had his cholesterol level. The HDL-cholesterol, the "good" cholesterol, had started to increase. For Bob, seeing the improved numbers was a great reinforcement (Sensing preference) to continue what he was doing.

Rachel, the INFJ

Rachel belongs to a local athletic club. Exercise videos by Jane Fonda and Denice Austin inspired her. She wanted to have a body like theirs, and could even see herself with a new figure (iNtuiting preference). Fortunately the club had equipment on which she could work individually. She didn't want a group-participation class (Introversion preference) like aerobics.

Rachel did circuit training, first warming up on the treadmill and then working out on the weight machines (Judging preference). Lastly, she did some aerobics on the stair-stepper or stationary bicycle, depending on her mood. The more definition she got to her body, the more inspired she was to go to the club. Her body actually *was* beginning to look like Fonda's and Austin's.

Henry, the ENTJ and Millie, the ISFP

Henry appreciated that exercise was a necessity if he was to control his blood sugar (Thinking and Judging preferences). His doctor reminded him that the extra pounds he had put on were contributing to his insulin resistance. By losing weight, he would promote a more efficient uptake of glucose into his cells, using the insulin that his pancreas was able to produce. He might even be able to stop taking his medication at some point. With Henry being a Judger, scheduling exercise was not a problem. That wasn't quite the case for Millie, the Perceiver, who didn't want to get that committed in case something else came up. However, most of the time they would walk together.

The Healthy Habit of Relaxing

Jennifer, the ENFJ

You can imagine how stressful it was for Jennifer when she learned she had breast cancer. At that moment, she felt her days were numbered. It didn't matter that her doctor told her that they had caught it early, and that with chemotherapy and radiation treatments, they could probably cure it.

All she could think about was what would happen to her young family if she didn't make it (Feeling preference).

Jennifer is a wife and the stay-at-home mom of two toddlers. Picking up after them, making sure they don't get into trouble, feeding and entertaining them were additional stressors in Jennifer's life. She needed to find a way to cope. Her husband would tell her she needed to take time for herself. However, that seemed unrealistic to her with two toddlers to look after.

She often felt as if she were going through postpartum blues, but knew that couldn't be the case. Her youngest was already 1½ years old. Not until she found out her personality type did she appreciate why she had a hard time dedicating a few moments to herself. It was time to nurture *herself.* Her first order of business was to find a sitter who would look after her kids each afternoon. Sometimes she would get together with friends to go shopping or see a movie. Other times she might stay home and enjoy sewing, knowing the kids were being watched. No interruptions. Just time for herself.

Bob, the ESTJ

Bob found that his greatest source of stress was his job. As a computer programmer, there always seemed to be tension in the air at work. If it wasn't racing to get the job done on time, he was reworking a glitch in the program. His boss expected him to be at work early every day and often wanted him to work late to get a project completed. Even though the atmosphere was fairly casual, the pace of work wasn't. The way Bob found to escape the pressures of work was to leave the computer and find someone with whom he could get into some lively debate. It definitely took his mind off work. Removing himself from his work area helped a lot (Sensing preference), and being with other people helped recharge his batteries (Extraversion preference).

Rachel, the INFJ

Rachel works at a place just right for her: an animal rights protection organization. It's a cause she strongly believes in. While her job can be stressful, what actually weighs heavy on Rachel's mind is her need to find the answers in life, her purpose for being here (iNtuiting and Feeling preferences). She never seems to be satisfied with life and is always looking for more. When she can, she closes her eyes and takes a "mental vacation," visualizing herself on the beach in the Mediterranean (iNtuiting preference). It can be so effective that she is surprised, when she opens her eyes, that she didn't get a tan or rack up any frequent-flyer miles!

Henry, the ENTJ and Millie, the ISFP

Being retired, Henry and Millie are able to take time for themselves. Oh, they do their share of babysitting for the grandchildren, which can occasionally be stressful. Then there are always the financial concerns about having enough money to see them through, so they don't become a burden on their children. They tend to do leisure things together, though Henry's purpose is often different than Millie's. Henry enjoys activities that involve strategy (Thinking preference), maybe even some competition. When he and Millie play cards or golf together, he is out to win, while she just plays to have a good time (Sensing and Feeling preferences). Fortunately, she doesn't mind his winning.

The Top Ten List of Healthy Habits

My clients helped create the following **Top Ten List of Healthy Habits.** Do you have any to add? Again, the list goes backward from 10 to 1, saving the best for last.

Top Ten List of Healthy Habits

10. Seek the help and knowledge of the experts.
9. Learn as much as you can about nutrition and fitness and find the ways to incorporate that knowledge in your daily life.
8. Believe in the adage "variety, moderation, and balance" as it applies to nutrition, exercise, and relaxation.
7. Find some sort of support network and use it on a regular basis—both for the good stuff and the bad.
6. Take time for yourself each day, focusing on relaxing.
5. Don't smoke, and if you drink, do so in moderation.
4. Realize that there are no bad foods, just bad diets.
3. Exercise and be physically active on a regular basis.
2. Use your personality type to find it within yourself to be the healthiest you can be.
1. Don't make up excuses. Just do what it takes.

It is not a hopeless situation. You can change your not-so-healthy habits. Of course, it won't happen overnight, nor should you even attempt to change all your habits at one time. You need to decide what is most important to you and your health, prioritizing your list. Then set to work, using your personality to make it happen.

5

Breaking Habits—Making Habits

The first step in breaking unhealthy old habits and making healthy new ones is deciding you want to change. The fact that you're reading this book leads me to believe you do. You've probably been through the "I'm thinking about it" stage, when you recognized there was a problem, but weren't yet willing to do what it might take to fix it. Now you're in the "I'm ready" stage, full of motivation and commitment. In Part II, you'll get to the "I'm doing something about it" stage.

Though most people don't think about it or realize it, decision making lies at the root of all the habits you have and all the changes you'll make. In fact, everything we do, no matter how simple or complex, requires a decision. When the alarm rang this morning and you were fast asleep in bed, the thought of sitting up and planting your feet on the floor preparatory to starting a new day probably didn't seem too appealing. You had to make a simple decision: "Do I get up or lie here a couple of more minutes?" Then there are the heavy-duty decisions, such as "I'm unhappy with my job. Should I quit? What would I do instead?"

We often overlook the fact that certain off-hand decisions we make have long-range effects. Let's say that about six months ago a friend asked you to join her for the afternoon coffee break. You followed her to the vending machine, where she got a candy bar. Not knowing what you really wanted, if anything, you also bought a candy bar to keep your friend company while she ate hers. The next day, the same situation occurred and again, you bought a candy bar. Now, six months later, it's become second nature to go to the vending machine, plunk your money in, select a candy bar, and start eating. You probably rarely stop and ask yourself whether you really need or want the candy bar. Yet, by not taking the time to make a decision, you're allowing your habits to rule your existence, with the chance of those habits ruining your existence. We all need to make decisions more consciously and conscientiously, as well as take the results more seriously.

By consistently making the same decisions in particular situations, you establish ways of acting and doing things that become habits. Once that happens and the situation arises again, you no longer feel compelled to make a decision about it. You do whatever it is without thinking. That's great if what you're doing is healthy. However, we all know there are many things we do that aren't good for us.

When you appreciate that different people make different decisions given the same situation and conditions, you can begin to understand the involvement our personalities have in the decision-making process. Our priorities are different, and what is a good decision for one person may not be for another. It's important to determine where you're headed and then make the decisions accordingly. In making those decisions, we may use only a part of our personality when we really should be using all the preferences within our type.

One of the major benefits of identifying your personality type is becoming aware of who you are, what makes you tick, what you need to make your life run smoothly. When you start to consciously use personality typing in your daily life, you almost become a spectator, watching yourself to weigh your behavior, consider what you're thinking, and notice your feelings. The more you understand your actions, the easier it is to change those actions that aren't working for you. Remember when you were little and your mother reminded you to "Stop, look, and listen" before you crossed the street? The same applies here, with an emphasis on the word *STOP!* Take the time to be an astute observer.

Who's in Charge Here?

Let's look at how the preferences within your type interact and work together to make your personality so dynamic. As in an orchestra, where the conductor leads the musicians, in life you need something within you to lead your thoughts and actions. Can you imagine trying to gather information, make a decision, and take action all at the same time? Something has to be done first. That's where your **dominant preference** comes in. It takes charge, helping to orchestrate what goes on in your mind. Your dominant preference is the one you trust most, the one you go back to time and time again because it feels comfortable. The preferences that can be dominant are Sensing, iNtuiting, Thinking, or Feeling.

Dominant Sensors put their greatest emphasis on the present moment and the concrete facts and realities that can be learned from it. Knowing what has worked in the past serves as a good yardstick for them. They don't like to make decisions that go against the facts as they have experienced them.

Dominant iNtuitives want to continually explore the unknown to find alternative ways of doing things, find new meaning and significance in things, discover the relationship and connection of things. Their decisions are often based on a "gut" feel.

Dominant Thinkers have a need for structure and end up making logical decisions that can then be affirmed by collecting the appropriate data. If you ask them, they will have no difficulty explaining why they made the decision they did.

Dominant Feelers, on the other hand, would have a hard time explaining why they make certain decisions other than that they want to be sure everyone, including themselves, ends up happy. They seem to have an inner monitor for determining what is good or bad, right or wrong, even though to Thinkers it may not seem like a logical system.

Figure 11 shows you which preference is the dominant one for each of the 16 types (it's the letter that is bolded and larger

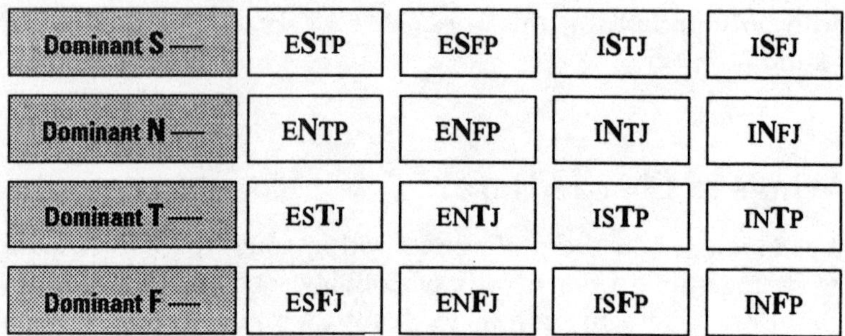

Dominant S —	E**S**TP	E**S**FP	I**S**TJ	I**S**FJ
Dominant N —	E**N**TP	E**N**FP	I**N**TJ	I**N**FJ
Dominant T —	ES**T**J	EN**T**J	IS**T**P	IN**T**P
Dominant F —	ES**F**J	EN**F**J	IS**F**P	IN**F**P

Figure 11. Dominant Preferences

than the rest). Knowing the preference that's in charge will be a tremendous help when you set out to break those unhealthy habits.

The Support Team

Don't expect the dominant preference to do all the work all the time. It does need some help. That's why one of the other preferences within your type serves as the **backup preference.** It complements the dominant preference, provides balance, and keeps you from being one-sided in dealing with life. When the dominant preference comes from the "What's significant to you" category (Sensing or iNtuiting), then your backup preference must come from the "How you make decisions" category (Thinking or Feeling). In the same way, if your dominant preference is either Thinking or Feeling, your backup preference will be either Sensing or iNtuiting.

Visualize the dominant and backup preferences as if they were officers in a big corporation. There's the president, who is equivalent to the dominant preference, and then there's the vice president, who serves as backup to the president, sometimes even taking over if necessary.

Looking at the same basic table again, let's see what your backup preference is. It's the underlined letter. The dominant preference is still the bold letter. (See Figure 12.)

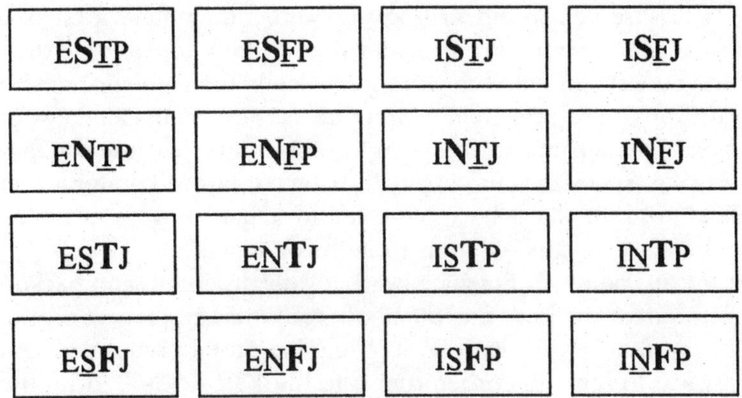

Figure 12. Backup Preferences

What You Shouldn't Forget

I don't want you to forget, as you look at your type, that you have Sensing, iNtuiting, Thinking, and Feeling at your disposal (even if you don't see their letters in your type). For example, just because you have *dominant* Sensing and *backup* Thinking preferences doesn't mean that you can't call on your less-favored preferences, iNtuiting and Feeling, when needed. Using the Sensing and Thinking preferences will be more natural to you, while using the iNtuiting and Feeling preferences will require more of a conscious effort. They are not as well developed and pose a challenge we'll be working on throughout this book.

It is easy to ignore the input from your less-favored preferences because your dominant and backup preferences already represent the "What's significant to you" category (Sensing or iNtuiting) and the "How you make a decision" category (Thinking or Feeling). These alone are sufficient to make a decision. Yet, without the contribution of your less-favored preferences, the decisions you make may not be the best ones.

In Chapter 2, I discussed what it would feel like, after an accident involving the arm of your dominant hand, to have to write with your other hand. Now I want you to try something. On a piece of paper, first write your name with your dominant hand. Then write your name with the other hand.

I'm sure you found writing with your other hand a bit of a struggle. Your signature probably doesn't look very good either. But you were still able to write some semblance of your name. I want you to keep that feeling in mind as you start to change your habits. Change may not feel comfortable at first because you may be using aspects of your personality (the less-favored preferences) that haven't had much exercise. Yet those parts of your personality hold some valuable tools to help you change.

At this point, you now know what your dominant and backup preferences are. Let's find out about your third and fourth preferences—that is, your least-favored and least-used preferences. An easy way to remember the order is to think "1–2–3–4," with the dominant preference being #1 and your least-favorite preference being #4. In Table 5, find your type and then read across to see what is your 1–2–3–4 order.

You may want to go back to Chapter 2 and reread the sections on the various preferences to better understand the contribution each makes to the decision-making process. Please note that Extraversion and Introversion and Judging and Perceiving influence the decision-making process but aren't directly involved in the process.

What Is the "Best" Decision?

Before I go into how to make the best decision, we need to agree on what it means to make the "best" lifestyle habit decisions. It's not a matter of my judging you and saying that the decision you made was or wasn't a good one, based on the knowledge and experience I have as a nutritionist. If that were the case, I would need to be with you every minute of the day. No. You're the one who needs to become knowledgeable, responsible, and accountable for the decisions you make. In Part II, I will help you become more *knowledgeable* about what are healthy habits and how to achieve them. The *responsible* and *accountable* parts of decision making are up to you. And your motivation and commitment to your goal will influence how responsible and accountable you want to be.

In my opinion, the measure of the "best" decision you can

TABLE 5. **Your Type's 1–2–3–4 Order.**

To recognize the different preferences in the table:

#1 preference (Dominant)	= Capital letter in bold
#2 preference (Backup)	= Capital letter with underlining and no bolding
#3 preference	= Capital letter in italics
#4 preference	= Small letter in italics

Most Favored Preference ⟶ **Least Favored Preference**

TYPE	#1		#2		#3		#4
ESTP	**S**	→	T	→	*F*	→	*n*
ESFP	**S**	→	F	→	*T*	→	*n*
ISTJ	**S**	→	T	→	*F*	→	*n*
ISFJ	**S**	→	F	→	*T*	→	*n*
ENTP	**N**	→	T	→	*F*	→	*s*
ENFP	**N**	→	F	→	*T*	→	*s*
INTJ	**N**	→	T	→	*F*	→	*s*
INFJ	**N**	→	F	→	*T*	→	*s*
ESTJ	**T**	→	S	→	*N*	→	*f*
ENTJ	**T**	→	N	→	*S*	→	*f*
ISTP	**T**	→	S	→	*N*	→	*f*
INTP	**T**	→	N	→	*S*	→	*f*
ESFJ	**F**	→	S	→	*N*	→	*t*
ENFJ	**F**	→	N	→	*S*	→	*t*
ISFP	**F**	→	S	→	*N*	→	*t*
INFP	**F**	→	N	→	*S*	→	*t*

make is one that moves you toward your *life vision.* Setting goals to change certain habits gives you something to shoot for, a direction in which to head. Whatever actions you take, preceded by the decisions you make, will either move you toward your goals and *life vision* or away from them. Every time you do something that moves you away—perhaps saying "just this once," as you do so—you are being untrue to yourself. When you've made the "best" decision, you should be happy with it, having no regrets or self-doubt.

Of course, circumstances can affect what makes a good decision. For example, let's say your goal is to lower your blood cholesterol. However, you have been stranded on a desert island and all there is to eat is ice cream. (Darn!) You know that ice cream is high in calories and contains damaging saturated fat. Should you eat it? The circumstances pretty much dictate that the best decision you can make is to eat the ice cream.

You're going to have to be pretty creative to come up with an excuse like that on a daily basis to allow yourself to eat and act in a way that is counterproductive to a healthy lifestyle. Most people don't have to be told what they're doing wrong. They know. If they don't, then they need to be responsible and seek out the knowledge they're missing. Ask questions. Become a detective. When you can justify and support a decision with sound information, not rationalize and make up excuses for it, you've probably made the best decision.

The Optimum Way to Make the Best Decision

The optimum way to make a decision is to employ each preference one at a time. That way, one preference won't interfere with the others, and you can really focus on the characteristic approach of each preference.

There is also an optimum order for using the preferences:

1. Use the Sensing preference first to gather concrete facts and data. It gives you a realistic picture of the situation, what is going on, who is involved, what everyone is doing, and whether you have experienced anything similar. Of course, data alone cannot solve a problem.
2. Employ your iNtuiting preference to pinpoint the possibilities associated with the situation, the meaning of the data, and the relationship it has with past experiences. It will help you get the big picture and identify some potential changes. Again, you'll still have only input at this point.
3. Present the information you have gathered with your Sensing and iNtuiting preferences to your Thinking preference.

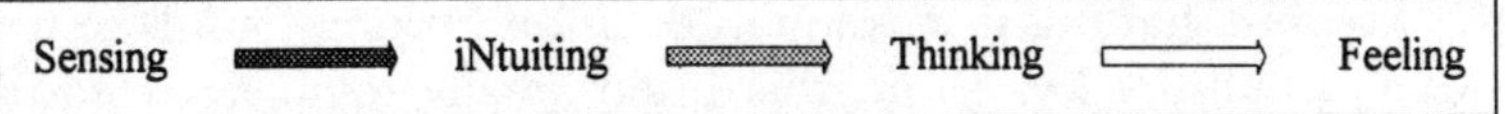

Figure 13. Diagramming the Decision-Making Process

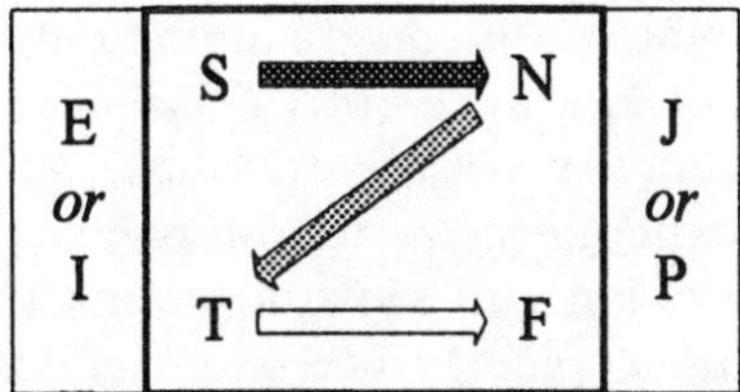

Figure 14. The *Z* Pattern of Decision-Making

It will give you an impersonal analysis, consider the consequences of the alternatives presented, both good and bad, factor in the cost-benefit considerations, and examine any logical misgivings and support you have for the alternatives.

4. Put all of this through your Feeling preference, allowing it to weigh your personal feelings about the matter. Consider the temporary and permanent gains and losses to you, as well as how the decision will affect others.

When you have gone through each of these steps, you should have a well-thought-out decision. It should be truly the best decision you could make, because you have collected as much information as possible and processed it as thoroughly as you can. You've also done it in the order that is scientifically sound—first gathering the information, then making decisions. Too often we make a decision and only *then* seek out information to support or justify our decision.

If we were to diagram the process, it would resemble the example in Figure 13.

Another way to look at it is in a *Z* pattern, as shown in Figure 14.

With this idealistic *Z* pattern (which doesn't exist in real life, as you will soon see), there is no dominant preference to sway the direction of the process. Each preference is equally weighted, providing as much input as possible without favoritism or bias.

I realize that this discussion of decision making sounds somewhat simplistic. I've done this intentionally to make it easily understood and put into action. In actuality, our minds are such miraculous machines that many of the preferences are working simultaneously and so quickly that it would be almost impossible to diagram. To some of you, diagramming the process may also seem like an effort to reduce every decision to a simple black-or-white choice. But, as you make decisions, you'll become aware of how your past experiences, relationships, and personal attitude all color the discussion and move it beyond the realm of any mere black-or-white choice. Just be sure you don't take the first response that comes into your mind. Put it through the full decision-making process.

Your Type's 1–2–3–4 Decision-Making Process

While I want you to keep the idealistic *Z* pattern in mind, you need to be true to your type if you're to change your habits successfully. In reality, your dominant, backup, and less-favored preferences are not weighted equally. In fact, they influence the outcome according to their weight. Your dominant preference tends to have the most influence. Your #4 preference has the least. Yet your #4 preference has much to offer. By using all the preferences within your type and giving each its say, you allow yourself a checks-and-balances approach to decision making that leaves nothing out. Your habits are then no longer governed strictly by your dominant preference, the preference that has probably been responsible for some of the unhealthy habits you have.

Figures 15 and 16 show graphically your type's 1–2–3–4 order of decision making. Notice the difference from the *Z* pattern.

Getting into Trouble

We get into trouble when our dominant preference (#1) takes over and ignores the input from the other preferences. We then

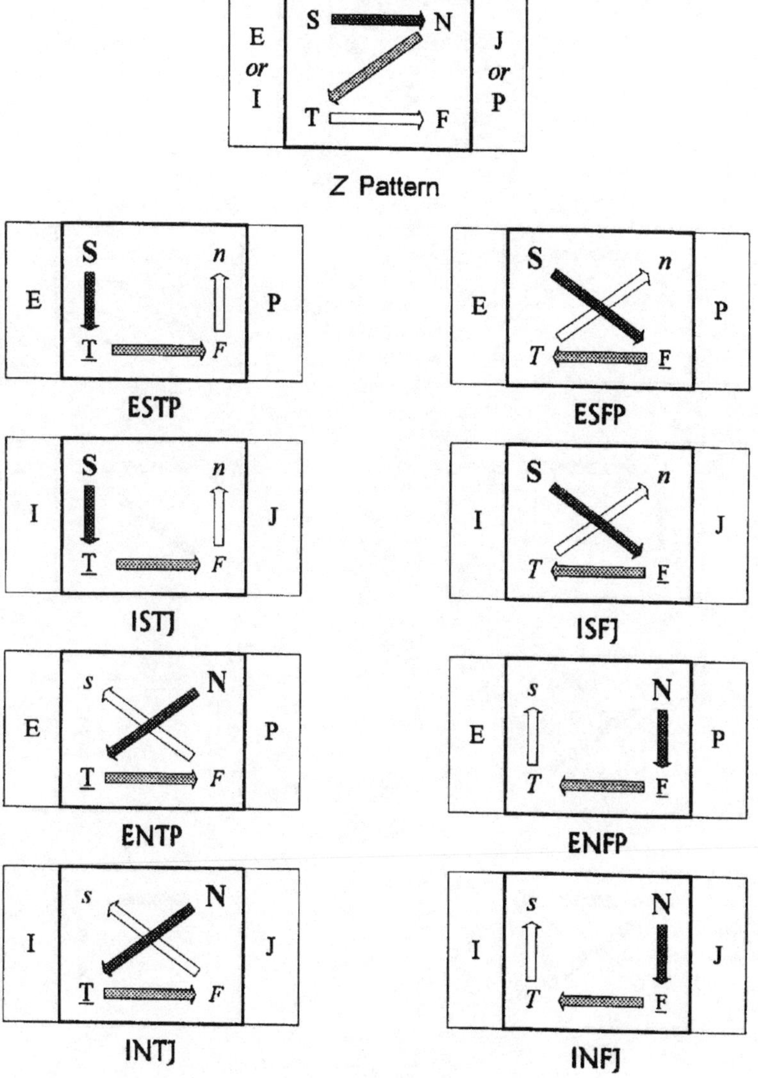

Figure 15. Your Type's 1–2–3–4 Order

make decisions based on inadequate information and/or processing. Dominant Sensors may accept the first solution presented to them as being the best, ignoring the possibility that there are better alternatives. Dominant iNtuitives may ignore the facts and

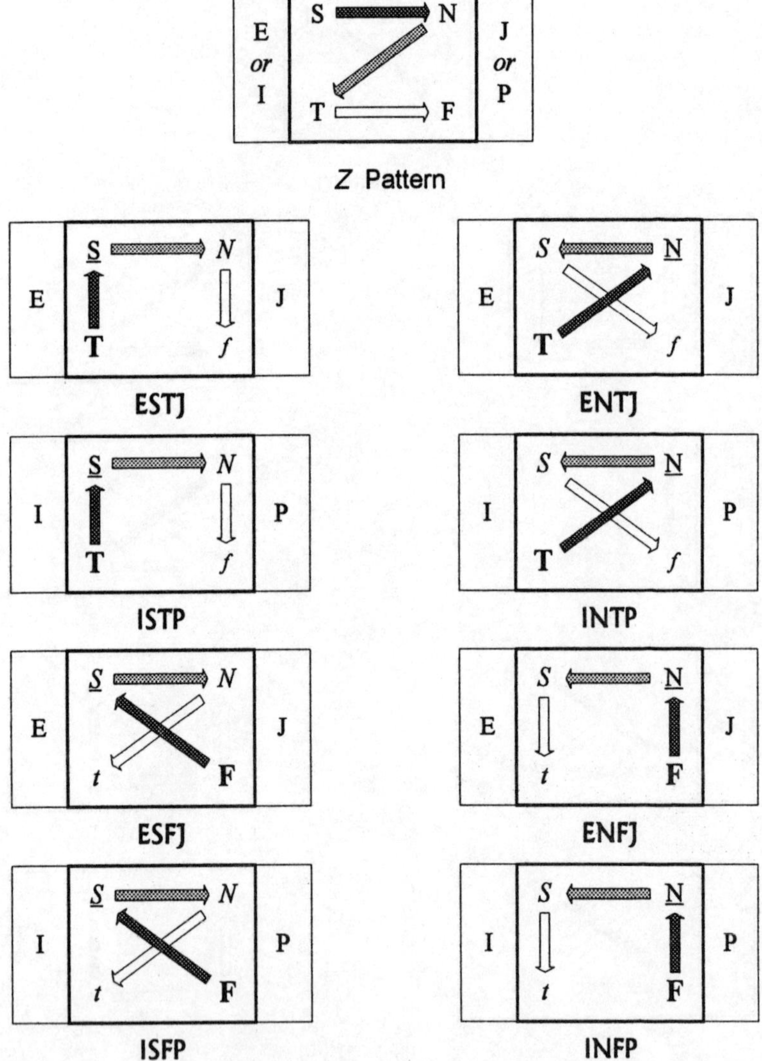

Figure 16. Your Type's 1–2–3–4 Order

data that the Sensing preference can provide, rushing to make decisions solely on their impression of future possibilities. Dominant Thinkers will tend to ignore the human aspects of a decision and dominant Feelers may ignore the consequences of a decision,

TABLE 6. **Not Using All Your Preferences.**
The shaded area shows you the input that you are partially or completely missing.

Most Favored Preference ⟶ **Least Favored Preference**

Type	**#1**	⟶	**#2**	⟶	**#3**	⟶	**#4**
ESTP	**S**	⟶	T	⟶	*F*	⟶	*n*
ESFP	**S**	⟶	F	⟶	*T*	⟶	*n*
ISTJ	**S**	⟶	T	⟶	*F*	⟶	*n*
ISFJ	**S**	⟶	F	⟶	*T*	⟶	*n*
ENTP	**N**	⟶	T	⟶	*F*	⟶	*s*
ENFP	**N**	⟶	F	⟶	*T*	⟶	*s*
INTJ	**N**	⟶	T	⟶	*F*	⟶	*s*
INFJ	**N**	⟶	F	⟶	*T*	⟶	*s*
ESTJ	**T**	⟶	S	⟶	*N*	⟶	*f*
ENTJ	**T**	⟶	N	⟶	*S*	⟶	*f*
ISTP	**T**	⟶	S	⟶	*N*	⟶	*f*
INTP	**T**	⟶	N	⟶	*S*	⟶	*f*
ESFJ	**F**	⟶	S	⟶	*N*	⟶	*t*
ENFJ	**F**	⟶	N	⟶	*S*	⟶	*t*
ISFP	**F**	⟶	S	⟶	*N*	⟶	*t*
INFP	**F**	⟶	N	⟶	*S*	⟶	*t*

being more concerned with maintaining harmony. Table 6 shows what's happening when you're not using all of your preferences.

If you believe a decision you've made is not the best one you could make, think about what's really bothering you about the decision, what information you're ignoring or missing. For example, if you're trying to lose weight, you might be worried what people will say if you eat something fattening. If you eat it anyway, you are disregarding your Feeling preference's concerns. If you realize that something fattening doesn't fit into your diet and you eat it anyway, you have ignored the input from your Thinking preference. If the sight or smell of food "forced" you to eat something, you're allowing your Sensing preference to take over.

If you can't concentrate on what you're eating because you're already planning what else you should have, your iNtuiting preference is working overtime.

Find Your Opposite

By now you probably get the point that by tapping into all of your preferences, you can make better decisions. At first, having to go through all of the preferences each time you have a decision to make may seem laborious. Yet the awareness it will bring and the help it will give you in establishing healthier habits makes it worth the time. It's like learning to play an instrument or master a sport. If you want to be the best you can be, you can't leave any of the steps out, even if they're not always fun. Playing an instrument requires understanding chords and practicing scales. Becoming a figure skater requires perfecting your edges and turns. Living a healthier lifestyle requires learning to make healthy decisions.

If you're struggling with your less favorite preferences and not being able to get much from them because your dominant and backup preferences are so strong, I have a suggestion for you. Find someone whose dominant preference is that of either your #3 or #4 preference. Ask them what they would do in a particular situation. For example, if your dominant preference is Sensing, it means your #4 preference is iNtuiting. So find someone with a dominant preference of iNtuiting.

The Sensor may be very good at considering pertinent facts of a situation, but could use the iNtuitive's ability to see the possibilities inherent in a situation. The reverse holds equally true: that is, while the iNtuitive is seeing the possibilities inherent in a situation, he could use the Sensor's ability to consider the facts. Sensors look to their previous experiences when trying to solve a problem. Yet they might benefit from the insight, the "gut feel" for what's the right thing to do, that the iNtuitive has to offer. Sensors focus on the joy of what's presently happening but could take advantage of the iNtuitives' ability to open a window to the joys that the future might hold.

Thinkers will analyze anything and everything to determine

the consequences of a situation. They often lack Feelers' ability to consider how others will be affected by a situation. Thinkers will be too critical, always looking for flaws. They could take a lesson from the Feelers who know how to praise, looking for what is positive in others and things. Thinkers may be very good at creating systems. However, if those systems involve people, they often overlook their needs. Feelers should be consulted to help Thinkers learn how they could create a harmonious working environment, to focus more on human-centered values.

Again, in all these situations, the reverse holds true. You might want to go back through the last couple of paragraphs and reread them as if you were a dominant iNtuitive or dominant Feeler. As you can see, each type offers much to the other if each is willing to listen and try.

We're Similar but Unique

Someone with the same type as you may not always come up with the same decision. That's partly due to the strength of your preferences. Remember in Chapter 2, when you drew a bar graph of your type? If someone else with the same type has a bar graph that looks different from yours, it means the strength of his preferences is different from yours. Therefore, he or she might respond differently in the same circumstance. Also, your past experiences aren't the same, and this will influence the decisions you both make because you are each bringing different information to the process.

You may find that other types are making similar decisions as you. That's normal. It may be, though, that they came to their conclusions via a different route or preference. If everyone uses all of their preferences as recommended in this book, there should be a greater chance that the results will be the same . . . hopefully in the direction of healthier habits!

A Call for Decisions

Throughout the remainder of this book you'll be faced with decisions to make. Whenever I mention that you need to make a decision, I want you to remember what we discussed in this chapter. Go through the steps according to your type, and then you should be able to say to yourself, "This is the best decision I could make."

To help you do that, I've created a Decision Road Map to guide you on your journey. (See Figure 17.) We'll be considering such questions as: "Am I going to eat now, even though I'm not hungry?" "Am I going to eat more, even though I'm full?" "Am I going to skip exercising today?" "Am I going to let your remark ruin my day?" If your dominant or #1 preference says "no" to these questions, great. You've made a healthy decision and you needn't think about it any more. However, if your #1 preference responded in its habitual way, telling you "yes," you need to move on to your #2 preference. Maybe it can help you out by telling you why the decision of your #1 preference isn't the best one. Of course, there's no guarantee that your #2 preference is going to save the day. Since most of our habits come from our #1 and #2 preferences, you may have to continue on the Road Map to your #3 and #4 preferences. Once you've reached a "no" decision, one you can support without regrets, you'll know you're changing your habits.

If you consistently find yourself answering "yes" with your #1 and #2 preferences, you might find it beneficial to go directly to the #3 preference on the Road Map and start enlisting the help of your less-frequently-called-on preferences.

In the following chapters are Decision Road Maps to help you learn to:

1. Eat only when you're hungry.
2. Stop as soon as you are satisfied.
3. Exercise or engage in physical activity on a regular basis.

Note that the Road Maps may vary slightly for each of these.

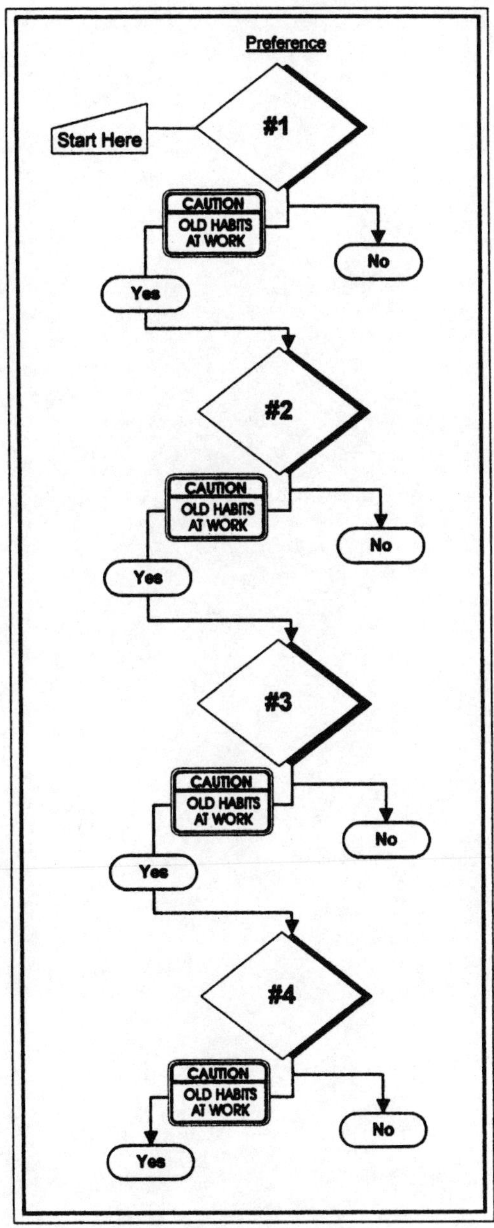

Figure 17. Decision Road Map

PART II

HEALTHY HABITS MADE EASY USING YOUR PERSONALITY

6

Making It a Habit #1: Achieve Your Life Vision

We have now arrived at the point where it's time to take action, and use your personality to help you improve your lifestyle habits. In this part of the book you'll learn the necessary skills to become healthier, feel better, and have more energy—and in turn, to reach your *life vision.* If you're an iNtuitive, the destination of your journey may be important, but don't forget that the journey itself is every bit as important (Perceivers and Sensors would vouch for that). However, iNtuitives have a slight advantage over Sensors because, while the Sensors are concentrating on short-term goals, iNtuitives are thinking, "How can I make this change last a lifetime?"

This concept of *life vision* may be difficult for you _S_Ps and _S_Js to grasp since you tend to live in the present moment. You're probably wondering how anyone can see that far into the future. However, it's living in the present moment with no concern for where your actions may lead you that often gets you into trouble. Your _S_Ps' impulsive nature has you saying, "Why not?" to many opportunities that may not fit into a healthy lifestyle. Your _S_Js are somewhat resistant to change. Are you doomed to failure? Not at all. You just need to tap into your other preferences. The Feeling preference can show you what a *life vision* means in terms of your family and yourself. Tapping into the Thinking preference will provide a logical analysis and the benefits of having a *life vision.* Fortunately, the steps to reaching a *life vision* are taken in the here-and-now, something that *does* appeal to you _S_Ps and _S_Js.

Measuring Your Progress

Do Your Goals Need to Be Measurable?

For Thinkers and Judgers, the answer to this question would be "yes." How else would you know what progress you're making or when you've arrived at your destination? You don't even mind setting a date to accomplish your goals. For Perceivers, measurements mean "too much structure" and don't leave room for changes if and when they become necessary; you Perceivers might be willing to set some guidelines as long as you don't have to establish a timeframe for achieving the goals. How long you will adhere to the guidelines is the question.

The Oracle Known as the Bathroom Scale

As I mentioned previously, your weight can serve as a measuring tool for seeing how well you're doing in changing your habits. But your weight should not be your goal. Changing your habits is the goal. I am often reluctant to recommend using a bathroom scale. Too many people end up worshipping the scale and seeing it as an oracle in their lives. They get on the scale in the morning praying for it to tell them what they want to hear: "You have been good, so I will be nice and show you that you have lost one pound." When the reading shows no loss—or worse, shows a number larger than yesterday's—they hear, "You have been bad and will have to repent." To many that means having to starve and employ that destructive thing called willpower. Any time a value judgment ("You are bad") is put on the results of your weighing in, your Feeling preference has been at work. The Thinking preference, on the other hand, responds to an increase on the scale by analyzing what might have caused the increase so as to avoid the problem again.

The bathroom scale can be motivating for some, but for most of us it tends to sabotage our efforts. Depending on the results, the Feeling preference will set an emotional tone for the day. You may either be floating on cloud nine or wallowing in your depression. It can degrade your confidence in yourself by weighing your self-esteem rather than your body weight. The scale becomes the controller and you, its subject. One of the major messages of this book is that *you* are in control of you.

Use the scale sparingly as a measuring tool, keeping in mind that the numbers you see are not a very good measure of your weight, anyway. Retained fluids look no different on the scale than extra fat. That's why body composition analysis to determine body fat percentage, done about every six months until your weight is stabilized, is a much better measurement. Having it performed is not as convenient (you'll have to go somewhere for a reading) and is more expensive than just jumping on your bathroom scale in the morning. It's still worth doing. Choose from the three standard methods: (1) bioelectrical impedance analysis (where a very slight electrical impulse is sent through you to measure the amount of fluid versus fat in your body); (2) measurements by calipers (pinchers that measure thickness of skinfold); or (3) hydrostatic weight measurement (in which you are weighed underwater).

Using a tape measure to measure your hips, waist, thighs, and chest is also an effective way to monitor changes to your body fat or muscle mass. Don't ever lose track of the reason you are taking these measurements, though. You are headed toward a *life vision,* not a beauty pageant.

Other Numbers

Your blood cholesterol, blood sugar, and blood pressure can also provide valid measurements of change. As we discuss the various habits, you'll find that changes in each can be measured to determine how you're doing. For example, the number of calories, the percentage of fat, protein, and carbohydrates, and the grams and milligrams of vitamins and minerals can all serve as a way of monitoring your diet. Exercising includes its own numbers:

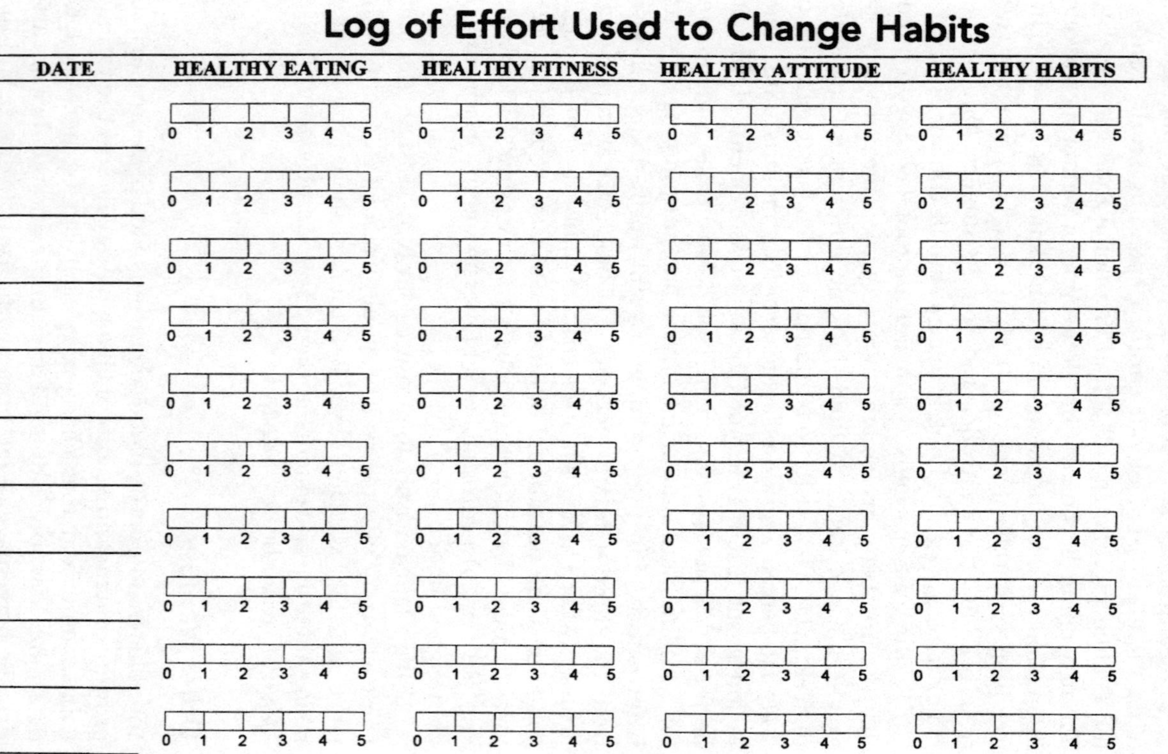

Log of Effort Used to Change Habits

DATE	HEALTHY EATING	HEALTHY FITNESS	HEALTHY ATTITUDE	HEALTHY HABITS
	0 1 2 3 4 5	0 1 2 3 4 5	0 1 2 3 4 5	0 1 2 3 4 5
	0 1 2 3 4 5	0 1 2 3 4 5	0 1 2 3 4 5	0 1 2 3 4 5
	0 1 2 3 4 5	0 1 2 3 4 5	0 1 2 3 4 5	0 1 2 3 4 5
	0 1 2 3 4 5	0 1 2 3 4 5	0 1 2 3 4 5	0 1 2 3 4 5
	0 1 2 3 4 5	0 1 2 3 4 5	0 1 2 3 4 5	0 1 2 3 4 5
	0 1 2 3 4 5	0 1 2 3 4 5	0 1 2 3 4 5	0 1 2 3 4 5
	0 1 2 3 4 5	0 1 2 3 4 5	0 1 2 3 4 5	0 1 2 3 4 5
	0 1 2 3 4 5	0 1 2 3 4 5	0 1 2 3 4 5	0 1 2 3 4 5
	0 1 2 3 4 5	0 1 2 3 4 5	0 1 2 3 4 5	0 1 2 3 4 5
	0 1 2 3 4 5	0 1 2 3 4 5	0 1 2 3 4 5	0 1 2 3 4 5

Figure 18. Log of the Effort Used to Change Your Habits

how far you can stretch, how much weight you can lift, the percentage of maximum heart rate at which you are comfortable exercising.

Rating Your Effort

Another way of measuring your progress is to monitor how much effort you expend in trying to change your habits. If you're not seriously doing anything, how can you expect any results? There is a direct relationship between your effort and your success. As you learn new habits, I want you to record your progress in the amount of effort you put forth. You'll be rating your effort on a scale of 1 to 5, with 1 being very little effort and 5 being the most effort of which you are capable. I have provided you with a log for keeping track of your effort. (See Figure 18.)

Here's how one person filled in the log. She felt she was giving it almost all her effort and so logged in 4½ on the scale.

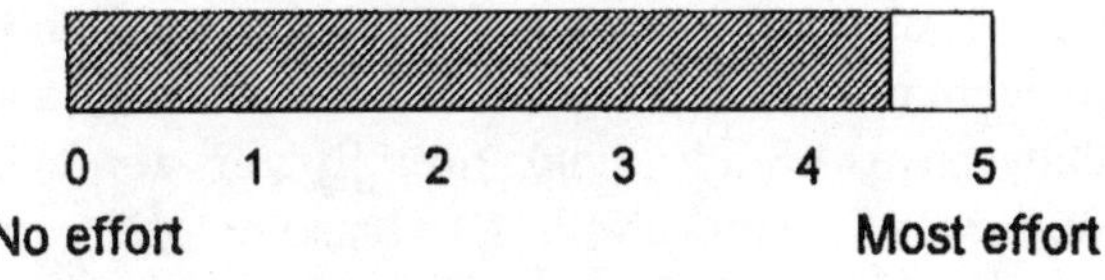

Figure 19. Rating Personal Effort—An Example

I can already hear some of you Perceivers balking at having to keep a log. Being so structured isn't in your nature. If, after giving it a try, you find you don't feel comfortable actually recording your effort, just think about it and register it in your mind. Those of you who do log in your effort are going to find this measurement very enlightening. After several weeks of tracking your effort, a quick look at the log will show you your problem areas, if there are any. Then you'll need to dig deeper to determine why you're not expending enough effort in a particular area.

Giving Yourself a Time Frame

You need to have a time frame to achieve your goals. Without a time frame, it's too easy to slack off and tell yourself, "One of these days I will . . ." (as a Perceiver or iNtuitive might say). This is where your personality is really going to show itself. Some people can handle long-term goals, while others prefer short-term goals.

Those of you who are Judgers will be working on a plan long before we finish the book. You'll feel very comfortable setting a time frame, scheduling things as necessary. Perceivers, on the other hand, may feel pressured by having to set a time frame. You may do it, but will probably abandon it at some point. If you are also Feelers, you'll probably feel guilty afterwards for abandoning it. I don't want Perceivers or anyone else to feel guilty about the approach they take to changing their habits. It just may be that Perceivers will have to look to another preference within their type to push them onward if the Perceiving preference is holding them back.

(Perceivers, please do not think that I'm picking on you when I point out what might be considered by Judgers to be a weakness. You actually have the advantage over Judgers for being more flexible and therefore more willing to try some of the new things I'm suggesting in this book. By the way, remember that I'm an ENFJ, and the last thing I want to do is hurt anyone's feeling by attacking any personality type.)

Because you Sensors are here-and-now people, asking you to set long-term goals may be asking too much. Consider setting a series of smaller goals, each of which you can accomplish in a shorter time period. Don't worry about the five-year plan. The six-month plan may be much more attractive to you. Setting a *life vision* may be even more difficult because it's too far in the future to have any sense of reality for you. If you're a Sensor, you may have to set your vision using either your analytical, Thinking preference, or your Feeling preference, placing your faith in it being the best thing for you. You are very aware of "what is," but have a harder time visualizing "what might be"—what isn't real and tangible. For you, long-term goals are pipe dreams. Short-term goals are more like puzzle pieces: As you acquire each piece, you can see the picture forming.

You iNtuitives, on the other hand, can see the whole puzzle completed. However, seeing the individual pieces can be a challenge. You have no problem imagining how things *could* be different, what potential may lie ahead. In fact, you spend most of your time thinking about how you can change things, how you can make things better. You are actually happier with long-term goals, since short-term goals are satisfied too quickly and leave you trying to figure out what else needs fixing.

If you are a Sensor and a Perceiver, you'll want the goal to have been completed yesterday. The _S_P combination tends to seek instant gratification. A weight-loss diet that calls for losing one to two pounds a week seems agonizingly slow. You can't imagine being able to hold out or stick with the diet long enough. _S_Ps tend to take care of things as they arise, an attitude incompatible with goal setting, which requires some degree of planning.

Fortunately for people with the _S_J combination, they have no problem planning, but they're not happy having to look too far into the future.

If you are an iNtuitive and also a Perceiver, you may often find yourself reluctant to act on goals because you figure that a better way will come along to accomplish them. Setting the goal isn't difficult, whether short or long-term, because you can well imagine how things might be different. But accomplishing it is something else. If you are an _NTP, you're always trying to perfect the way you'll go about it. Even when you reach your goal, you probably won't be satisfied. As an idealist, you believe things could always be better. _N_Ps are great at putting things off until tomorrow; they're the "diet-starts-on-Monday-morning" people.

iNtuitives who are also Judgers not only know how to set goals but also are able to schedule and plan how they'll go about achieving them. However, you _N_Js may ask unrealistic things of yourself unless you have some rules and guidelines.

Making Your Goals Proactive, Not Reactive

Your life should be the result of the decisions you make, not the conditions you have to react to. You can choose between being proactive or reactive. When you're being proactive, you have a feeling of positive energy. You can use phrases like "I choose to," I prefer," "I will," "Yes" and "No." It's having an idea where you want to go and determining ways to get there. You're in control. You're in the driver's seat.

Compare that to being reactive. Whatever happens, you have to respond to it; you aren't in control. You find yourself using such phrases as "I have to," "I can't," "I should," and "I must." Any energy you expend doesn't move you forward in the direction of your choice, but only away from something that is unacceptable. There isn't room for decision making, only response to the demands of the situation or the people involved.

There are two major elements to being proactive—being effective and being efficient. When you're effective you get results by "doing the right things." Efficiency is using methods that allow you to "do things right." Effectiveness and efficiency work hand in hand. Hopefully, by the end of this book you will have learned how to become more effective and efficient.

It's the Difference That Makes the Difference

Why are you willing to go through the effort of changing your habits? You must be discontent with the way things are *and* believe things could be better. Therefore, you recognize that a difference exists. How well you can visualize that difference is partially dependent upon your personality.

You Sensors are very aware of "what is," right now. If you aren't satisfied with that condition, you know something needs to change. Being actually able to picture what you will be like when you have brought about the change is another story. You iNtuitives, on the other hand, concentrate less on what you have right now, but have a great image of "what might be," and that moves you forward.

Whether you're a Sensor or iNtuitive, for you to take some action, there needs to exist a difference between "what is" and "what might be." The amount of that difference will be an essential factor in determining the drive you have to accomplish your goals. Let's say that right now you are eating a diet that contains 32 percent fat. Health experts tell us that our diet should consist of less than 30 percent fat. With only a little more than a 2 percent difference, you're probably saying to yourself, "If I get it down, great. But if I don't, it's no big deal."

On the other end of the spectrum, suppose you're eating a diet that contains 55 percent fat. Now you have a huge difference from the goal of less than 30 percent fat. How can you possibly shave off 25 percent of your fat intake? When people are faced with what appears to be an insurmountable goal, they often avoid it. By avoiding it, they figure they can also avoid the potential for failure. If they do attempt it, they may give up somewhere along the line because it's taking too long to see the fruits of their labor.

Your goal should be just out of reach, but not out of sight. It should stretch you but be realistic. It should be attainable in a reasonable amount of time and with a reasonable amount of effort. If it is set too high (too much of a difference), you have a ready excuse for not succeeding: "It's just too hard to achieve, no matter how much effort I put in." A goal set too low (too small a difference) doesn't give you a sense that you've accomplished something. As with the picture of the magnets in Figure 20, if "what is" and "what might be" are too far apart, there won't be much attraction or motion. If they're too close, there's not enough pull.

Please don't misunderstand me. I'm not suggesting that when a difference is large you should just ignore the problem. If your health demands that you make a tremendous change, you need to do it. Having to decrease your fat intake by 25 percent may seem difficult but it doesn't mean that you should just give up. It just means that you may need to break it down into a series of small goals. You could do it in increments of 10 percent, for example. Allow yourself the feeling of success when you accomplish that first milestone. Then the next 10 percent will seem achievable as well, and so on.

Time is another factor that must be considered. If the time frame is too short, you may figure it can never be done, so why even start. A time frame that's too long makes some people (especially Sensors) feel that there is no reality to the change so why bother trying. Perceivers won't get started until the last min-

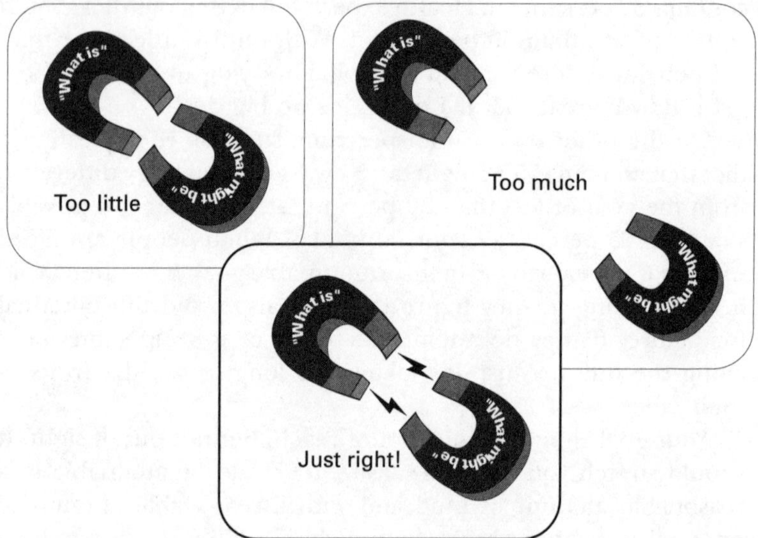

Figure 20. The Amount of Difference Makes the Difference

ute anyway. For them, too long a time frame just amounts to putting off the change.

Add a Generous Helping of Motivation

Motivation comes from recognizing that a difference exists between "what is" and "what might be" and putting a value on that difference with your Feeling preference. The fact that I want to see you make the necessary health changes isn't going to motivate you to do anything about it. *You* have to want to make the changes. How badly you want them is going to be the force driving you to accomplish your goal.

There are a number of factors involved in determining your motivation, many of which are based on your personality. You need to be aware of the long-term negative consequences of continuing the habits you presently have. Hopefully, Chapter 3 gave you that background. How are your habits going to affect your health and well-being? Thinkers will have an easy time analyzing this question from a medical and scientific point of view.

Feelers will decide on their goals based on the effect they have on others who are important to them or on themselves.

On the flip side are the long-term positive consequences of changing your habits. What's the payoff, what are the benefits, both to yourself and to others (another Thinking perspective)? How will you feel about yourself and how will others see you (the Feeler's perspective)? Your degree of motivation is intimately involved with your belief that you can accomplish your goals this time. Using your personality in order to change gives you a much greater chance of success than you might have experienced in the past.

It's easy to make an impulsive decision and say, "I've had it with myself. I'm changing my habits as of this moment." Actually, this sounds very much like a New Year's resolution. After getting aggravated with yourself for all the things you've done to your body for the past year, you proclaim that this coming year, things will be different. The problem with New Year's resolutions is that they are, at best, temporary, largely because they are reactive. ("I'm not going to sneak snacks anymore." "I'm swearing off chocolate.") You've convinced yourself that you're going to change, but you haven't thought through your motivation. Without a positive motivation for change ("I'll have more energy when I start exercising regularly"), where will your commitment come from? Without both motivation and commitment, the likelihood of success is quite low. They are measures of your readiness to change.

Take a moment:

Having decided on your *life vision,* you need to consider how motivated you are to reach it. On a scale of 1 to 10, with 1 being very low motivation and 10 being very high motivation, how would you rate your true motivation to reach your *life vision?* (A rating of 1–5 isn't strong enough to pull you forward. A rating of 6–7 means you're warming up to the idea. A rating of 8–10 tells you that you're ready and willing to do what it takes.) Be honest! If you're not in the 7–10 range, you may want to wait until you are truly ready. Otherwise, you'll be using willpower to get you through, which won't take you all the way to your *life vision.*

When you start setting goals, you will also need to think about how motivated you are to achieve each one, remembering that they are the stepping stones to your vision.

No Finger-Pointing

Everyone is capable of changing. You must believe that in order to successfully change. Some people refuse to accept responsibility and accountability for achieving their goals. If they fail, they figure they can always point the finger at someone or something else (circumstances, fate, their genes, luck) that got in their way. But that's too easy an out and gets you nowhere.

There are some personality types who are "just-tell-me-what-to-do" people. And there's nothing wrong with looking for advice and suggestions from others. Problems arise, though, when we refuse to accept responsibility for the results, placing blame instead on the giver of the information when things don't work out as planned. We must realize that *we* are responsible for making the decisions about what methods to use to change our habits, as well as carrying out those methods. As discussed in Chapter 5, your personality will be instrumental in helping you reach those decisions.

Success feeds on itself. With every goal you reach, the stronger will be your belief that you can reach your vision. When you think there are too many obstacles in your way, just remember:

> *Obstacles are those things you see when you take your eyes off your goal.*—Hannah Moore

Take a moment:

What do you think are going to be the challenges or obstacles to achieving your goals? Are these insurmountable? How do you think you would handle them? (Don't forget what you learned in Chapter 5 about decision making. It is also the format for problem solving.)

Your Personality Guidelines for Setting Your Goals

As you set your goals and *life vision,* keep in mind the characteristics of your personality type, as shown in Table 7. It will be easier for you to set goals if you abide by your dominant and backup preferences. However, you should also consider what contribution your #3 and #4 preferences can make to maintain balance.

Use the contract form in Figure 21 to set your *life vision* and goals. Make a copy of it so that if you want to set other goals later on, you'll have a blank form from which to work. By the way, I'm aware of the fact that you Perceivers aren't too keen on doing something as structured as filling in a contract, whereas you Judgers will find it a natural way to organize your approach to your vision. And I appreciate that you Extraverts would rather just tell the world about it than write it down. However, please give it a try. Don't forget, you do have all the preferences within you. You may just have to work a little harder on the preferences that aren't your dominant or backup ones to get you through this. Of course, maybe they can also help you develop an alternative!

TABLE 7. **Personality Guidelines for Setting Goals**

Personality Type	Tend To	Need to Consider
Extroverts	• Talk their goals over with others.	• Putting their goals in writing to make them more concrete.
Introverts	• Sign a contract with themselves. • Share their goals with others only after they've been determined.	• Getting input from others when setting goals.
Sensors	• Set goals that are practical and down-to-earth (for example, losing weight vs. becoming more beautiful). • Have an easy time making the goals measurable. • Set a realistic time frame, preferably short term. • Determine what their goals are going to do to their everyday life.	• The big picture—where their goals are leading them.
iNtuitives	• Set goals that are long term. • See the big picture and the far-reaching impact of achieving their goals. • Consider different and out-of-the-ordinary ways to reach their goals.	• The practical side of their goals, so that something tangible and realistic is accomplished. • The present and the pitfalls it holds.

Thinkers	• Look for the cause and effect of the decisions they make regarding their goals. ("I realize that my high blood-sugar level is the result of poor diet and lack of exercise. By watching my diet and including exercise in my life, I hope to have more energy and less dizziness.") • State their goals objectively, concisely, and clearly. ("I want to gain more control over my blood-sugar level by increasing the amount of fiber I eat to 30 grams a day, decreasing the amount of sugar I eat to 10 percent of my daily calories, and upping my exercise to five times a week.)	• How they personally will deal with their goals, how their goals will affect others, and how they will deal with the reactions of others.
Feelers	• Set goals based on the effect those goals have on themselves or others. ("Sam says he's worried about how little energy I have. It seems I can't keep up with him, so I'm going to try getting out and walking more.") • Soften the deadlines on goals or their approach to them if that's affecting someone else. ("I know I was supposed to eat only six servings of starch a day, but because it's your birthday, I'll indulge myself.")	• The logical consequences of their goals, especially when those goals were based on meeting others' needs.

TABLE 7. **Continued**

Personality Type	Tend To	Need to Consider
Judgers	• Set goals quickly and get on with it. ("My doctor told me that my cholesterol is too high. He recommended I see a dietician, and I've already made the appointment.") • Set goals according to some sort of structure to make them easier to attain.	• Slowing down the goal-setting process to be sure enough information has been collected. • Consider alternatives.
Perceivers	• Consider and reconsider, evaluate and reevaluate their goals. • Consider alternatives that give them some flexibility in achieving their goals. ("The best way to lose weight is. . . . If that doesn't work, I could try. . . .")	• Imposing some structure on their goals so they don't let spontaneity negatively influence the attainment of their goals.

MY *LIFE VISION* CONTRACT WITH MYSELF

On ______________________ (today's date), I have determined my *life vision* to be *(include your level of motivation, using a scale of 1 to 10, 1 being the lowest and 10 the highest):*

____

____

____

I plan to work toward my *life vision* by completing the following goals *(include measurement guidelines, time frame, and level of motivation, using a scale of 1 to 10 for each goal):* ______________

____

____

____

____

Using my personality type of ________________, the following are points I will keep in mind as I set my goals. ________

____

____

____

I believe the following are obstacle(s) or challenge(s) I will face on my path to my *life vision.*

____

____

____

____

Signature

____

Signature of Witness(es) (if desired)

Figure 21. *Life Vision* Contract

7

Making It a Habit #2: Eat for the Right Reasons

It's amazing how many different reasons people give when asked, "Why are you eating when you're not hungry?" Here are some of them:

1. "My friend made this cake for me—how could I not have some?"
2. "I may never get to try this again."
3. "I'm waiting for someone to meet me here, and I'm just filling time."
4. "I was passing the bakery. The aromas drew me in, and then I couldn't resist the cupcakes."
5. "When I can't afford to doze off, food keeps me awake."
6. "I deserve it as a reward for being so good."
7. "I needed a break from work. It's so boring."
8. "I'm so frustrated and angry, I could chew a nail in half. The next-best thing would be a candy bar."
9. "When I'm cooking something, I need to sample it often to be sure it tastes just right."
10. "Just a little taste won't do any harm."
11. "Everyone else is eating."
12. "It's lunchtime."
13. "I always have popcorn when I go to the movies."
14. "I didn't even realize I was eating."

15. "It was there."
16. "It was free."
17. "If I don't eat now, I may get hungry later."

Do any of these reasons sound familiar? Do you have any of your own to add? It's interesting how creative we can be in finding reasons to eat, other than for reasons of genuine hunger. Can you imagine a lion in the wild eating for any of these reasons? Since it has to expend a great deal of energy and effort to bring down a zebra, gazelle, or other four-legged creature, it's not going to eat unless it's really hungry. Our problem may be that food is so readily available or is so often consumed for reasons other than hunger, that we no longer associate food solely with nourishment. In fact, if you go over the list of reasons, you won't find one having to do with physical health. We eat in response to many other triggers: environmental cues, people, our emotions, our attitude, the time of day, our established habits.

Tracing the Personality Element

Let's review those reasons for eating again and see how they show personalities at work. It's normally one or two preferences in our personalities, most often our dominant or backup, that create such habitual responses.

1. "My friend made this cake for me—how could I not have some?"
   - *What's going on here?* The Feeling preference doesn't want to hurt your friend's feelings. So eating the cake seems a good way to preserve harmony.
   - *Try this instead:* Let your Thinking preference tell you the illogic of eating something because of someone else. Your body doesn't need the calories. If you really want the cake, that's another story. Then your decision is whether to eat it despite the fact that you're not hungry and, if so, how much to eat. Your iNtuiting preference could tell you that you could take a couple of bites and save the rest for later. Your Sensing preference could tell

you whether it tastes good; then your Feeling preference could determine if the taste is really worth the calories.

2. "I may never get to try this again."
   - *What's going on here?* Being future-oriented, the iNtuiting preference is questioning when this opportunity will arise again. Not seeing an answer readily available, it has quickly decided that it would be best to eat it now.
   - *Try this instead:* Using your Thinking preference, how did you determine that this opportunity may never come up again? Is it a veiled excuse to eat something when you know you shouldn't if you're not hungry? Let your Feeling preference determine how important it is to try this food. Will you always regret not having tried it, or is it not that big a deal? You could take a bite or two, let your Sensing preference register the taste and lock it into memory, and forgo the rest.
3. "I'm waiting for someone to meet me here and I'm just filling time."
   - *What's going on here?* Eating in this situation is serving as a transition activity between what you've just been doing and your expectation of meeting your friend. Your Sensing preference is very much into the here-and-now, "what can I do with myself?" mode.
   - *Try this instead:* I'm sure your iNtuiting preference can come up with many other transition activities that don't involve food. Then you can allow your Thinking preference to tell you that there is no logical connection between waiting and eating. If you need to fill your time, consider the alternatives iNtuiting has offered. If your Feeling preference really cares about you, it will confirm that eating is not being good to yourself.
4. "I was passing the bakery. The aromas drew me in, and then I couldn't resist the cupcakes."
   - *What's going on here?* Very much influenced by sights and smells, the Sensing preference has succumbed.
   - *Try this instead:* Just because you smell or see something good, is not grounds for eating it. Yet that's what gets many people into trouble. They're on the "see-food" eating plan—they see food, they eat it. But when do

they call it quits? Instead, try using your Thinking preference to analyze the consequences of your "see-food" diet. Done only occasionally, it wouldn't be a problem. However, is eating whenever you see something appetizing becoming a habit? Your iNtuiting preference could help by coming up with a way that you could "have your cake and eat it too." Why not buy the cupcake now and save it for later when you get hungry and can truly enjoy it to its fullest? It does mean, though, putting off instant gratification, and saving your Feeling preference from feeling guilty about eating when you know you shouldn't.

5. "When I can't afford to doze off, food keeps me awake."
   - *What's going on here?* This is consequential thinking very typical of the Thinking preference. If I eat something, I'll stay awake. While it is a poor excuse for eating, it appears logical on the surface.
   - *Try this instead:* Your iNtuiting preference could offer some alternatives to eating, whether it's getting some fresh air or having a cup of coffee. Next time, you could eat less for lunch so more of your blood would be circulating in your head rather than in your stomach for digestion. Listen to your Sensing preference and realize that, try as you may to stay awake, your level of alertness is impaired and you would be better served by taking a quick nap (even if it is just putting your head down on your desk).
6. "I deserve it as a reward for being so good."
   - *What's going on here?* How you reward yourself for accomplishing something is a personal decision based on what your Feeling preference believes makes you feel good. Your Sensing preference is a diary of past events, a history of receiving candy or cookies for being good, that may seem worth repeating.
   - *Try this instead:* You need to start thinking of alternative rewards by using your iNtuiting preference. With your Thinking preference, you should remind yourself that food is for nourishment and should not carry the emotional baggage of being considered a reward. This is

not to deny food's pleasure, just the labels you attach to it.

7. "I needed a break from work. It's so boring."
   - *What's going on here?* The Feeling preference has put a value on the work being done and hopes to use food as an avoidance activity.
   - *Try this instead:* The Sensing preference is realistic and appreciates that food is not the answer. It may change its mind when exposed to food, though. Let the iNtuiting preference suggest some alternatives: take a walk; go talk with someone; come up with a more creative approach to doing the work. Your Thinking preference should be analyzing why you are finding the work boring. Is there someone else who could do the job while you use your talents elsewhere? It should also be explaining to you that there is no logical connection between eating and boredom other than food serving to take your mind off a boring task.
8. "I'm so frustrated and angry, I could chew a nail in half. The next-best thing would be a candy bar."
   - *What's going on here?* Emotional turmoil can be making you feel sorry for yourself. Your Feeling preference, in a self-nurturing mode, wants to "take care of you" with food.
   - *Try this instead:* Your Thinking preference knows that eating when angry is only a stopgap measure; eventually you have to face up to the problems causing your anger. Besides, food is not well digested when eaten during an emotional upheaval. The iNtuiting preference can certainly come up with some nonfood alternatives, such as taking a walk, airing your problem with a friend, or working on a hobby.
9. "When I'm cooking something, I need to sample it often to be sure it tastes just right."
   - *What's going on here?* Cooking involves the use of all of one's senses. The Feeling preference wants to be sure it's cooked right because of concern over how others will receive the dish or how it will be personally enjoyed. Yet, sampling often becomes a meal before the meal!

- *Try this instead:* The Thinking preference can point out that eating samples of the ingredients before they are even mixed into the dish is not a necessary component to cooking. Sampling continuously doesn't make sense when it takes some time for the flavors to meld and let you know whether the dish needs any adjustments. You may want to tap into your iNtuiting preference to make suggestions as to what you could do with your time while the dish cooks, such as setting the table, reading a book, or watching television. There's always a timer to remind you to check the pot. Just remember, "A watched pot never boils."

10. "Just a little taste won't do any harm."
    - *What's going on here?* Your Sensing preference is seeing the food, smelling it, and being tempted by it. From the Thinking preference's perspective, it would seem that logically, a little taste can't hurt. (The trouble is that most "little tastes" lead to more!)
    - *Try this instead:* Who are you kidding? Few people are able to stop at just a little taste. Remember the potato chip commercial slogan, "Bet you can't eat just one"? Why place temptation in your path? Your Feeling preference should be honest and admit that it has a difficult time dealing with temptations and look to the iNtuiting preference for some creative ways to avoid them. Maybe it's best never to bring the goodies into your house. Or you could allow yourself the goodies, just put how much you think you should eat on a plate and then put the package away.
11. "Everyone else is eating."
    - *What's going on here?* Studies have shown that people eat more when in a group than when alone. This would be especially true for the Extravert who is energized by the group and the Feeler who doesn't want to make others uncomfortable not joining in or feels cheated not having something.
    - *Try this instead:* Your Thinking preference can explain to you logically that it makes no sense to be eating just because others are. What's the benefit to you? You can

enjoy their company just as well without food. Why eat when you're not hungry? To address the Feeling preference that's experiencing discomfort, consult your iNtuiting preference for ideas. Maybe you could just order a beverage or a small dinner salad. If you don't have anything to eat, you can carry on the conversation while the others do. (After all, they shouldn't talk with their mouths full!)

12. "It's lunchtime."
    - *What's going on here?* Scheduled and organized, you Judgers are clock-driven people. Your eating when the noon bell rings has become somewhat of a conditioned response, possibly even stimulating gastric juices that can mimic true hunger.
    - *Try this instead:* Where did this habit come from? If it arose out of necessity, because of your job or life situation, ask your Feeling preference whether it's a habit you're happy maintaining. You may need to make the rule "Don't eat unless you're hungry" a part of your life before your clock-driven actions change. Do you believe the rule is a good one to follow? If so, give your iNtuiting preference a chance to solve this problem for you. Maybe for a week you could avoid wearing a watch or looking at clocks, eating only when you can honestly sense hunger.
13. "I always have popcorn when I go to the movies."
    - *What's going on here?* The Sensing preference is the holder of traditions. Once the connection between popcorn and movies has been established, it is hard to break the habit. These two activities have become one. Your Feeling preference feels comfortable with traditions so you need to find strength from some other preference to be willing to part with them.
    - *Try this instead:* This is the time to bring in your Thinking preference to analyze whether you are going to the movies for the food or the movie. If it's for the movie, eating can be distracting. Your undivided attention can't be on the movie. If it's as much for the food as for the movie, then at least plan ahead with your Judging

preference and don't eat before you go. You might want your Feeling preference to consider the effect you are having on other people when eating, possibly bothering them with the noise of munching and the strong smell of popcorn.

14. "I didn't even realize I was eating."
    - *What's going on here?* When you are engrossed in something else, such as watching television, eating can become an unconscious act. Even though both eating and watching television are Sensing-preference stimuli, the message to your brain from the stimulus of food on your taste buds is being buried by the sights and sounds of television. You will never be aware of your hunger level when your attention is engaged elsewhere.
    - *Try this instead:* Your Thinking preference can tell you that the only logical solution to this problem is not to be doing anything else while you're eating. You need to have your undivided attention on the task at hand. If you're not hungry, apply all your attention to whatever else you're doing. If you're not willing to honor eating only when you're hungry, your Feeling preference will need to determine which is more important to you: the activity at hand or eating.
15. "It was there."
    - *What's going on here?* Extraversion and Sensing have paired up here, where your attention is on things outside yourself. You have not made a determination of hunger or a decision of any kind. At this point, it might be difficult to figure out where the habit got started or why. However, that's not really important. Making some changes is.
    - *Try this instead:* You definitely need to rev up your conscious decision-making process. You need to be aware of what you're doing, using your Thinking and Feeling preferences, so that you can actively decide whether or not to eat something.
16. "It was free."
    - *What's going on here?* As a society, we are easily taken in by the word "free." The Feeling preference is particularly

turned on by getting something for free and by the thought that you can get away with eating "fat-free" foods.

- *Try this instead:* Are you really getting something for nothing? Of course not. You need the consequential thinking typical of the Thinking preference to measure the cost to your body of eating when you're not hungry. Your iNtuiting preference might suggest that you take the food and save it for later. You could even consider that, since it's free, you can pass it up without worrying that you spent good money for something you won't be eating.

17. "If I don't eat now, I may get hungry later."
    - *What's going on here?* This is definitely the look-into-the-future person speaking. His iNtuiting preference is not sure whether food will be available at a time when he might be hungry. Eating now, according to the Thinking preference, seems like the logical answer. Or is it?
    - *Try this instead:* This is an example of how the preferences can be used both in a negative and positive way. Your Thinking preference can see the "logic" of the statement, but it also realizes it's illogical to think you can fill up now and avoid hunger at a later time. If that were true, we would never stop eating, "just in case." Your iNtuiting preference might suggest that instead of eating now, you could carry a snack bar or piece of fruit with you so you'll have something available if you do get hungry.

Life's Obstacles to Eating "Only When Hungry"

It's idealistic to ask people to eat only when they are truly hungry. It's a great goal to shoot for and one I hope you'll work on, but I appreciate that it's impossible to meet it 100 percent of the time. The problem arises when people resort to making excuses for eating when they're not hungry, so they don't have to go through the decision-making process and consciously decide the healthy thing to do. Then habits rule their lives.

Besides the situations previously mentioned, what circumstances can you think of that you would consider valid reasons for eating when you're not hungry? (Let me warn you, every reason can probably be countered with an alternative that allows you to be more responsive to hunger.)

- "I have to be at work early in the morning and I must eat breakfast before I go."
  Suggestion: You could eat the not-so-portable foods, such as cereal or eggs, before you go and save your fruit for a midmorning snack. Or you could even pack yourself a sandwich to eat at the office.
- "The company I work at has a set lunch hour."
  Suggestion: You could use your lunch hour to buy your meal and save it to eat during your afternoon coffee break.
- "My friend has made us a special dinner."
  Suggestion: Not wanting to hurt your friend's feelings, you'll probably eat. However, you *are* in control of the quantity you eat.
- "I was on a long flight, and I had to eat the meal when it was served even though I wasn't hungry."
  Suggestion: Most of the time, airline meals are not something you can save for later in the flight when you do get hungry. Therefore, bring some fruit and/or cut-up vegetables with you or consider stopping at one of the food kiosks in the airport before you board. Save these and the roll that comes with your meal to eat later. Ask the stewardess for a carton of milk to round out your snack.
- "It's important to me that we eat together as a family. However, trying to get my children fed early enough to get them to bed means I'm eating before I'm hungry."
  Suggestion: You could just sit with your children, have a cup of coffee or tea, and then eat your meal later. However, if you feel it's better to set a good example of healthy eating by eating with your children, serve yourself small portions.

Knowing Whether or Not You're Truly Hungry

Let's make sure we agree on what true hunger is. What signs should you look for that tell you your body needs nourishment? I'm not talking here about imagined hunger or appetite, but true bodily sensations. Many people experience one or more of the following sensations depending on how hungry they are:

Signs of Hunger

- Stomach growls or grumbles
- Having an empty feeling
- Stomach pain
- Being light-headed or shaky
- Being slightly irritable
- Lack of energy
- Having difficulty concentrating
- Having a headache
- Feeling slightly faint

When I say "stomach growls or grumbles," I'm not referring to the sounds of indigestion or the sloshing of liquid as it makes its way down through the intestine. The sounds of true hunger normally don't occur an hour after you finished eating a decent meal.

On the other hand, there are the people who often wait so long past their original sensations of hunger, either not recognizing them or ignoring them, that they feel faint and light-headed. Many naively think that by ignoring their hunger pangs they can eliminate those calories they would have if they responded to their hunger. They may try to "fill up" on calorie-free drinks or celery sticks. This may make them feel full temporarily, but doesn't answer the body's need for fuel. At this point, they are set up for overeating. People's lives are often so hectic that it becomes easy to ignore the hunger signals until they find themselves cramming in food.

People who never experience typical hunger signs will have to consciously tune in to their body regularly throughout the day, trying to recognize the changes they experience that denote their personal hunger signs. After eating, does the feeling go away? Some people never allow themselves to become hungry enough to let the hunger signs reveal themselves. Because they fear how out-of-control they can get when hungry, they avoid hunger by eating constantly.

What Is True Hunger?

Your body produces hunger signals for a reason. They are a message to tell you that your immediate fuel supplies are beginning to drop to levels that need refilling. Your body would appreciate your providing some food to bring the fuel supplies back up to normal. When your body requests nourishment, it is not only for its immediate needs but to ensure that some of that intake can be put away for later use.

If It Isn't Hunger, What Is It?

Many people confuse appetite with hunger. Appetite is the "desire for food," as opposed to hunger, which is the "physiological need for food."

Signs of Appetite

- Sight and smell of food
- Pleasure principal
- Parties and socializing
- The environment
- The clock
- Thirst
- Cravings
- Pleasant memories
- Coping and handling emotions

Our appetite for certain foods is often a matter of habits that have been formed over the years. They start in our youth and are continually added to over time. The content and quality of the food, its sensory factors, how it was served, who was serving it, the environment in which it was eaten, all helped develop our appetite for certain foods. The appetite center is found in the brain, where our conditioned reflexes are formed.

Think about the conditioned responses you have to certain foods. Sometimes the sight or smell of food can get you to eat when you're not hungry. It could be the sounds associated with the preparation of a meal—the clatter of dishes, the sizzle of oil, the whistling of a tea kettle. Sometimes a situation, like a party, can do it. Even the colors of the room, the position at the table where you normally eat, and the table settings play their part in your appetite. The clock can also play a part. It is amazing how many people eat when they are actually thirsty, when water or some other liquid would be more than sufficient. Whether cravings are physiologically induced or are merely mental creations, few cravings occur simultaneously with true hunger signals. Maybe the emotional impact of certain situations stimulates you to eat particular foods, or you eat certain foods that you know will make you feel better (calmer or more alert). In all cases, your personality comes into play by determining which stimuli will be the strongest and most influential for you.

Sights and Smells

ESTPs and ESFPs with their dominant Sensing preference, and ISTPs and ISFPs, with their backup Sensing preference, will be most attuned to the sight and smell of food as cues to their appetite. It's a here-and-now, external cue. The problems of following impulses and seeking immediate gratification are typical of _S_P types. This may make them even more influenced by the sensory stimulation of food.

Considering that nutrition is a necessary part of survival, it would be naïve to say that iNtuitives have no interest in the sight and smell of food. They just don't tend to spend as much attention or time on the sensory aspects of eating, unless they intentionally devote some energy to the process. When iNtuitives find themselves becoming obsessed with the sight and smell of food, they probably are experiencing something stressful in their lives. People who are under stress often use their least favorite preference. For the iNtuitive, that would be the Sensing preference.

Parties and Socializing

Extraverts will be especially vulnerable to the kinds of appetite stimuli associated with parties and social occasions. Studies have shown that people tend to eat more when they're with others. In fact, the amount they eat goes up according to the number of people in the group.

ESFJs and ENFJs, with their dominant Feeling preference (and the fact that they're Extraverts), and ISFJs and INFJs, with their backup Feeling preference, will find that their appetite is often stimulated by the people around them. My grandmother was a good cook and a fantastic baker. Because I'm an ENFJ, just knowing we were having dinner at Nana's house used to stimulate my appetite.

The Environment

Restaurants have done much research on color and how it influences appetite. That's why McDonald's color scheme is orange and yellow. It stimulates the appetite. Compare that to eating in a room decorated with greens or greys, which depress the appetite. (Those of you who want to lose weight or diminish food's hold on you might consider redecorating!) Be careful about the number of candlelight dinners you have. Candles, flowers, and soft music playing in the background can stimulate the appetite.

You may find that, after consistently sitting in the same place at the dinner table, switching positions will decrease your appetite. Having to reorient yourself, your attention is diverted from the food.

The Clock

People who plan to retire soon look forward to calling their time their own. Being able to set their own schedules, rather than being ruled by a clock, is freedom to them. Yet when they finally retire, they find themselves still *eating* by the clock rather than in response to their hunger level. "If it's noon, I should be eating lunch," they think, believing themselves hungry even though the physiological basis for hunger (low blood sugar and a high level of free fatty acids in the blood) is not present.

What they are feeling is the gastric secretion that has now been paired with certain times of the day. The Russian scientist Ivan Pavlov did an experiment that proved this. He fed a dog every thirty minutes. After conditioning had taken place, Pavlov removed one of the half-hour feedings. The dog still salivated at the half-hour even though no food was presented.

While we ourselves may be responsible for this pairing of time and eating (Judgers are very good at this because of their need for scheduling), our response is now conditioned. To eliminate a conditioned response, it's necessary to perform differently. To accomplish that, someone who always eats at noon should try eating at 11:00 A.M. one day and then at 1:00 P.M. the next day. Once the old pattern is broken, it will be easier to start focusing on hunger, not the clock.

Mistaking Hunger for Thirst

Your internal barometer for thirst is quite precise; your body knows when the fluid level in and out of your cells is not in balance. A dry mouth is accepted as a sign that we are thirsty (though, as we get older, the signs aren't as apparent) and yet many people respond by eating, rather than by drinking water or other fluids. Granted, most foods contain some amount of water, and eating does stimulate the salivary glands to moisten the mouth. However, the calories from that food are not needed or wanted by your body. It's important to learn to recognize whether you are truly hungry or merely thirsty.

Cravings

Where do cravings and food urges come from? One minute, you're thinking about something completely unrelated to food, and the next, you're completely overtaken by a strong need for chocolate, a doughnut, Chinese food, or whatever. Some people try to defend their cravings by saying that their body is crying out for certain nutrients. That's rarely the case. However, there is a large psychological and mentally derived component to cravings, often with an addictive quality.

The challenge is how we deal with cravings. Deriding ourselves for having cravings (a favorite pastime of many Feelers) gets us nowhere, since it won't remove them. We need to start recognizing the signs that an "attack" is approaching by using our Sensing preference. Does it start as a little pebble of a thought, slowly growing into a boulder, or is it like a roaring locomotive that seems to hit you right between the eyes? Once you start to recognize what to look for, you can come up with alternatives by putting your iNtuitive and Thinking preferences to work. You could go for a walk, read a book, or see a movie before the attack does its damage.

Your Emotions

How many times have you felt guilty about turning to food when you're upset, angry, bored, or even elated? Some foods seem to be the elixir for whatever bothers us or excites us. There's good reason for that. There are chemicals in foods that, once in the body, are converted to neurotransmitters that are mood enhancers. In the next chapter, I'll go into more detail about these neurotransmitters and the foods that enhance them. The point to be made here, though, is that because of our bodily reaction to certain foods, we become conditioned to those that give us a certain feeling. Chocolate, for some, is a remedy for stress, anxiety, depression, and anger. With its sensual mouthfeel, it is also the food of love. Cookies are always good as a reward or even a bribe. Hot chocolate and bread can be comforting. Meat can be energizing.

The guilt you feel when you turn to food for solace is actually telling you something; it means you sense that you have stepped over some kind of boundary of behavior you've set for yourself. If you don't handle it correctly, your self-esteem and inner strength can come into question. Feeling guilty can become quite destructive when you not only experience it while eating for emotional reasons, but then eat more to punish yourself for feeling that way. You have two options: (1) reset the boundary, or (2) reassess what's making you feel guilty and try to do something more constructive. What can you do that doesn't involve food?

It's hard to imagine a celebration without food. It's especially hard to imagine a birthday without cake. My dad used to say that it was bad luck if everyone didn't have a piece of cake on someone's birthday. As a little girl, I believed him. When I got older, I realized he just said that so he didn't have to feel guilty about having some himself. Of course at this point, he set up a conditioned response in all the members of my family. If you're celebrating, let there be cake!

It is clear from Oprah Winfrey's book, *Make the Connection,* that her personality was playing a large part in her weight problem. Her personal trainer, Bob Greene, pointed out to Oprah that she always seemed to be celebrating something, going out with her friends at least once a week. He wondered why she was eating foods she knew she shouldn't, and found out that she felt pressured to eat and drink with her friends. (Oprah's type is most likely ESFP.) The Extravert in her is energized by her friends (and audiences). The Feeling preference is what would make her want to please other people and, therefore, she goes along with the group. This same preference is the basis for her using food as a coping mechanism, something that has comforted her when problems seemed too big to handle.

It is very important for you to tune into your body's signals and learn to distinguish between true hunger and emotional hunger. If you're not hungry, try to find something else that will take care of your emotions—talking to a friend, exercising, reading a book, going shopping.

An important note: Just remember, we possess all the preferences in our type. Pointing out the aspects of the dominant or backup preferences doesn't mean that the less-favored preferences aren't involved. While a Sensor is strongly affected by sights and smells, an iNtuitive is still aware of external inputs. Even though it is typical for a Feeler to eat something because it was made by a significant other or friend, it doesn't mean a Thinker wouldn't eat it for the same reason.

It's Just a Matter of Making a Decision

If your body is telling you it's hungry by alerting you with true hunger signals, you don't have to go through any decision-making process to determine if you should eat. Your body needs food. The decision you need be making at this point is *what* to eat—an issue we'll tackle in the next chapter.

It's when you are confronted with all the circumstances we've just been discussing—your appetite, other people, the environment, the situation, your habits, and so on—that you have a major decision to make. Should you eat, whether it be a sample bite or a platefull? Wrapped up in the answer to that question is another question: How is eating going to help you reach the goals you set in the previous chapter? You must not lose track of where you're headed, and why.

When you have an eating decision to make, look at the following lists to decide whether it's hunger or appetite.

Signs of Hunger	Signs of Appetite
Stomach growls or grumbles	Sight and smell of food
Having an empty feeling	Pleasure principal
Stomach pain	Parties and socializing
Being light-headed or shaky	The environment
Being slightly irritable	The clock
Lack of energy	Thirst
Having difficulty concentrating	Cravings
Having a headache	Pleasant memories
Feeling slightly faint	Coping and handling emotions

Ideally, you should always begin by consulting your Sensing preference (the first step of the *Z* pattern) to determine if you're really hungry before making a decision to eat. Let your Sensing preference help you determine if you are hungry by listening to your "body talk." Remember, Sensing is the here-and-now preference and it's in the best position to tell you what your body needs. Keeping in mind what true hunger signs are for you, use the Hunger Gauge in Figure 22 to decide if and how hungry you

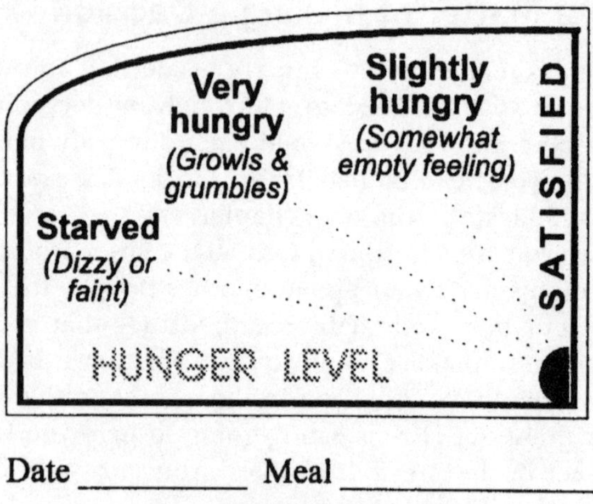

Date __________ Meal ______________

Figure 22. Hunger Gauge

are. Do you feel *satisfied,* with no hunger signs, or are you *slightly hungry,* with a somewhat empty feeling, *very hungry,* with stomach growls and grumbles, or *starved,* to the point of being dizzy or faint? By the way, if you're down to the *very hungry* or *starved* level, you've waited too long to consider eating, and there's now a greater likelihood that you will overeat.

If you decide to follow your 1–2–3–4 order instead of the *Z* pattern to decide whether to eat when you're not hungry, you will find the Hunger Decision Road Map (see Figure 23) helpful. Read about each preference's contribution to this decision-making process to make it easier for you to make the right decision—not to eat when you're not hungry.

It's often very tempting to come up with the decision you want (that is, to eat when you're not hungry), and then find information that appears to support your decision. But when you do that, you're only fooling and hurting yourself. However, if that is what you want to do, do it consciously, take responsibility for the results of your actions, and understand the effect your actions will have on your ability to reach your goal. No moaning later that, "I can't believe I ate that" or, "I'm going to be sorry tomorrow."

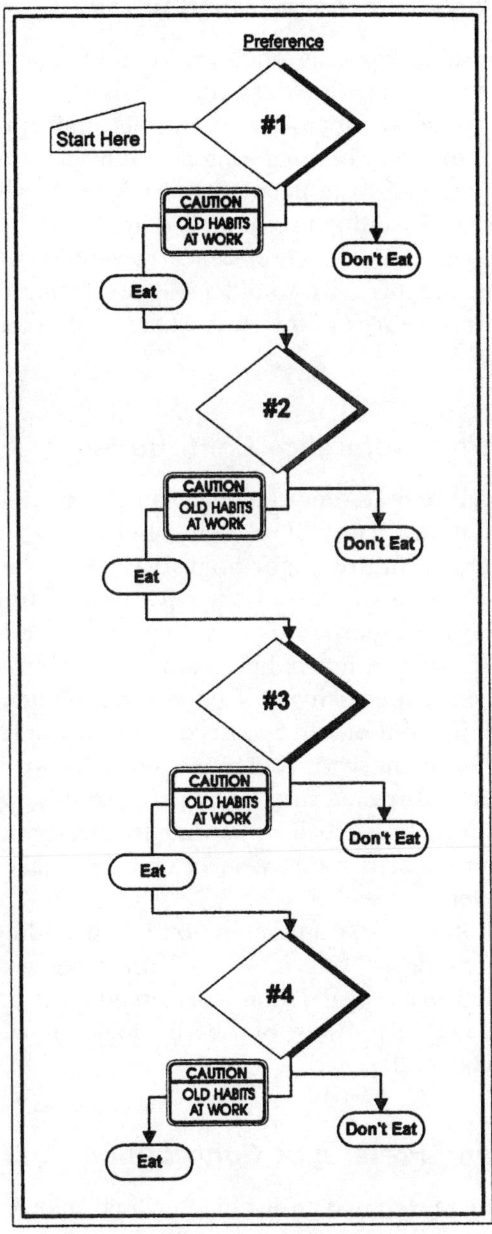

Figure 23. Hunger Decision Road Map

The Sensing Preference Contribution

If you're considering eating when you're not hungry, your Sensing preference can provide facts and details about the situation that may convince you not to eat. It can collect information about the situation that may be triggering an eating response, such as the environment and the people involved. It can also find out how many calories and grams of fat are in the food you want to eat so that your Thinking preference can evaluate the consequences of eating this food. Your Sensing preference can remember similar experiences to this one, what you did, and what the results were.

The iNtuiting Preference Contribution

Let your iNtuitive preference paint you a picture of where you're heading when you eat without being hungry. It sees the big picture, what the future might hold. It can see your *life vision* and possible obstacles in your way. With such insight, it can help you consider alternatives to eating. If you're looking for nurturing, consider a hot bubble bath or a dip in the jacuzzi, listening to music or talking to a good friend. Snuggle up with a good book in front of a fire or decorate your home with fresh flowers. If you're angry with someone, consider writing a letter to that person expressing your feelings (but don't mail it!). Play a game of tennis, racquetball, or bowling to release your tensions. If you are bored, start a new project or hobby, take a walk, or play with a pet.

Look at Table 8. Take a moment to fill it in, adding your own reasons for eating as well. Now you'll have some alternatives available when an eating decision is presented to you. This list will be especially helpful for those of you who do not have iNtuiting as your dominant preference.

The Thinking Preference Contribution

The Thinking preference involves impersonal analysis using generally accepted rules. One important rule is that you *eat only when your hunger level registers below Satisfied on the Hunger Gauge.* (See

TABLE 8. **Reasons (Excuses?) for Eating When You're Not Hungry**

Reasons for Eating When Not Hungry	What You Can Do Instead of Eating
SITUATIONAL REASONS	
Smell/sight of food	
To avoid doing something	
Food available	
Mealtime	
While cooking	
Others eating	
Social event	
Transition activity	
EMOTIONAL/MENTAL REASONS	
I'm bored	
I'm unhappy; lonely	
I'm upset; frustrated	
I'm happy	
Thought of food	
My reward	
To avoid hunger later	
PHYSIOLOGICAL REASONS	
I'm cold/hot	
I'm tired; I need a pick-me-up	
My mouth needs refreshing	
I'm thirsty	

Figure 22.) This rule is only logical, since the calories you eat when you are not hungry are not needed immediately and go into storage. If you have too much going into storage, you know what the results are: extra fat in all the wrong places.

If you're at the *satisfied* level, you should analyze the alternatives that your iNtuiting preference has come up with. What are the pros and cons of each? Can you use them in the situation that's presented itself? What if you don't eat?

Your Thinking preference is very valuable in keeping an eye on your appetite. As we discussed earlier, appetite is simply the "desire to eat"; it doesn't involve true hunger. Using your Thinking preference to analyze your appetite, go back through the section If It Isn't Hunger, What Is It? beginning on page 157, and review the reasons you eat when you're not hungry. Remember, this is a logical analysis that must be based on concrete facts and an understanding of the consequences. When I ask my clients to do this exercise, they quickly realize how often they've given themselves lame excuses without a logical basis, and usually have a good laugh over it.

The Feeling Preference Contribution

When Feeling is your dominant preference, you can all too often make a decision before all the information is in from the Sensing preference and before it's been analyzed by the Thinking preference. Without considering whether you're hungry, your decision to eat might be based on your personal value system, your wanting to maintain harmony, or your desire to make yourself feel good. You might eat because everyone else is eating or because someone cooked or offered you something. Or you might eat because you feel you deserve it, you're feeling unhappy, or you're rewarding yourself.

It's so important that those of you who have a dominant or backup Feeling preference *not* make a decision until all the other preferences have been consulted. Then your Feeling preference can put its stamp of approval on the decision, ensuring that you'll have no regrets later about your actions.

Record Keeping

The Hunger Gauge in Figure 22 can be a valuable tool for keeping track of whether or not you're eating only when you're hungry. Consider making copies of the gauge so you can have them with you whenever there's an eating opportunity. Mark on the gauge where you believe your hunger is before you start to eat. You'll find that reviewing the gauges is helpful in determining how often you're eating when you are not truly hungry.

Judgers probably won't have much of a struggle with this because it's an organized and structured process. For Perceivers, on the other hand, it could be a problem. If you're a Perceiver, see if you can do this exercise for a little while, even if not on a regular basis. Just trying it will be very helpful. Maybe you can turn to your Thinking preference to give you a hand. At the very least, try to have the gauge with you so that you can be thinking about the process.

Questions to Consider for the Hunger Decision Road Map

If you have taken a hunger reading and you are hungry, by all means eat. However, if you aren't hungry and you're thinking about eating, then it's time to use the Hunger Decision Road Map in Figure 23. But first, have a look at the list of questions in Table 9. They should help you consider many aspects of the situation so that you don't fall into your usual trap of eating when you're not hungry. Do your answers lead you along the path to "Don't Eat" or "Eat"? Keep in mind that the objective is to keep you from eating when you're not hungry so that you can attain your *life vision.*

Let me give you an example of how to use the Hunger Decision Road Map in Figure 23. David, who is an ISTP, is thumbing through the newspaper and finds a coupon for 50 percent off an entrée at a new restaurant he's been wanting to try. Unfortunately, he's had a big lunch and an afternoon snack before finding the coupon. So he's not the least bit hungry. Yet the coupon is only good for today. What decision will he make?

TABLE 9. **Hunger Decision Questions**

Preference	Questions to Consider
Sensing	• Am I hungry? Are my eyes bigger than my stomach? • Is it the sight and smell of the food that is getting to me? • What happened the last time I was in this situation? • How many calories and grams of fat do I think this contains? • Who else is eating? • What is happening at the moment?
iNtuiting	• If I eat now, am I going to be full for the next meal? • Is eating now going to help me reach my *life vision?* • Are there other alternatives to eating? • Am I using food for other reasons than nutrition? • Am I eating now to avoid being hungry later? What other planning could I do?
Thinking	• Is this my appetite showing? • What are the pros and cons of eating when not hungry? • Will this treat fit into my daily calorie and fat allowance? • Isn't eating when my hunger level registers *satisfied* against the rules? • Am I eating this because it's free? • Is it logical to eat when I'm not hungry?
Feeling	• Am I eating just because "I want it"? • Am I using food as a reward? • Am I eating because others are eating? • Am I eating because someone gave it to me and I don't want to hurt his feelings? • Am I eating because I'm bored, unhappy, angry, or avoiding something? • Don't I care enough about myself to realize what I am doing to myself? • Am I eating this because I don't know how to say "no"?

David's #1 preference is Thinking. Looking at the Thinking questions, these are his thoughts:

- "I know that eating another meal out today is only going to sabotage my efforts to lose weight. Also, the rule says to eat only if I'm hungry. But, the restaurant is offering a 50 percent discount. That gives me the opportunity to try it at quite a good deal. Think of how much money I can save."—*Decision:* Eat.

Because David's decision is to eat, he must continue to his next preference to see if it can help him out. (Remember, the purpose of the Road Map is to keep prompting you to question your reasons for eating when you're not hungry. Some preference in your personality will be able to give you grounds for making the healthy decision. You just have to keep probing until you find it.) His #2 preference is Sensing. These are his thoughts using his Sensing preference:

- "The coupon is only good for tonight. I remember the last time I wanted to try a new restaurant and missed out on the opportunity."—*Decision:* Eat.

It seems that David's old habits are kicking in. He's using his preferences in his habitual way. At this point, he is willing to eat at the restaurant even though he isn't hungry. Let's see if his #3 preference, iNtuiting, can save him:

- "Leaving aside the fact that the dinner will be cheaper tonight, I can eat at that restaurant any time. Besides, I have this image of a slim me that isn't going to happen if I keep coming up with reasons to eat when I'm not hungry. Maybe I could go by the restaurant and pick up a menu to see what they have. Then I could plan ahead what I should eat during the day to allow for the extra calories and fat."—*Decision:* Don't eat.

Now David has a reason *not to eat* that makes sense to him. He should have no regrets, and he can feel good about himself because he allowed his personality to work for him, not against him.

Susie, an ESFP, admits that her biggest downfall is walking past a bakery, hungry or not. The sweet buttery smell of the croissants and cookies drifting out of the store is extremely tantalizing. She looks in the window to see trays of danishes, loaves of crusty bread, elegant dark-chocolate cakes, and mounds of cookies.

- Allowing her #1 preference, Sensing, a chance at the Hunger Decision Road Map, turns out to be a problem. It's so captivated by smells and sights, that the choice is quickly made.—*Decision:* Eat.

Time for Susie to pass the decision baton on to her #2 preference, Feeling. Her first inclination is to say that she should have something as a reward for having lost ten pounds. On further consideration, however, she realizes she's just trying to rationalize her old bakery habit.

- Wanting to feel good about herself and her weight-loss success, and anxious to maintain that loss, she vows to look to rewards that come in shapes other than food. What about getting a new dress or going to a show? she thinks.—*Decision:* Don't eat.

You can use your own preferences in different ways—ways that can sabotage your healthy good intentions or promote them. Never forget where you're headed and why you want to improve your habits.

8

Making It a Habit #3: Eat Smart (And Still Get Your Favorite Foods)

Are you wondering how you can eat smart and still have your favorites? You're probably saying to yourself, "She should only know what my favorites are. They wouldn't fit into *any* diet." As far as I'm concerned, there are no "bad" foods, only bad diets. A cheeseburger, a pizza, or a steak, for example, are not bad foods. They are all good sources of protein, albeit high in fat. The cheese on the cheeseburger and the pizza is a good source of calcium. The tomato sauce on the pizza provides a cancer-preventing compound. The hamburger bun and pizza crust are made of complex carbohydrates. However, pizza for breakfast, a cheeseburger for lunch and a steak for dinner makes for a bad diet. So repeat after me: "There are no bad foods, just bad diets." All foods should be legal unless you have a specific health problem that dictates what you can and cannot have.

Note that when I use the word *diet* I mean what you eat each day. If I mean what to eat to lose weight, I will say *weight-loss diet.* To most people, a "diet" means sacrificing, using willpower, or feeling guilty when overstepping the boundaries of self-imposed or external restrictions. Since the purpose of this book is to change your lifestyle habits in a way that is personally agreeable, suffering "on a diet" is not part of the approach.

Just think about it: If you never have to deprive yourself of something, you never have to use willpower to avoid it. If you never have to crave something because you can always eat it, then you never have to overindulge for fear of never eating it again. If you never feel guilty about eating something, then you never have to "sneak" it or feel the need to punish yourself afterwards.

You can be at peace with food. However, in exchange for this peace, you have to be willing to understand and incorporate into your daily life the reason for eating: to promote a healthy life. First and foremost, food is nutrition for your body. Its purpose is to provide the energy and nutrients necessary for you to live. With such an abundance and variety of food available, there is no reason that you can't find foods that you enjoy *and* are good for you.

How Much Do You Already Know?

Eating should not be like a game of craps, in which you hope the dice will roll your way. You are in control of what you put into your body. If you know the benefits and drawbacks of the foods you choose, you'll be eating smart.

To find out what you need to learn, let's see what you already know. Select only one answer for each question.

1. Which has more fat?
   a. McDonald's Big Mac
   b. KFC Extra Crispy Thigh

2. About how many teaspoons of sugar (or equivalent) are there in a 12-ounce can of cola?
   a. 5
   b. 7
   c. 10
   d. 13

3. Which of these fruit juices is a good source of vitamin C (assuming no vitamin C has been added)?
   a. Grape
   b. Apple
   c. Prune
   d. Pineapple

4. Which of these has the most fiber per serving?
   a. Cooked oatmeal
   b. Lentils
   c. Corn
   d. Dried prunes
5. Which of these is lowest in the antioxidant beta-carotene?
   a. Zucchini
   b. Broccoli
   c. Kale
   d. Winter squash
6. Which of these meats has the least amount of fat?
   a. Extra lean ground beef
   b. Ground turkey breast
   c. Ground turkey
   d. Ground chicken
7. The *Nutrition Facts* label on a package of food shows the percent Daily Value for fat is 25 percent. That number tells you the percentage of fat in a serving of the food.
   a. True
   b. False
8. Which of these vegetables is not a source of calcium?
   a. Kale
   b. Broccoli
   c. Green beans
   d. Collards
9. Brown rice is higher in fiber than white rice.
   a. True
   b. False
10. Which is *not* the best source of the antioxidant vitamin E?
    a. Wheat germ
    b. Nuts
    c. Vegetable oils
    d. Green leafy vegetables
11. Butter has more calories than margarine.
    a. True
    b. False

12. Corn oil has fewer grams of the healthy monounsaturated fat than olive oil.
    a. True
    b. False

13. What is the recommended serving size for meat?
    a. 8 ounces
    b. 6 ounces
    c. 5 ounces
    d. 3 ounces

14. Skinless chicken has no cholesterol.
    a. True
    b. False

15. Which food has the highest amount of sodium per serving?
    a. Canned tomato soup
    b. A beef frankfurter
    c. Cottage cheese
    d. One-fourth of a medium pizza with sausage topping

16. Skim milk has more calcium than whole milk.
    a. True
    b. False

17. Which food has the highest amount of cholesterol?
    a. 3 ounces shrimp
    b. 1 tablespoon butter
    c. 3 ounces porterhouse steak
    d. 3 ounces beef liver

18. What is the minimum number of servings of vegetables you should have per day?
    a. One
    b. Two
    c. Three
    d. Five

You'll find the correct answers at the end of the chapter. So how did you do? Don't be too concerned if your score wasn't as high as you would like. By the time you reach the end of this chapter, you'll be able to answer each question easily.

Misconceptions

It is amazing how many preconceived notions and misconceptions people have about food. As the number of these goes up, the enjoyment of eating goes down. Do any of these sound like something you've said or thought about before?

- Bread is fattening.
- Sweets are bad for you.
- There are good foods and there are bad foods.
- The only way to lose weight is not to eat any fat.
- You shouldn't eat before you go to bed.
- There's no room in a healthy diet for junk food.
- Healthy food doesn't taste good.
- Most snack foods have too many calories.

The Nutrition Facts

The Building Blocks

If you were to build a house, what supplies would you require? Concrete for the foundation, wood for the structure, plenty of nails, and so on. What if, instead of building a house, you were building your body? What would you require? First, you would need **proteins** to make almost everything structural in you: muscles, cells, tissues, hair, nails, glands, enzymes, and hormones. Then you would need **carbohydrates** (sugars) for energy, the basic fuel on which your brain, central nervous system, red blood cells, and muscles rely. Even though **fat** in the body has a bad reputation (especially when it's around your hips and thighs!), you still need a certain amount of it to insulate you from the environment, provide shock absorption for your organs, build membrane structures, transport fat-soluble vitamins, and provide energy. We can't forget to include **water** since it accounts for about half the average adult's weight. The more muscle mass you have and the less fat, the greater proportion of your weight is water. Water is found everywhere in your body from your muscles to your bloodstream. It serves as cushioning for your organs and joints, helps regulate your body temperature, affects your blood pressure, and influences energy metabolism. Lastly, you'd have to include many **vitamins** and **minerals** to be a part of your structure and orchestrate the many chemical reactions that occur throughout your body.

Your body is constantly in flux, with cells being made and cells dying, bone being made and bone being reabsorbed, proteins being made and proteins being destroyed. There has to be a constant supply of fresh materials with which your body can continue to build and maintain itself. What your body can't *make,* it must *take* from the food you eat. That's where your diet comes in. Anything that passes your lips is influencing how well your body can perform its job. Therefore, your choices and decisions about what you eat are very important. So let's take a closer look at what's in the food you eat.

Protein

Amino acids are the building blocks of protein. Of the 20 kinds of amino acids, your body can make 11. That means you must get the other nine from your food, making them *essential amino acids.* If you did not supply these essential amino acids, your body would have to break down its own protein to obtain them.

Protein Quality

A protein is considered *complete* when it contains all the essential amino acids in about the proportions the body requires. Meat, fish, poultry, cheese, eggs, and milk are examples of foods that contain complete proteins. Some proteins—most notably plant proteins, such as grains, dried beans, seeds, nuts, and vegetables—may not contain all the essential amino acids or may have some in limited amounts, making them *incomplete* proteins. The exception to this is soy protein.

When you eat a variety of plant and animal foods, essential amino acids missing in some foods will be made up for in other foods. Then your body will have all the ingredients for making complete proteins. Even vegetarians who eat no meat can get enough protein in their diet.

While your body seems to be largely protein, your diet need contain only 10 to 15 percent of its calories from protein to provide a sufficient amount. Many proteins in the body are recycled. For example, the cells sloughed off from the lining of the intestine are reabsorbed into the body and used for protein.

Side Effects of Too Much Protein

The body does not store excess protein. Therefore, eating a diet that is too high in protein forces your body to get rid of any excess. It does so by breaking the protein down into a nitrogenous waste product and carbohydrate. The waste product is excreted in the urine, which can put a burden on your kidneys. Excess dietary protein may also promote the loss of calcium in the urine. This can increase your risk for osteoporosis (weakening of the bone).

The carbohydrate is recycled and used for energy. Consider that a pound of meat (a good source of protein) is much more expensive than a pound of grain (a good source of carbohydrate). Therefore, eating an excess amount of protein that ends up being used for its carbohydrate content is hard on the pocketbook as well as taxing to the kidneys. Also, protein-rich foods tend to be high in fat. For all these reasons, your objective should be to eat only the amount of protein your body will use for protein purposes.

Don't take amino acid supplements in the hope of building bigger muscles. Muscles get larger by being used. Unless you are a professional athlete, a normal diet should provide you with all the protein you need. The body uses proteins in certain proportions. Just because you provide an abundance of one particular amino acid doesn't mean the body will use it completely. The body must maintain the correct proportions and will dump any excess. It makes more sense to let your body do what it knows how to do best. Give it a balance of proteins, in moderate amounts, and allow it to take what it needs.

Mood Food

Protein isn't just for structural purposes. It is also the precursor of chemicals called *neurotransmitters* that send messages and information between cells. A couple of these, dopamine and norepinephrine, are considered the "alertness chemicals." When there is enough of these in your brain, you can think and react more quickly, your attention span is better, and your motivation to do things is greater.

Are there times during the day when you seem to have a lull, when your brain seems to be asleep? If that's the case, you need to look at the meal you had before this feeling overcame you. If you're finding that you are dragging around 10:00 in the morning, consider whether breakfast was too heavy on the carbohydrates (cereal, fruit, toast and jam, sugar in your coffee). If so, try eating some of your daily protein allowance for breakfast (a turkey sandwich, an egg) and save your carbohydrates for the evening, when you might appreciate calming down. Note that for the protein to have its fullest effect, the meal needs to be low-fat. Fat slows down the absorption of protein so it takes too long to get to your brain and create the appropriate neurotransmitters.

Protein Choices

Check Appendixes A and B at the end of this book for a listing of protein sources organized according to fat content. Circle the choices that you enjoy eating. As you look over the list, you'll find lower-fat alternatives to what you might normally eat. For example, if you love prime rib roast, you might decide to try a porterhouse steak, which has less fat.

Protein Tips

- When most of your protein is coming from high-fat meat sources, it is easy to get too much fat in your diet. Be sure to check out the lists in the appendixes for lower fat sources.
- While cooking meat with the fat on it keeps it from drying out, you should be sure to trim the excess fat before eating it.
- Consider meat not as the main event, but as a side show.
- Select a beef grade labeled USDA Select for cuts that are lower in fat and calories than choice or prime grades.

- Stir-fries and casseroles are good ways to decrease the amount of meat you eat without feeling you're being deprived. Just add more vegetables or starch, and you'll never miss the meat.
- Chill stews and soups to remove the fat that will harden on the surface.
- Legumes and dried beans are a good source of protein. A serving has about the same amount of protein as one ounce of meat.
- When making a hamburger, cook it thoroughly throughout, with no blood showing, to guarantee you have eliminated any potentially harmful *e.coli* bacteria. You can cook steaks rare, but be sure the outer surfaces, where bacteria can lurk, have been well cooked.
- To remove as much fat as possible from your hamburger, first brown the meat in a frying pan. Then transfer it with a slotted spoon to a plate lined with several sheets of paper toweling. Pat off as much fat as possible. Transfer the meat to a colander and rinse with hot water. Allow to drain. Then stir into your dish and reheat.
- Consider buying your meat in three- to four-ounce serving-size portions.
- When purchasing ground turkey or ground chicken for making burgers, chili, or meatloaf, make sure it is breast meat, which has even less fat than extra lean ground beef.
- Use stronger-flavored cheeses so that you can use less and thereby eat less fat.
- Try boiled shrimp in place of breaded and fried shrimp.
- When you're trying to decide whether to eat a chicken breast with or without skin, keep in mind that a 3-ounce serving of roasted chicken breast with the skin on has 8 grams of fat, while the same roasted chicken breast without the skin has only 4 grams.

Carbohydrates

Carbohydrates should provide the bulk of the calories in your diet—from 55 to 60 percent—with most of that amount coming from the complex carbohydrates found in grains, dried beans, and vegetables—not from simple carbohydrates, which is another word for sugar. The average American is not eating enough complex carbohydrates. How about you? The *Healthy Eating Index* survey conducted by the Department of Agriculture in 1995 found that fewer than one in five people was getting the recommended number of servings of grains, fruits, and vegetables every day.

Getting Enough Carbohydrates

One complaint often made is that it takes too much time and is a nuisance to wash, trim, and cut up vegetables. But now you can go into the produce section of your supermarket and find everything from baby carrots to cut-up broccoli and cauliflower, to salad-makings already prepared. Fruits come naturally packaged in one-serving portions. So "inconvenience" is no excuse.

Many people aren't sure what counts as a serving and so may underestimate their intake. Serving sizes aren't as large as you think. People sitting down to a plate of spaghetti don't realize that one serving is only one-half cup of pasta. When was the last time you had only one-half cup of spaghetti? Similarly, a whole bagel is considered two servings. You may actually be doing better than you think.

Grains, fruits, and vegetables can be very filling. If you tried increasing your intake of these foods, you'd probably find that you were eating a lower-fat diet overall and were very satisfied. Carbohydrates contain only 4 calories per gram, as compared to fat, which has 9 calories per gram. Just think how much more bread, bagels, rice, cereal, carrots, celery, apples, berries, and bananas, you can eat for the same number of calories as an ice cream sundae!

Simple Carbohydrates

Part of the problem with our typical diet is that it contains far too many simple carbohydrates, most notably sugar. However, most people don't even realize how much sugar they're eating since it goes by many aliases—sucrose, dextrose, glucose, fructose, levulose, invert sugar, high-fructose corn syrup, maltose, molasses, fruit juice concentrate, corn sweetener, and honey.

It seems that our preference for sweet things starts as early as the day we're born. Newborns prefer sugared water to plain water. Even cultures that don't normally have sugar available to them (for example, the Inuit of northern Alaska) easily adapt to and enjoy sweet foods when introduced to them. Scientists have therefore concluded that there is a genetic component to the desire for sugar. Yet they have also found a strong environmental influence. If your parents ate cake for dessert every night, you'll probably do the same. If you were given cookies as a reward, you'll probably continue to want cookies when you've been "good." We also look to sugar to give us that quick pick-me-up. It may do that, but because of the reaction in the body, it produces as quick a roller-coaster ride down.

Considering the genetic and environmental components, it would be foolish for you to try to avoid sweets altogether. Talk about grounds for a binge! What you need to do is learn how to make sweets something special and not a major part of your diet. Less than 10 percent of your daily caloric intake should be from simple carbohydrates, since they supply little more than calories and contribute both to tooth decay and to rapid blood sugar swings. Consider having a piece of fruit—or even dried fruit, which is sweeter—when you have a sweet-tooth attack. Even though fruit is also considered a simple carbohydrate, it gives you vitamins, minerals, fiber, and other beneficial elements you don't get from table sugar.

Complex Carbohydrates—the Staff of Life

It's the complex carbohydrates that are so beneficial to your health. They are called "complex" because they have a bunch of sugar molecules hooked together, somewhat like the branches of a tree. These are the starches found in grains (wheat, rice, oats, barley, corn, millet, rye), legumes (dried beans), potatoes, and vegetables. They have a wealth of vitamins, minerals, fiber, energy, antioxidants and phytochemicals—compounds that have recently been strutting their stuff in the news. Depending upon the foods you choose, complex carbohydrates can be very low-fat sources of energy.

Mood Food

These are the comfort foods—and for good reason. First of all, the smell of fresh bread baking has always meant nurturing, love, and a friendly environment. I'm sure you Feelers can relate, since you're often the givers of comfort.

Second, and more important, the carbohydrates in these foods help trigger neurotransmitters in your brain to make *serotonin,* the calming chemical. Depending upon what time you eat a generous helping of carbohydrates, you could find yourself dozing when you need to be alert. A breakfast of basically carbohydrate foods may not be the best thing to eat when you have a midmorning meeting to attend. A pasta lunch may come back to haunt you some time around 2:00 in the afternoon, when you have a project to get done. On the other hand, after a hard day at work, a little calming down doesn't hurt, and what better way than with carbohydrates (better than a drink). This would be a good time for that pasta meal. It doesn't take much carbohydrate to stimulate serotonin. However, if your carbohydrate source is loaded with fat, you're going to slow down the absorption of the carbohydrate as well as its mood-enhancing capabilities.

Your Mother Was Right—You Should Eat Your Vegetables

Make your mother feel good and tell her she was right. Vegetables are nature's wonderful arsenal against diseases, and phytochemicals are fast becoming our number-one weapon. While the term *phytochemical* sounds terribly complicated, it simply means chemicals that are found in plants (*phyto*). All vegetables, fruits, and grains contain phytochemicals. A hamburger with onions, tomatoes, and lettuce on a whole-grain bun, along with a cup of coffee or tea and a piece of fruit, is a phytochemical smorgasbord. Make that a soybean hamburger, and you've just increased the number of phytochemicals working for you.

The antioxidants—beta-carotene and vitamins E and C—are just one form of the phytochemicals that protect the body from free radicals (those molecules I told you about in Chapter 3, Killer Habits, that can be very destructive to cell structures). Then there is the army of chemicals that go by such names as *indoles, coumarins, sulforaphane, genistein, saponin, isothiniocyanates,* and *lycopene.* Scientists believe these compounds can do many things: (1) help prevent or lower your risk for heart disease by reducing blood cholesterol levels; unclog arteries and protect them from damage; (2) reduce the risk of cancer by preventing cancer cells from forming or, once formed, from moving on to their next stage of development; (3) boost your immunity to block infectious diseases; and (4) best of all, possibly even age-proof your body.

It's interesting to look at various ethnic groups to see the effects phytochemicals are having. It's thought that the phytochemicals found in wine may be involved in the so-called French paradox whereby, despite a relatively high-fat diet, the French don't seem to experience the high rate of heart disease that Americans do. Then there are Asian females, who experience much less breast cancer than American women because of their low-fat, high-soybean based diet. Mexicans rely heavily on hot peppers, which contain *capsaicin*, a phytochemical that appears to be heart-healthy by helping to reduce cholesterol in the blood. People from India use a great deal of curry powder in their cooking. It contains the phytochemical *curcumin*, found in turmeric (one of the spices that make up curry), which appears to help prevent cancer.

As better and better ways of detecting phytochemicals are discovered, the list of phytochemicals continues to grow. With tens of thousands of phytochemicals available in nature's bountiful food supply, it may be some time before the scientific community has analyzed, categorized, and determined how they all function. Yet we don't need to wait until then to reap the benefits. Just eat your vegetables, fruits and grains, and let your body do the rest. Keep in mind that scientists are beginning to believe that the power of phytochemicals rests in their interaction with each other within the whole food. So don't look to supplements to do the job in order to avoid eating your vegetables.

Phytochemical star performers: Broccoli, brussels sprouts, cabbage, cauliflower, carrots, citrus fruits, dark green leafy vegetables, garlic, kale, onions, peppers, soybeans, squash, tea, tomatoes, whole grain foods, yams, and yellow and orange fruits and vegetables

Not only do these foods provide phytochemicals, they also are packed with vitamins and minerals.

Have You Had Your Roughage Today?

Compare eating an apple with drinking a 6-ounce glass of apple juice. They both contain about 80 calories and are almost 100 percent carbohydrates. But the whole apple gives you about 3 grams of fiber toward a recommended 25–30 grams per day. When apples are processed into apple juice, the fiber is removed. In addition, the apple takes longer to eat and gives you more mouth satisfaction. You feel as if you've really had something to eat, while the juice is gone in several swallows. (Of course, if you're simply trying to quench your thirst, fruit juice is better than soda.) The fiber in the apple slows down the absorption rate of the sugar in the apple. It acts like a time-release mechanism to help maintain a fairly consistent blood sugar level. This means you will not get hungry again as quickly.

There are so many fruits and vegetables to choose from that could help you achieve the daily goal of 25–30 grams. (The average American eats only about 11 grams of fiber per day.) The important thing to know is that there are two types of fiber, soluble and insoluble, that can work wonders for you. Soluble fiber is so named because, with water, it forms a gel. This gel helps trap cholesterol and carcinogens in the intestine so they can be flushed out of the system without being absorbed. It also causes the stomach to empty more slowly, helping you to feel full longer and not overeat. It promotes a slower absorption of sugars. Soluble fiber can be found in fruits, vegetables, legumes (dried beans), and oats.

Insoluble fibers are just as beneficial as the soluble fibers. Because our bodies can't digest these fibers, they pass quickly through the intestines. As they go, they act like brooms, sweeping out carcinogens along the way. The faster these carcinogens are excreted, the less risk there is of their causing colon cancer. Also, insoluble fiber increases fecal bulk, making the walls of the intestine work harder. (It's almost like weight-lifting for the intestinal muscles.) As people get older, constipation can become a problem. The bowel gets lazy without much work to do, with the result that digestive disorders can develop. That's why it is even more important as we get older to be sure we get enough fiber. Don't forget to drink plenty of fluid—at least eight cups a day. The fiber will absorb water in the intestine. If you don't provide enough fluid, you're bound to get bound up! Insoluble fiber is in many of the same foods as soluble fiber (vegetables, legumes, and fruits), but the best sources are whole-grain products.

As long as you eat a variety of foods and achieve the recommended 25–30 grams of fiber per day, you'll have no problem getting enough of both the soluble and insoluble fibers. If you have been eating a very low-fiber diet, you might want to gradually increase the amount of fiber-rich foods you include so as to prevent flatulence and bloating. It sometimes takes the body a little while to adjust to fiber. If you follow the Food Guide Pyramid recommendations found toward the end of this chapter, you shouldn't have any problems.

By the way, fiber is found only in plant sources. (See Table 10.) Even though you may eat a piece of meat that is quite tough, it isn't dietary fiber that you're having difficulty chewing, just a poor cut of meat.

Label Watching

	% Daily Value*
Total Fat 8g	**13%**
Saturated Fat 3g	**17%**
Cholesterol 130mg	**44%**
Sodium 1010mg	**42%**
Total Carbohydrate 22g	**7%**
Dietary Fiber 9g	**36%**
Sugars 4g	
Protein 25g	

The Food and Drug Administration requires that food manufacturers include three carbohydrate values on the label: *Total Carbohydrate, Dietary Fiber,* and *Sugars.* You might notice that adding the grams of *Dietary Fiber* and *Sugars* doesn't equal the grams of *Total Carbohydrate.* What's missing are the grams of complex carbohydrates. If you add the grams of *Dietary Fiber* and *Sugars* and then subtract that value from that for *Total Carbohydrate,* you'll find out how many gramsof complex carbohydrates you're eating.

Check Appendix C for a list of carbohydrate sources organized according to fat content. Circle the choices you enjoy eating.

Carbohydrate Tips

- To increase the amount of vegetables you eat, try adding more vegetables than are called for in the recipe and removing some of the meat in such dishes as stir-fry, casseroles, and soups.

TABLE 10. **Dietary Fiber Star Performers**

Food	Quantity	Grams of Fiber
Kidney beans	½ cup	7 grams
Lentils	½ cup	5 grams
Raisin Bran cereal	1 cup	5 grams
Oatmeal cereal	1 cup	4 grams
Prunes	3	3 grams
Apple or orange	1 medium	3 grams
Green peas	½ cup	3 grams
Corn	½ cup	3 grams
Banana or pear	1 medium	2 grams
Carrot	1 medium	2 grams
Popcorn	3 cups	2 grams
Whole wheat bread	1 slice	2 grams
Granola bar	1 bar	1 gram

- Try sprinkling some bran or wheat germ on your cereal, or using them as a topping for a casserole.
- Be adventurous, and try some new types of grains: amaranth, bulghur, couscous, quinoa.
- Check out the produce department. Many vegetables are available already cut up, cleaned, and ready to eat.
- The darker the color of the vegetable or fruit, the more nutritious it usually is. For example, romaine lettuce has more nutrition than iceberg lettuce. Dark-orange vegetables like carrots and yams have a good deal of vitamin A (beta-carotene). Dark-green vegetables, such as broccoli and spinach, are a good source of vitamins A (beta-carotene) and C, calcium, and iron.
- Try adding an assortment of vegetables to your sandwiches besides the usual tomato and lettuce. Sliced carrots, sprouts, zucchini, and bell peppers can give your sandwich pizzazz.
- To increase your fiber intake, add legumes like beans, lentils, and peas to soups and casseroles and use other legumes like garbanzo beans, kidney beans, peas in dips and salads; buy whole-grain breads and crackers (look at the label for the whole grain to be listed first); eat whole-grain cereals like

shredded wheat, bran, and oatmeal (corn flakes and many specialty cereals are not whole grain).

- Tofu is a healthy soy product. Try incorporating it in dips, soups, casseroles, and salads.
- Think "color" when you plan your meal, mixing oranges, greens, and yellows for a more nutrient-dense meal.
- To eat more fruit, add some to cereal, muffins, and pancakes at breakfast. At lunch, try a peanut butter and banana sandwich or just pack a whole fruit in your lunch bag. At dinner, consider adding pineapple to coleslaw, apples to pork, apricots to chicken. Raisins make a great portable snack.
- Top your potatoes with steamed vegetables, a sprinkling of grated parmesan cheese, and a squeeze of lemon juice.
- Eat a variety of grains, vegetables, and fruits. It makes your meals more interesting, and you'll also be getting a variety of nutrients.
- For more fiber, select whole fruits instead of juice.
- Use applesauce or prune puree as a fat replacement in some baked goods.
- Carbohydrates such as bread and potatoes are not fattening. It's what you put on them that makes the difference.
- Try whole wheat toast with jam instead of a fruit-filled Danish pastry.

Fat

The American Heart Association, the American Dietetic Association, and the American Diabetes Association all recommend that less than 30 percent of our total daily calories come from fat, because diets with more than that increase our risk for heart disease, cancer, and diabetes. The percentage figure refers to the total diet, not to individual foods. A high-fat food can be averaged out with a low-fat food. Trying to eat only foods with less than 30 percent fat would mean absolutely no oil, shortening, and margarine, since they are all 100 percent fat.

Fat Phobia

Do you suffer from "fat phobia"? Because of everything we hear and read, many of us have become afraid of fat and are turning to fat-free products with a passion, figuring that fat-free products must be good. "It says 'free,' doesn't it?" they say. "That means I can have an unlimited amount." Not really. Next time you have a fat-free product, look at the label. Take note of the calories. They can be as high as the regular-fat version of the food, and many of those calories come from the sugar that's been added to give the product flavor.

Don't be afraid of fat. You do need some in your diet, and besides, fat gives food flavor. However, you have to keep in mind that one gram of fat contains nine calories, whereas one gram of carbohydrate or protein contains four calories. Fat is like a double-edged sword. Not only does it contain more calories, it can be digested, absorbed, and metabolized using fewer calories than are needed to do the same with protein and carbohydrates.

Interestingly, many of my clients who learned to wean themselves off the great amount of fat they used to eat have found that fat has actually lost its appeal. It's just too greasy for them now. As hard as it might be to imagine, the mouthfeel and the lingering flavor from the fat are no longer pleasurable to them.

The average American is getting 34 percent of his or her calories from fat. While this overall figure is not very far off the ideal percentage per day—30 percent—it's the *type* of fat we are choosing to eat that is the problem.

Saturated Fat

The three types of fat in the foods we eat range from healthy monounsaturates to unhealthy saturated fats. Most saturated fats come from animal products such as meat, butter, cheese, and milk. They're also found in tropical oils, such as coconut oil and palm oil. An easy measure of how highly a fat is saturated is whether it is solid at room temperature. Compare a cube of butter and a cup of olive oil; the butter is definitely more highly saturated.

Remember, even though saturated fats are not the healthiest of the fats, it doesn't mean you can't have some in your diet. You simply have to budget how you will spend your saturated fat "allowance." Studies have shown that people tend to eat less saturated fat for breakfast and snacks than for dinner. Therefore, dinner may be the meal you need to keep an eye on.

Polyunsaturated Fat

You'll find polyunsaturated fat in vegetable oils such as corn oil and safflower oil. What distinguishes polyunsaturated fat from saturated fat is that it is liquid at room temperature. Too much of it in the diet raises the level of both the bad LDL cholesterol and the good HDL cholesterol. The amount of HDL may not be enough to cancel out the amount of LDL, but it is definitely better than eating too much saturated fat. On the downside, however, too much polyunsaturated fat can increase one's risk for cancer. All fat should be eaten in moderation.

Polyunsaturated Fat's Shining Star

There is one particular type of polyunsaturated fat you should definitely seek out—omega-3 fatty acids, which are found in fatty, cold-water fish such as salmon, tuna, and sardines, and to a lesser extent in canola and soybean oils. This polyunsaturated fat is protective against the inflammation from arthritis and the blood clotting associated with heart disease and stroke. One of the problems in heart disease is atherosclerosis, a hardening and narrowing of the arteries. If a blood clot gets stuck in this narrowed passage, it can block blood flow, causing a heart attack or a stroke. Eating fish twice a week and/or cooking with canola or soybean oil can help avoid this problem by keeping the blood thinner and less sticky.

Monounsaturated Fat—Another Shining Star

Good sources of monounsaturated fat are olive oil and canola oil. Monounsaturated fat raises the good HDL cholesterol without raising the LDL cholesterol level. As scientists study different diets around the world and their effect on health, the Mediterranean diet keeps surfacing as a heart-healthy one. A particular noteworthy feature is that even though the diet includes almost 40 percent of calories from fat, most of it is from monounsaturated fat sources. The Mediterranean diet also differs from the typical American diet in emphasizing generous amounts of fresh produce and fish, while including relatively little meat and dairy foods.

Trans Fatty Acids

Trans fatty acids have recently been taking center stage in the media. They start out as polyunsaturated fats, but end up looking and acting more like saturated fats, thanks to hydrogenation. Hydrogenation is the process of forcing hydrogen atoms into a polyunsaturated fat, causing it to go from a liquid state to a semisolid state. Margarine is a good example of a food with a substantial amount of trans fatty acids. Look at the list of ingredients: right up there in first or second position is "hydrogenated vegetable oil." The more hydrogenation, the firmer the fat. For example, a stick of margarine has more trans fatty acids than a tub of margarine.

With all this talk about trans fatty acids, I'm often asked the question whether we should skip the margarine and go back to eating butter. Since a teaspoon of each provides the same number of calories, your decision will have to be based on their fat content. With trans fatty acids acting like saturated fat in your body, your decision will be based on how you want to spend your saturated fat allowance. Butter contains a total of 2.6 grams of saturated fat and trans fatty acids per teaspoon compared to margarine, which contains 1.1 grams.

A Word about Cholesterol

Your body needs cholesterol for cell membranes, hormones, vitamin D, and bile acid production. But since the body can make all the cholesterol it needs, your diet doesn't have to contain any. If you are a vegan, you are not eating cholesterol and you are not missing anything. Cholesterol is found only in animal products.

Let me clear up one potential source of confusion. You will recall that there is the "bad" cholesterol, known as low-density lipoprotein (LDL) cholesterol, that clogs arteries by building up plaque deposits, and the "good" cholesterol, known as high-density lipoprotein (HDL) cholesterol, that acts as a vacuum

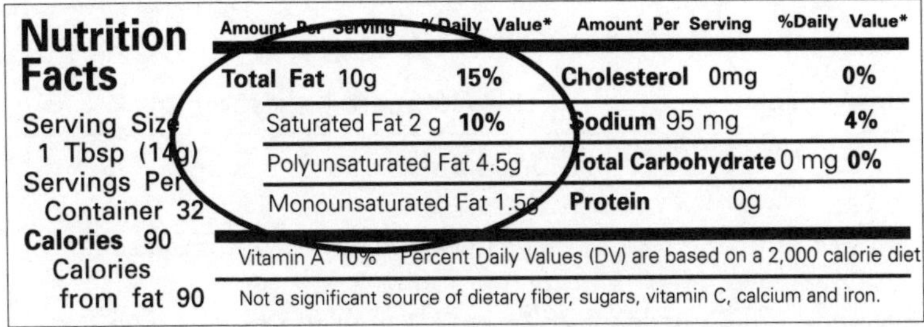

Figure 24. Label for Margarine

cleaner sweeping up some of the cholesterol left behind by the LDL. Many people assume that if there is good and bad cholesterol in the body, there must be good and bad cholesterol in food. Not so. There is only one type of cholesterol in food, and it is neither good nor bad. After your body absorbs food cholesterol, it decides whether it will become "bad" LDL or "good" HDL cholesterol.

You can elevate your blood cholesterol by eating too much dietary cholesterol or even worse, too much saturated fat, which stimulates the liver to make cholesterol. The American Heart Association recommends that each of the different fats—saturated, polyunsaturated, and monounsaturated—contribute less than 10 percent of your total calories and that your diet contain less than 300 mg of cholesterol.

Label Watching

When the Food and Drug Administration introduced their new food labeling some years back, they stipulated that only the total fat and saturated fat content had to be included. When you see polyunsaturated and monounsaturated fats mentioned on the label, it's because the food manufacturer has decided to put it there. Few manufacturers include the level of trans fatty acids. The only way you can find out how much is in the food is to add up the grams of monounsaturated, polyunsaturated, and saturated fats and subtract that amount from the *Total Fat* grams listed.

In the example shown in Figure 24, the listings for *Saturated,*

TABLE 11. **Label Lingo**

The Words	The Numbers (per serving)
Fat-free	Less than 0.5 grams of fat
Low-fat	3 grams of fat or less
Light or Lite	Product has ⅓ fewer calories *or* 50% less fat per reference amount
Reduced	At least 25% less fat than the comparison food
__% fat free	If the product meets low-fat requirements (3 grams or less); the percentage is based on the amount of fat, **by weight,** per 100 grams of food. For example: Serving size: 100g Total fat: 5g 5g ÷ 100g = 5% fat Therefore, food is 95% fat free (100% – 5% = 95%)
Lean	*Total Fat*—less than 10g *Saturated Fat*—less than 4g *Cholesterol*—less than 95 mg
Extra Lean	*Total Fat*—less than 5g *Saturated Fat*—less than 2g *Cholesterol*—less than 95 mg

Polyunsaturated, and *Monounsaturated Fat* add up to 8 grams for one tablespoon of margarine. Subtracting that from the 10 grams of Total Fat gives you 2 grams of trans fatty acids.

It pays to check the label to find out how much fat is in the food you plan to eat or in the ingredients you'll be using in a recipe. It's surprising how much fat can hide in foods without your realizing it's there. It may be obvious when you look at a piece of well-marbled meat. It isn't quite as obvious when you have a dish of chocolate pudding or macaroni and cheese. How about those old family recipes from a time when no one knew the dangers of dietary fat?

Label Lingo

Table 11 lists some important words to look for on the label and what they mean in terms of the amount of fat you'd be eating.

TABLE 12. **Daily Intakes for Various Calorie Levels**

Calories	Total Fat *(grams)*	Total Fat *(calories)*	Saturated Fat *(grams)*	Polyunsat. Fat *(grams)*	Monounsat. Fat *(grams)*
1200	40	360	13	13	13
1600	53	480	18	18	18
2000	65	600	22	22	22
2400	80	720	27	27	27
2800	93	840	31	31	31

Translating Numbers into Practice

What does it mean to you when the American Heart Association recommends that healthy individuals get less than 30 percent of their total calories from fat and that the various fats (saturated, polyunsaturated, and monounsaturated) each contribute less than 10 percent of daily total calories? How can you make use of this information?

For _S_Js, it's a numbers game. They want the facts they can use in some structured way. Counting grams of fat or calories is quite a natural approach for them. So, to save you _S_Js from having to do all the math, I've created a simple reference tool. (See Table 12.)

Now, when you read a label, you can consider how much of your daily allowance for fat grams and calories that food represents. (A little later you will be determining your specific calorie requirements; then you can come back to this chart for the fat gram and calorie recommendations.)

Most _S_Ps and _NF_s are less captivated by numbers because numbers mean structure and food diaries and calculations. It's sufficient for them to have some general ideas to keep them on track. That's fine. It's why I have included tips throughout this section. Some of my clients have successfully lost weight just by going generally low-fat and saving the high-fat foods for special occasions.

Fat Tips

- Use nonfat and low-fat products whenever possible.
- Use monounsaturated fats (olive oil, canola oil) whenever possible in place of other vegetable oils.
- Use cooking sprays on baking pans and pots when you can.
- Try low-fat plain yogurt in place of mayonnaise in dips and spreads.
- Have your salad dressing on the side, dipping your fork into the dressing first before you spear the lettuce leaves.
- Try using herbs to perk up flavors in food rather than using fat.
- If you want butter, consider making it the whipped variety or add butter-flavored seasonings.
- Use stronger-flavored oils (olive, sesame, walnut) so you can use less.
- Switch from whole or 2 percent reduced-fat milk and milk products to 1 percent low-fat or skim milk and milk products.
- Broil meat or poultry on a rack to keep it out of the fat drippings.
- Remove the skin from chicken to save on some cholesterol.
- Organ meat (liver, kidneys, etc.) has the highest amount of cholesterol per serving, followed by shellfish, then beef, and lastly butter (probably because there is less butter in a serving).
- When having pie, skip the crust, since that's where much of the fat resides. (Okay, those of you who eat pie for the crust: consider having just a couple of bites of the crust—not the whole slice.)
- Make cheese a special treat rather than a daily or regular event. If you want it more often, go for the low-fat varieties.
- If you want to lower your cholesterol intake, substitute two egg whites or one-fourth of a cup of egg substitute for one whole egg.
- Try the low-fat versions of hot dogs, sausages, bacon, and deli meats. (Just remember that they are still very high in sodium.)

Vitamins and Minerals

We don't need a lot of vitamins and minerals, yet without them, many processes in the body could not happen. Since your body can't make most of the vitamins and minerals you need, *you have to get them from your diet.* It amazes me that people expect top-notch performance from their bodies when they don't supply it with top-notch nutrition. Just think what would happen to your car if you didn't put water in its battery or gas in its tank. It wouldn't run very well—and eventually, it wouldn't run at all.

There are two types of vitamins: water-soluble and fat-soluble. Water-soluble vitamins are easily flushed out of the body through the kidneys and thus are not stored in the body to any great extent. These vitamins must be replenished regularly. On the other hand, fat-soluble vitamins are stored in the liver and fatty tissues. To avoid the risk of toxicity, it is best to get these vitamins through a balanced diet rather than through supplementation. The exception to this rule is vitamin E, which doesn't seem to have the toxicity problems of the other fat-soluble vitamins.

Vitamins serve many functions, but among the most important is protecting us against free radicals. Free radicals are molecules that are hungry for hydrogen. To satisfy themselves, they attack healthy cells and steal hydrogen from them. Of course, this leaves the victimized cells in need of hydrogen, making *them* free radicals. Antioxidants, such as vitamins C and E and beta-carotene, offer themselves up as hydrogen suppliers without becoming free radicals as a result.

As for minerals, we don't need a lot of them. However, without them, our bones and teeth would be weak, our blood pressure would be out of control, we wouldn't be able to make red blood cells, our metabolism wouldn't work, there would be no carrier for the oxygen in our blood, and we'd have very little immunity. And those are just a few of the consequences. Since our body can't make minerals, it's essential that you get them from your food.

See Appendixes D and E for the primary functions and food sources of the major vitamins and minerals.

A Shaky Habit

Are you one to reach for the salt shaker before tasting your food? For some people, that might not be a problem. However, for those who are salt sensitive or have heart disease, too much salt in the diet can be harmful, potentially contributing to high blood pressure. While we do need some sodium (about 200 mg per day), just about one-tenth of a teaspoon of it is sufficient. The sodium that naturally occurs in foods is more than enough to meet our requirements. Most of the sodium in our diet comes from salt added at the table and in processed foods. Canned soup is very high in sodium, as are many luncheon meats, pickles, cheeses, salted snacks, pizza, hot dogs, and condiments. The American Heart Association recommends that our diets contain less than 2,400 mg of sodium per day—that's about one teaspoon of salt (both added and naturally occurring). The average American is getting closer to 4,000–8,000 mg.

An interesting note: You cannot interchange the words *salt* and *sodium* because they don't describe the same thing. Table salt is sodium chloride (40 percent sodium and 60 percent chloride). So one teaspoon of salt is not equal to one teaspoon of sodium.

Salt Tips

- Check food labels for salt content.
- Rely more on herbs and spices for flavoring, so you don't have to use as much salt.
- You don't have to add salt to your water when making cooked cereal or pasta.
- Instant hot cereals have more sodium than regular hot cereals to make them cook faster.
- There are light salts that provide about half the sodium of regular salt.
- When salting foods, shake the salt into your hand first so you can see the actual amount you are adding.
- If you can't shake the salt shaker habit, try mixing one-third

of a cup of sugar with two-thirds of a cup of salt in your salt shaker.

- Condiments are very high in sodium, especially soy sauce and pickles. Go lightly.
- Eat lean roast meats, poultry, and fish more often than cured or processed meats (ham, bacon, luncheon meats, frankfurters) that contain more sodium. Meats from the deli department might have salt added to them, so consider making your own.

Boning Up on Calcium

You have until about the age of 24 to set down the maximum amount of bone structure you will have for a lifetime. That is why it is so important that you get enough calcium as you are growing up. You also want to make sure you keep that structure by continuing to supply your body with the necessary materials. You should also do weight-bearing exercise that promotes the uptake of calcium and other minerals into the bones. Otherwise, you're on the road to osteoporosis—bones that have too little mass and are porous like Swiss cheese. When this happens, the risk for hip, spine, and wrist fractures increases.

Dairy products are very good sources of calcium, but you can find it in some vegetables, in fish canned with the bones, and in tofu processed in calcium. Interestingly, skim milk has slightly more calcium than whole milk. Have a look at Table 13 for sources of calcium.

Lactose Intolerance

Lactose is the sugar in milk. There is an enzyme in our intestine, lactase, for breaking down lactose for absorption into the body. However, many people have difficulty digesting lactose because of a deficiency of lactase. If the body can't break down the sugar, it continues on through the small intestine into the large intestine. There, bacteria feast on it, putting out large amounts of gas and multiplying. The body fights back with a bad case of diarrhea. Fortunately, there are digestive enzyme products that can either be taken orally when eating dairy products or can be added to milk to break down the lactose.

TABLE 13. Sources of Calcium

HIGH SOURCES OF CALCIUM
200 mg +

Food	Portion
Cheese—Mozzarella (part skim), Swiss, Cheddar	1 oz
Macaroni and cheese	1 cup
Milk—nonfat, low-fat (1%), reduced (2%), whole, low-fat chocolate	1 cup
Yogurt—low-fat or nonfat	1 cup

GOOD SOURCES OF CALCIUM
100–190 mg

Food	Portion
Almonds	¼ cup
Bok choy	½ cup
Broccoli	1 cup
Canned fish with bones (salmon, mackerel)	2 oz
Dried beans or peas	1 cup
Frozen yogurt	½ cup
Ice cream—regular, low-fat	½ cup
Kale	1 cup
Mustard greens	1 cup
Nonfat or low-fat cottage cheese	½ cup
Refried beans	1 cup
Tofu processed with calcium	½ cup

There are some other things you can try. Start with just a small amount of lactose foods and gradually add more as they can be tolerated. Drink milk with other foods to make the lactose easier to digest. Stick to hard cheeses and yogurt. During the processing of the cheese, about half of the lactose is removed. Select yogurt that contains "active cultures," allowing the resident bacteria in the culture to digest the lactose for you.

Caffeine and Your Bones

Bones are living tissue that are constantly having minerals added to and removed from them. The object is to keep what you started with in your youth. Caffeine acts as a diuretic, pulling calcium from the bloodstream and wasting it through increased urination. Lose too much calcium this way and your bones are going to have to donate some of their calcium. When you're having your coffee, add about one to two tablespoons of milk. Maybe even try a latté, the espresso drink with foamed milk. If you're drinking a lot of sodas that contain caffeine, think about making one of those sodas a glass of milk.

Are Supplements a Good Idea?

Even if you eat a balanced diet, there might be justification for taking supplements of vitamin E, folic acid, calcium, iron, and zinc. However, trying to make up for a poor diet by taking supplements is a bad idea, since there is much more in the foods we eat than can be put in a pill.

Vitamin E

Vitamin E is a powerful antioxidant that works in the fatty areas of cell membranes. It's difficult to get from diet alone the higher levels of vitamin E that research studies are showing effective in protecting against heart disease. Because the major source of vitamin E is vegetable oil, you would need to be eating a very-high-fat diet to get the 300 IU to 400 IU of vitamin E used in the research studies. *Note:* If you do take a supplement, take no more than the studies have shown to be effective. More is not necessarily better.

Folic Acid

There is now proof that a deficiency of folic acid when a woman conceives can cause neural tube birth defects such as spina bifida. Evidence also points to folic acid as a factor in lowering the risk of heart disease, especially in people with higher than normal levels of the amino acid, homocysteine, in their blood. Unless you are eating fortified foods, look to a multivitamin that supplies 400 mcg of folic acid.

Calcium

Look again at Table 13. Do you think your diet supplies the recommended 1000 to 1200 mg of calcium per day? If so, there's no need for a supplement. *Note:* If you eat only 1200 calories per day, you may find it difficult to get enough calcium-rich foods. You might want to consider taking a supplement.

Iron and Zinc

Women generally do not eat enough iron-rich and zinc-rich foods. The best approach is to focus on foods rich in these minerals (check out the list in Appendix F), but taking a general multivitamin/mineral supplement containing no more than 100 percent of the Recommended Dietary Allowance (RDA) is safe. Supplements that are greater than 100 percent of the RDAs can be dangerous for those with an inherited iron disorder that promotes heart disease.

Water

You can survive a long time without food. The same cannot be said about water. There are many functions in your body that depend upon water. Try to drink about eight glasses (about 64 ounces) each day. If you're exercising, you should drink more. Drinks such as coffee and cola don't count toward your water intake. The caffeine in them needs all the fluid to flush the caffeine out of the body.

It's interesting that thirst is not always an indicator of your need for water. In fact, as people get older, their thirst mechanism doesn't work as efficiently, so they need to make a conscious effort to get enough water. One way to guarantee that you get your daily water requirement is to fill a half-gallon container with water and put it in your refrigerator. If by the end of the day there's still water in the container, you've got some catching up to do.

How's Your Type Handling All This So Far?

You Sensors should be satisfied with all the facts, details, and concrete data presented. However, I appreciate that there is one important element missing—a step-by-step, hands-on approach to dealing with these facts. We'll get to that shortly. You iNtuitives are probably already starting to put these pieces of the jigsaw puzzle together, trying to create an overall scheme for it, and looking for the hidden meaning behind the facts. You Thinkers are pleased that some rules have been provided (for example, the percentages of each nutrient to eat), so you can start to analyze the facts and consider the consequences of certain food selections. I will be giving you some more rules soon. You Feelers are pleased, I hope, that you were allowed to select the foods you enjoy (from the lists in the Appendix), yet you may be reserving judgment until you see how you'll be using the facts presented so far. You Judgers are looking for some structure into which you can file all this information. It's coming. You Perceivers are trying to figure out how you can keep your food choices spontaneous and not be too tied down by all this. You'll be happy to know that you'll be free to choose as you like.

The Figures

Discovering Your Nutrition Needs (NN) Numbers

So far I've shared basic nutrition information with you. However, that's not enough to help you make personal eating decisions. You still don't know what your individual needs are. The purpose of this book is not only to help you change your lifestyle habits according to your personality, but also to help you personalize your lifestyle habits. That means knowing more about what your nutrition needs (NN) are.

Even though all foods are allowed, it doesn't mean that you can have unlimited quantities of everything. To maintain a healthy weight, your NN numbers dictate how many calories and grams of fat, protein, and carbohydrate you should eat, as well as how many servings of various foods are right for you. A 5-foot, 4-inch woman who weighs 120 pounds knows what will happen if she eats the way a 6-foot, 2-inch man weighing 195 pounds does. Since there's no way she can add inches to her height, the only direction she can change is from side to side! Your frame size, body composition, age, gender, activity level, and even family background will help determine how much you can eat.

To determine what your NN numbers are, you'll need to take a couple of measurements: your height, weight, and wrist circumference. Be honest with the measuring! Otherwise, your calorie calculations are going to be off. (By the way, rest assured that I'm not going to require anyone to count calories unless they want to. For most people with busy lives, that is asking too much. However, you need to know how many calories you can eat to determine how many servings of various foods you should have.)

Measuring Up

- What's your height?_________ inches *(without shoes)*
- What's your weight?_________ pounds *(without clothes)*
- What's the wrist measurement of your writing hand? _________ inches *(To measure your wrist, find the bony protrusion or bump on the outside of your wrist. Place a cloth tape measure on your wrist between that bone and your hand and take that measurement.)*

Your Body Mass Index (BMI)

Most people have come to rely on the bathroom scale to tell them how healthfully they are eating. They figure that if the scale gives them numbers that make them feel good, they must be doing okay. Of course, what the scale *isn't* telling them is how much of that weight is muscle versus fat. There are methods to find that out—hydrostatic weighing, bioelectrical impedance, and caliper measurements as discussed in Chapter 6. Since you may not have access to those forms of measurement, the next best thing is *body mass index* (BMI), which gives you an idea of

TABLE 14. **Calculating BMI**

Your Weight (inches)	Your Multiplier
58	0.21
59	0.20
60	0.20
61	0.19
62	0.18
63	0.18
64	0.17
65	0.17
66	0.16
67	0.16
68	0.15
69	0.15
70	0.14
71	0.14
72	0.14
73	0.13
74	0.13
75	0.13
76	0.12
77	0.12
78	0.12

your body composition. It doesn't tell you what percentage body fat you have, but it does give you an idea of whether your level of "fatness" is in a healthy range or not.

There are two ways to determine your BMI. You can either calculate it or look it up in a table (see Appendix G). The quick calculation method, which I'll explain in a moment, is more accurate, but either way is fine.

A Quick Calculation

Females and males should calculate their BMI the same way. In the first column of Table 14, find your height (in inches). Then multiply your weight by the number in the second column. Round off your answer to the nearest whole number.

TABLE 15. **BMI Health Table**

With a BMI of:	**18.5–24.9**	**25–29.9**	**30 and above**
Your body composition is:	Normal	Overweight	Obese
and			
Your level of risk is:	Healthy and generally acceptable	May be at risk for health problems*	Increased risk for health problems**

Recommendations by The National Institutes of Health (June 1998):
*Weight loss is recommended when there are two other weight-related risk factors such as high blood pressure, high blood cholesterol, diabetes, impaired glucose tolerance, and a waist circumference of 40 inches in men and 35 inches in women. If you do not have any of these risk factors, further weight gain should be prevented.
**Weight loss is required to decrease risk.

For example, Jerry is 5 feet 8 inches tall (68 inches), so his multiplier is "0.15." He weighs 150 pounds, so he multiplies 150 x 0.15 = 22.5 (which he rounds up to 23).

Once you have an answer, look for that number in Table 15. Jerry's BMI of 23 is in the "normal" weight range and, at that weight, he is not at risk for health problems. What's your BMI and body composition? Are you at risk?

What if Jerry were 200 pounds? Then his BMI would be 30, and he would be in the "obese" range.

Looking It Up

If you prefer to find your BMI on a table, look at Appendix G. Locate your height along the left-hand column. Then run your finger to the right along that row until you come to the weight that's closest to your own. Look up to the top of that column. The number you see is your BMI. For example, if you are 5 feet 6 inches tall and weigh 155 pounds, you have a BMI of 25, a number that puts you in the "overweight" category.

Healthy Weight or Need to Lose?

Did your BMI number tell you that you are in the healthy weight range? If so, then proceed to the section, *Taking Your Activity into Account,* on page 208. If not, and you need to lose weight, you have one more step to do: determine a healthy weight for yourself. This step is not meant to create a diet mentality so that you are constantly saying to yourself, "I need to lose ______ pounds." It is strictly to give you a basis for meal planning.

A Quick Calculation

I'm going to present two different ways for you to determine your healthy weight. One of the ways uses the BMI, the other, your frame size. You decide which approach appeals to you. (Some people are very curious about their frame size.) If you try both ways, the answers you get may vary slightly, but not enough to matter.

Method 1

Refer to the BMI Table in Appendix G. Find your height in the left-hand column. Run your finger across that row to the weights stated for BMIs of 19 to 24. Those values give you a normal weight range for your height. For example, if you're 5 feet 4 inches tall, a normal weight range for you would be 110 to 140 pounds. Keep in mind that staying in the lower to middle portion of that range would be healthier than getting too close to the top end. Write the range here for future reference: ________ pounds.

Method 2

Using your height and wrist measurement, determine your frame size. It's an easy calculation. Just divide your height by your wrist measurement.

____________ in. ÷	____________ in. =	____________
Height	Wrist measurement	Frame Size Value

Your frame size partially determines your weight. It makes sense, since the amount of bone will influence total weight. That's

TABLE 16. **Frame Sizes**

Frame Size Value Females	Frame Size Value Males	Frame Size
Greater than 11.0	Greater than 10.4	Small
10.1–11.0	9.6–10.4	Medium
Less than 10.1	Less than 9.6	Large

Source: From L. Kathleen Mahan and Marian Arlin's *Krause's Food, Nutrition, and Diet Therapy*, 1992, Appendix 18, page 823.

probably why we would all like to say we have large frames! Find your frame size value in Table 16. Look across that row to see what your frame size is.

Now look at Appendix H for the Metropolitan Height and Weight Tables. Make sure you're using the correct table for your gender. Locate your height, then look across the row to the frame size you found on the previous table. The weights you see there give you a **healthy range.** Write it here for future reference: ________ pounds.

Research is showing that when you are overweight or obese, losing as little as 10 to 15 percent of your body weight will bring dramatic changes in your health and the way you feel. It can help lower a high blood cholesterol count and high blood pressure. Some people find that, no matter how conscientiously they diet and exercise, they can never attain the table's *prescribed healthy weight* or, having attained that weight, maintain it for long. Their metabolisms may have been altered by one too many diets; their genetic background may also be playing a role. If you are one of those people, you should lose 10 to 15 percent of your body weight and then try maintaining that new weight for about three times the number of months it took you to lose it. For example, if it took you two months to lose 10 pounds, see if you can maintain that loss for six months. At that point, you can determine if it is medically necessary for you to pursue any more weight reduction.

Taking Your Activity into Account

When I say the word *calories,* what's the first thought that comes to your mind? Most people would say that they eat too many of them. Calories are not only a value assigned to the energy inside food. They are also a measure of how much energy you're using during the day to do your usual activities and exercise. Don't forget about the calories it takes for the basic functioning of your body at rest (heartbeat, digestion, metabolism, etc.).

Maintaining or losing weight is a numbers game. To maintain your present weight, it's just a matter of consuming the same number of calories your body uses for its basic functioning and physical activity. If you want to lose weight, you must eat fewer calories and burn more calories with physical activity than you have been doing. The question is: How active are you?

Which one of the following statements sounds most like you, even though you may do different activities?

1. "Most of what I do during the day requires me to be either sitting or standing. For fun, I play cards, watch television, or play an instrument."
2. "During the day, I'm up and about, climbing stairs to get to someone's office or doing housework. For fun, I like to golf, bowl, sail, or play table tennis. I try to walk or swim at least twice a week."
3. "My job is fairly active, as is my leisure time. If there's snow, I'm out there skiing. During the summer, I like to bike, play tennis, or jog at least three to five times a week."
4. "I feel like I'm on the go from morning to night. If I can, I'm out there exercising at least six or seven days a week, running, weight-training, participating in competitive swimming or some other active sport."
5. "I do heavy manual labor for a living."

If you think that statement #1 sounds most like you, then your activity level is **Very Light.** Statement #2 reflects a **Light** activity level; #3 is a **Moderate** activity level and statements #4 and #5 reflect a **Heavy** activity level. Now that you know how active you are, let's find out how many calories you get to eat.

Choosing a Meal Plan

Included in Table 17 (for women) and Table 18 (for men) are five Meal Plans from which to choose. Each is based on the

TABLE 17. **Meal Plans for Females**

Healthy Weight (in pounds)	Females—Activity Level			
	Very Light	Light	Moderate	Heavy
100–110	Plan A	Plan B	Plan B	Plan C
111–120	Plan B	Plan B	Plan C	Plan D
121–130	Plan B	Plan C	Plan C	Plan D
131–140	Plan B	Plan C	Plan C	Plan E
141–150	Plan C	Plan D	Plan D	Plan E
151–160	Plan C	Plan D	Plan D	Plan E+
161–170	Plan C	Plan D	Plan E	Plan E+
171–180	Plan D	Plan D	Plan E	Plan E+

+You are free to add from the various food groups after eating the recommended number of servings. Let your weight, hunger, fullness, and energy levels be your guide.

number of calories you should be eating. Find your healthy weight in the first column and then look across to the appropriate activity level. Make sure you're looking at the correct table, as the correct meal plan for you depends on your gender.

Applying the information from the tables is easy. First find the plan that coincides with your healthy weight and activity level. Then see the following list to see how many calories you need per day to maintain that weight. *Note:* If you're not sure what your healthy weight should be, consult Appendix G.

Plan A = 1200 calories
Plan B = 1600 calories
Plan C = 2000 calories
Plan D = 2400 calories
Plan E = 2800 calories

Those of you trying to lose weight have a decision to make. As you look at the Meal Plan tables, you have two choices:

1. You can eat according to the Meal Plan that corresponds to

Building a Healthy Meal Plan

The ancient Egyptians who built the pyramids were smart architects. They realized the advantage of having a broad, strong foundation upon which to construct, stone by stone, a structure that could stand the test of time. You can use the same principles to put together a healthy meal plan.

The U.S. Department of Agriculture believes that the pyramid structure is a perfect framework for its eating guidelines. (See Figure 25.) The Food Guide Pyramid is visual (something you Sensors should like) and general enough to leave room for choice (something you Feelers and Perceivers should enjoy). Notice which food group is the largest and which group occupies the least amount of space. That should give you an idea about the number of servings from each group.

Table 19 gives you an idea of the number of servings you can have from each of the food groups for your Meal Plan. (Sensors, we're starting to get to the hands-on stuff.) This is just a framework. (Remember iNtuitives, you have a part in creating a plan.) I don't want you to view this as a "diet," deviating from which means you've been bad. (Are you listening, Feelers?) Know that your body will be the better for eating according to the Pyramid. (It's only logical. Right, Thinkers?) Don't forget about that *life vision* you set in Chapter 6 as you choose your foods.

The major contributions from the *Bread, Cereal, Rice and Pasta Group* are complex carbohydrates, with a generous helping of vitamins, minerals, and fiber. The *Vegetable and Fruit Groups* provide the body with plenty of complex carbohydrates, vitamins, minerals, fiber, and phytochemicals. The *Milk, Yogurt, and Cheese Group* is a good source of protein, vitamins, and minerals (especially calcium, phosphorus and vitamin D) and some carbohydrates. The *Meat, Poultry, Fish, Dry Beans, Eggs, and Nuts Group* is the most generous contributor of protein, minerals such as iron and zinc, and the B vitamins.

Even though your body could survive quite well with little or nothing from the Fats, Oils, and Sweets section of the pyramid—they're not really considered a food group—many people feel that life just wouldn't be complete without them. Don't forget that fat and sugar lurk in many of the foods found in each of

TABLE 18. Meal Plans for Males

Healthy Weight (in pounds)	Males—Activity Level			
	Very Light	Light	Moderate	Heav
121–130	Plan B	Plan C	Plan D	Plan E
131–140	Plan C	Plan D	Plan D	Plan E
141–150	Plan C	Plan D	Plan E	Plan E+
151–160	Plan C	Plan E	Plan E	Plan E+
161–170	Plan D	Plan E	Plan E	Plan E+
171–180	Plan D	Plan E+	Plan E+	Plan E+
181–190	Plan D	Plan E+	Plan E+	Plan E+
191–200	Plan E	Plan E+	Plan E+	Plan E+
201–210	Plan E	Plan E+	Plan E+	Plan E+

+You are free to add from the various food groups after eating the recommended number of servings. Let your weight, hunger, fullness, and energy levels be your guide.

your healthy weight and appropriate activity level. Choosing this plan will bring about a slower weight loss, but you'll be learning to eat the way you should be eating the rest of your life.

2. You can select the Meal Plan that corresponds to the weight range one level less than your healthy weight, at the same activity level. In some cases, it may mean fewer calories.

Most dieters struggle with strict low-calorie weight-loss diets, finding them too restrictive. And the struggle doesn't end there, because once they've achieved their desired weight, they will have to add back some calories to maintain their new weight, and most people overdo it.

iNtuitives might feel comfortable with the slower-to-lose-it Meal Plan (the one that contains enough calories for their healthy weight) because they have the patience to look to the future and imagine the results. I'm just not sure _S_Ps could be that patient. I'll let you be the judge. When making your choice, go through what you learned in Chapter 5 about decision making, remembering to use all your preferences.

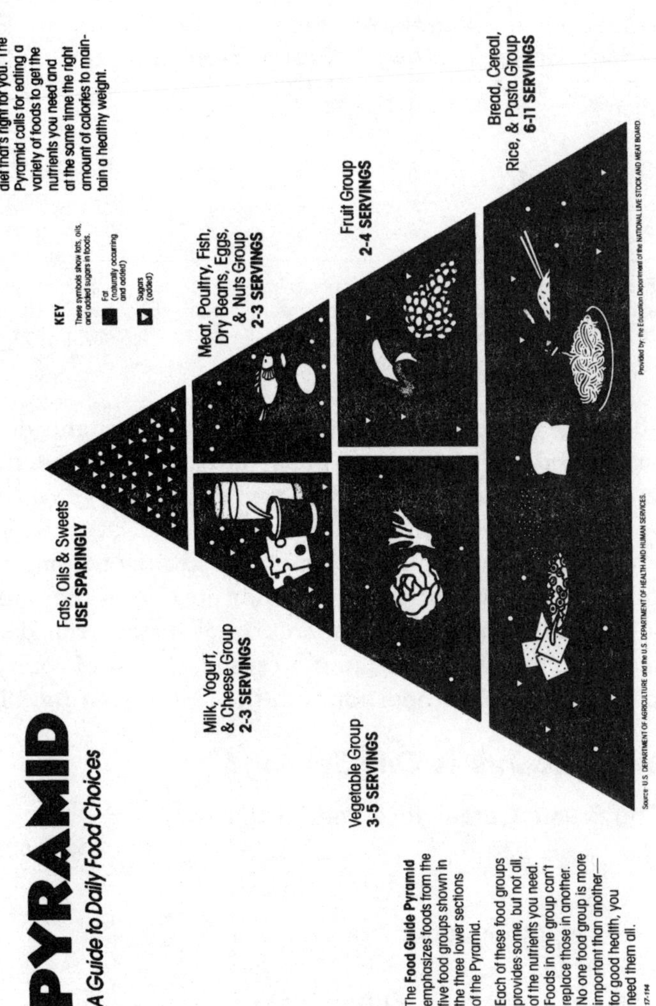

Figure 25. Food Guide Pyramid

TABLE 19. **Number of Servings for Each Meal Plan**

Meal Plan	Grains Group	Vegetable Group	Fruit Group	Dairy Group	Meat Group *(ounces)*	Extras Group
Plan A	5	3	2	2	5	50 calories
Plan B	7	4	3	2	6	100 calories
Plan C	9	5	3	3	7	150 calories
Plan D	10	7	4	3	8	200 calories
Plan E	11	8	4	4	9	250 calories

Extras Group: 1 tsp of fat = 45 calories/5 grams fat (butter, margarine, mayonnaise, salad dressing, sour cream, whipped cream, cream, chocolate); 1 tsp sugar = 16 calories/4 grams sugar (table sugar, candy, chocolate, jam, syrup, soft drinks)

the food groups. Even though Danish pastries and doughnuts are considered part of the *Bread Group,* they're loaded with fat and sugar. An apple pie may be part of both the *Bread Group* and *Fruit Group,* but again, it contains plenty of fat and sugar. You could drink chocolate milk and get a healthy helping of sugar. Maybe you're having sweet and sour pork from the *Meat Group,* a dish made with sugar. They all count toward your daily sugar and fat allowance. If you're not careful, the tip of your pyramid could get out of proportion with the rest of your food intake.

What Counts as One Serving?

The Bread, Cereal, Rice and Pasta Group

1 slice of bread
½ bagel
½ English muffin
1 tortilla
1–4½ inch-square waffle
1 small roll
½ cup cooked rice or pasta
½ cup cooked cereal
½ cup ready-to-eat cereal

The Vegetable Group

½ cup cooked vegetables
1 cup raw vegetables
1 cup leafy raw vegetables
½ cup vegetable juice

The Fruit Group

1 fruit (apple, orange, small banana, peach)
1 cup cubed melon
½ cup fruit juice
½ cup canned fruit
¼ cup dried fruit

The Milk, Yogurt, and Cheese Group

1 cup milk or yogurt
1 ounce cheese
2 tablespoons grated cheese

The Meat, Poultry, Fish, Dry Beans, Eggs, and Nuts Group

2½–3 ounces cooked lean meat, poultry, or fish
½ cup cooked beans (equal to 1 ounce lean meat)
1 egg (equal to 1 ounce lean meat)
2 tablespoons peanut butter (equal to 1 ounce lean meat)

How Nutritiously Are You Eating?

Do you know whether you're eating enough vegetables and fruits? Are you eating more meat than your body needs? Do you get enough dairy products in your diet?

The only way you can really answer these questions is to keep a Food Log for about a week. Only when you know what you have been doing can you know what is working for you and what needs changing. Some of you, especially the Judgers, should have no problem with keeping a log. Then there will be those of you who don't like to have that much structure and prefer something more graphic. That's why I've provided two types of Food Logs. (See Figures 20 and 21.) The first one allows you to write exactly what you eat. The second Food Log lets you check off a box when you've eaten a serving from a particular food group. When you review your log at the end of the week, it will be very clear which food groups you rely on too much and which you need to eat from more frequently. Just remember to eat as you normally would. Don't stop eating certain foods just so you don't have to log them in.

Consider doing this exercise again in about three weeks and then again a month later. The first time, it will be more a reflection of what you have been doing in the past. In three weeks, it will reflect a lot of what you have learned. You might even want to do this continuously as a way of keeping on track.

The Food Log examples in Tables 20 and 21 have been set up for Meal Plan A. When you set up your own log, fill in the number of servings you can have of each food group from Table 19. (*Note:* You can use the blank-log formats in Tables 22 and 23 when setting up your own log. Make enough copies of the format you prefer to last the week, and be sure to take one with you when you eat out.) Meal Plan A allows five servings from the *Bread Group,* three servings from the *Vegetable Group,* two servings from the *Fruit Group,* two servings from the *Milk Group,* and five ounces of protein from the *Meat Group.* Count off five boxes in the *Bread Group* row to correspond to the five allowed servings, and black out the other boxes. Do the same for the other food groups.

Now let's see how you would record a lunch on the two different types of logs. Let's say you are having a turkey sandwich, carrots, a glass of milk, and an apple. The sandwich is made with two slices of bread. If you refer back to the section *What Counts as a Serving?* you'll see that two slices of bread equal two servings from the *Bread Group.* There are about 2½ ounces of turkey meat on the sandwich, or one serving from the *Meat Group.* The one teaspoon of mayonnaise on the sandwich is equal to one serving from the *Extras category.*

TABLE 20. Example of Food Log (Type #1) Filled Out for Meal Plan A

Example					**MEAL PLAN *A***				**DATE ______**			
Bread, Cereal, Rice and Pasta Group	1 slice bread	1 slice bread										
Vegetable Group	½ cup carrots											
Fruit Group	1 apple											
Milk, Yogurt, and Cheese Group	8 oz skim milk											
Meat, Poultry, Fish, Dried Beans, Eggs, and Nuts Group *(Each square is equivalent to one ounce of meat)*	1 oz turkey	1 oz turkey										
Extras	1 tsp mayo											

TABLE 21. Example of Food Log (Type #2) Filled Out for Meal Plan A

Example					**MEAL PLAN A**				**DATE** ________			
Bread, Cereal, Rice and Pasta Group	●	●	○	○	○	○	○	○	○	○	○	○
Vegetable Group	●	○	○	○	○	○	○	○				
Fruit Group	●	○	○	○								
Milk, Yogurt, and Cheese Group	●	○	○	○								
Meat, Poultry, Fish, Dried Beans, Eggs, and Nuts Group *(Each square is equivalent to one ounce of meat)*	●	●	○	○	○	○	○	○	○			
Extras	●	○	○	○	○	○	○	○				

TABLE 22. Blank Food Log, Type #1

MEAL PLAN ______________									**DATE** ______________			
Bread, Cereal, Rice and Pasta Group												
Vegetable Group												
Fruit Group												
Milk, Yogurt, and Cheese Group												
Meat, Poultry, Fish, Dried Beans, Eggs, and Nuts Group *(Each square is equivalent to one ounce of meat)*												
Extras												

TABLE 23. Blank Food Log, Type #2

MEAL PLAN ____________									**DATE** ____________			
Bread, Cereal, Rice and Pasta Group	○	○	○	○	○	○	○	○	○	○	○	○
Vegetable Group	○	○	○	○	○	○	○	○				
Fruit Group	○	○	○	○								
Milk, Yogurt, and Cheese Group	○	○	○	○								
Meat, Poultry, Fish, Dried Beans, Eggs, and Nuts Group *(Each square is equivalent to one ounce of meat)*	○	○	○	○	○	○	○	○	○			
Extras	○	○	○	○	○	○	○	○				

The Decision

Factors Involved in the Decision about What to Eat

Good nutrition should be a major factor in deciding what to eat. That's why I shared the nutrition facts with you at the beginning of this chapter. Yet what seems to be more important to people is taste and convenience. Your mother may have told you liver was good for you, but that didn't make it taste good. However, with so many foods now available, you really don't have an excuse for not finding something that is both enjoyable *and* good for you.

There are other factors that influence people's eating decisions, including how readily available certain foods are, the information on food labels (nutritional content, calories), what's offered on the menu, the cost, what everyone else is having, food advertisements, customs and traditions, whether they are trying to lose weight, and habits.

Food Selection—by Flavor

Since taste and flavor are such a driving force in our food selection, let's talk about them first. Do you realize that if food had no flavor, we would probably all be thin? Foods that taste good tempt us to eat more, while those that lack flavor may only be eaten because we think they're good for us, or they're the only thing available. Flavor makes food interesting, appetizing, and appealing. Yet all flavors are not liked by all people. Just because you like spicy food doesn't necessarily mean I do. Our environment helps shape some of our food preferences (you probably like many flavors your parents liked). Your body chemistry also plays a part; the person who likes spicy food, for example, has a higher tolerance for the burning sensation that accompanies spicy food than the person who prefers milder foods. There is a reason, after all, why Baskin and Robbins has 31 flavors of ice cream. Not everyone likes chocolate.

There are many components to flavor—taste, mouthfeel or

texture, aroma, temperature, and appearance. They all work together to make a food taste to you the way it does. Something, that doesn't smell good to you—liver, for example—may not taste good either. If you like the crisp bite to raw or steamed broccoli, puréed broccoli will seem unappetizing.

Flavor Components

- *Taste*—You need to ask yourself each time you want to eat something, "What taste am I looking for—sweet? salty? sour? bitter? bland? fruity? spicy? tart? lemony? buttery?"
- *Mouthfeel*—What texture do you want from that taste—crunchy? crispy? chewy? juicy? light? creamy? soft? melt-in-your-mouth? flaky? tender? bite-size? full-mouth feel?
- *Aroma*—You may not consciously think about what aroma you want from a food. However, once you've determined what taste and texture you want, the food you select will have a particular smell that affects you. Is it pungent? floral? herbal? spicy? fruity? fresh? sweet? Aroma plays a big role in getting us to eat something even when we're not hungry. Think about walking past a bakery with its sweet, buttery, yeasty smells wafting out the door. It's like a magnet for *me.* What about you?
- *Temperature*—Not many people think about the temperature of the food they eat as playing a big part in eating enjoyment. An obvious exception might occur on a day when they've been freezing in the snow and are looking to "defrost" with some hot food, or on a very hot day, after they've been roasting in the sun and want cold food to help them cool down. Eating foods with contrasting temperatures can make each more enjoyable.
- *Appearance*—Even the appearance of the food sometimes makes a difference. Five-star restaurants pride themselves on presentation. Contrasting colors and shapes create interest.

When you start making eating decisions consciously, you need to consider what component of flavor you're looking for and what you are trying to satisfy. You Sensors should be really good at this. You tend to have strong preferences in flavors, textures, and colors. How many times have you eaten a cookie when actually what you wanted was something juicy and refreshing, such as a ripe peach or a fruit slush? If you had really taken into account that your mouth was dry, you might have considered something liquid. Because eating the cookie didn't satisfy what you really wanted, the chances of your scavenging in search of something else increase. When you feel a strong need to chew on something, ice cream or soup isn't going to do it. When you want to suck on something, eating carrot sticks isn't going to be satisfying (unless you plan to lick them!). If you can't decide what flavor component you want to satisfy, it may be that you really aren't hungry.

If you select something to eat and find you're not enjoying it, you have a choice whether to continue to eat it. With your Thinking preference you might think, "I paid for it. I can't waste it," but your Feeling preference might tell you, "I care about myself, and since I'm not enjoying it, this is a waste of my daily calorie allowance."

I've Got to Have It Now!

True cravings are great. They are the most defined desire for a particular flavor. Instead of having to ask yourself what you want, your body cries out for something specific. However, to determine whether this craving is for real and not just a mental creation, you should take a 20-minute time-out. Find something to do that is distracting—drink some water, read a book, write a letter. Did the craving pass? If not, then don't ignore it any longer or try to shut it up with carrot and celery sticks.

When you recognize it as a craving, treat it kindly but in moderation. If an ice cream sundae is just what you wanted, have it. However, it doesn't have to be the monster size. A little dish should more than satisfy the craving, since most cravings are not hunger-based. However, saying you are craving something just as an excuse to eat it "without guilt" won't work for long. Only you and your body will suffer in the end. Remember, cravings are not free foods. They still count toward your daily allowance of the different food groups.

Pleasure Seekers

Pleasure is a strong driving force in selecting foods. For example, I would rather have one bite of sinfully rich dark chocolate than a whole cheap chocolate candy bar. Those extra calories and fat have to be delicious or they aren't worth the eating. That's how I make *my* decisions. You may think otherwise. However, making personal decisions is what this book is all about.

The art of tasting: There are many people who don't really taste their food. The iNtuitives, who have their minds elsewhere, often don't consciously take note of flavors. They may be thinking about what they'll be having for dessert even before they've finished their meal. Sensors are probably better at tasting because they're more in the present than iNtuitives. Then there are those people who are in such a hurry that they seem to inhale their food, never giving it a chance to register on their taste buds.

Try this exercise and see how to really taste chocolate, or use another food if you prefer. Think about what wine tasters do:

1. *Look at the chocolate.* What kind of surface does it have—velvety, shiny, matte?
2. *Break the chocolate.* Does it give off a snapping sound or is the break slightly muted?
3. *Smell the aroma.* Is it a strong chocolate smell or a somewhat waxy smell?
4. *Experience the mouthfeel.* With your tongue, place the chocolate against the roof of your mouth. Do nothing but let it melt there. Does it have a velvety smooth finish or is it grainy?
5. *Experience the flavor.* Now allow the melted chocolate to roll around your mouth, letting it touch as many surfaces (the tongue, the cheeks, the lips) as possible. What flavors are you sensing? Is it a nutty, roasted flavor mingled with sweetness?

This exercise will demonstrate the importance of eating slowly to really experience and enjoy your food. Why have food that's tasty if you never give your taste buds a chance to find out? Besides, the slower you eat, the *less* you'll probably eat.

Chocolate tip: If you have a chocolate urge and want to avoid the fat, try having a teaspoon of fat-free chocolate syrup. Just slowly lick the spoon, allowing the chocolate to travel around your mouth before swallowing.

Many people no longer experience the pleasure of eating. They worry about the fat and cholesterol content; they fear they'll gain weight when they eat what they like. Worse yet, once they've eaten it, they feel guilty. It's time to throw away that kind of thinking. It will only end up destroying you and cause you to splurge, binge, or sneak food, which can only lead to destroying your self-esteem and ending your journey to a healthy lifestyle.

Food Selection—by Convenience or Availability

Because of the fast pace of life today, many people no longer have the time or the inclination to create meals from scratch. Although cooking from scratch gives you more control over your food selection, you can still eat well in a hurry. Your supermarket has many healthful items. Pick up your veggies already cut up from the produce department or go to the supermarket's salad bar. Most markets sell complete meals or prepared ingredients that you can just toss together. Then there are always frozen packaged single-serving meals. Or you can pick up a meal, complete with utensils and napkin, at a restaurant's drive-through window. Of course, there's always the option of eating out.

Plan Ahead

Do you know how to recognize the difference between a Judger and a Perceiver? Look in their refrigerator or pantry. The Judger has every shelf stocked. There isn't just one can of tomato soup but three or four. Every staple, such as mayonnaise, has a backup jar to the one in the refrigerator. There isn't enough room for another thing in the refrigerator. Now contrast that with the Perceiver, who probably has just one can of tomato soup on the shelf. If he runs out of mayonnaise, he figures he can always run to the store to get another jar. You can actually see the back wall of his refrigerator without removing anything.

Whether you are a Judger or a Perceiver, eating well must involve some degree of planning ahead. Perceivers should consider making a big batch of soup, stews or casseroles on the weekend. (The Judgers probably already have.) They can then be stored in meal-size containers in your freezer to be pulled out whenever you don't have time to cook. These meals can even be defrosted in your microwave if you didn't take them out in the morning. (Perceivers should be big fans of the microwave oven, which allows them to make last-minute decisions.) Listen to your Thinking preference and realize that it's logical to have something available for quick meals, it's certainly less expensive than takeout food, and batch-cooking uses your time more efficiently. Planning ahead comes down to good time management. If you find you never have enough time, maybe you should think about taking a time management class.

Make bag lunches the night before to avoid the hectic rush in the morning. Most sandwiches will stay fresh overnight in the refrigerator, as will cut-up vegetables and fruit when stored in zippered plastic bags. If you're worried about the lettuce wilting, pack it in a separate bag to slip into your sandwich at lunchtime. For those of you who need some variety, consider other breads besides sandwich bread, such as pita, tortillas, and Kaiser rolls. Think about different low-fat fillings for your sandwich, such as shredded cabbage mixed with chicken pieces and red peppers moistened with a light vinaigrette. Try cottage cheese seasoned with chili powder, or mashed garbanzo beans flavored with chopped tomatoes, cucumbers, parsley, and onions (if you won't be offending anyone!).

You Judgers and iNtuitives will probably do fine using this plan-ahead approach. If you're a Perceiver, you might put up a bit of a fight. I know you like to leave your options open, and making a bag lunch may be too much of a commitment. What if someone were to ask you to go out to lunch? You could always save your bag lunch for the next day.

Food Selection—by the Numbers

Whether you're eating out, bringing home ingredients to put a dish together yourself, or purchasing packaged meals, it's important to read whatever nutrition information is available. It's also important to consider what you've already eaten during the day to see how the options fit into your daily allowances. All the facts I presented at the beginning of the chapter should be included in the decision-making process. They are an especially important input from your Sensing preference, the keeper of facts.

There is other valuable information on a food label besides what I have already shared with you at the beginning of this chapter.

Percent Daily Value (%DV)

Too many people think the "% DV" listed on the label is the percentage of a particular nutrient in a serving of the food. It's not. Daily Value represents the total nutrient levels recommended for a 2000 calorie diet. When the Food and Drug Administration came out with their new labeling requirements in 1994, they wanted people to have an idea of what contribution a food made to their overall daily intake. Since there isn't enough room on the label to show the percentage for the various calorie levels, they set 2000 calories as the standard. They figured that 2000 calories would cover the average person's needs. *Your* calorie intake, however, may be more or less. That's why I've created a % Daily Value Converter, which you'll find in Appendix I. Whatever your calorie intake, you can adjust the % DV on the label to that number.

However, even if the % DV on the label doesn't exactly represent your calorie intake, it gives you a way of comparing one food product to another.

Some rules of thumb:

- Foods with a 5% DV or less are considered *low* sources of the nutrient.
- Foods with a % DV of 6 to 19% are considered a *good* source of the nutrient.
- Foods with a % DV of 20% or greater are considered a *high* source of the nutrient.

If you're trying to lower your fat intake, it's best to look for foods with 5% DV or less. When attempting to increase your intake of, say, fiber, look for a 20% or more DV.

Calorie Watching

Many years ago calorie counting was a popular way to lose weight. We knew that to lose weight, more calories had to be expended than consumed. Considering that you must burn or decrease your calorie intake by 3500 calories to lose one pound, calorie counting seemed the best approach. However, most people don't have the patience to look up each food in a calorie book, decide if it will fit into their day's allowance, and keep a running balance. So the method was pretty much discarded, except by those with the personality that enjoyed the challenge and the number crunching.

A newer and perhaps better approach is to start ''calorie watching.'' With so many people eating more packaged foods, they no longer have to carry a calorie book around. The calories per serving are written right at the top of the Nutrition Facts on the label.

Calories still count, whether the food is fat-free or not. In fact, it's the fat-free foods that are getting people into trouble. They think if it is fat-free, they can have an unlimited quantity. Yet fat-free foods have calories, and sometimes can have as many calories as their full-fat cousins because of the addition of sugar for flavor. Your body is more than happy to convert those extra calories into body fat for possible later use. So consider the number of calories as just another bit of information you'll need when the time comes to make a decision about what to eat.

Food Selection—by Impulse

Shopping in the supermarket can be quite an adventure, especially when you spend too much time in the aisles. That's where you'll find many of the high-fat processed foods. If you go to the perimeter of the store, you'll find more of the five food groups in their natural state. There are some high-fat foods here, but most of them are not highly processed. Be careful at the end of aisles or at the cash register. (Are you listening, _S_Ps?) That's where the store puts impulse items and individual packages of crackers and cookies. Then there's always the candy rack you seem to have too much time to study while the person in front of you pays for his or her groceries.

To avoid buying things you don't need just because they look appetizing, it's best to eat before you go. A grocery list also helps decrease impulse shopping. Moreover, it guarantees that you have included foods from the five food groups. (I can just hear you Perceivers saying that that would take away all the fun and spontaneity in grocery shopping. I recommend that before something that is not a necessity makes its way into your shopping cart, you put it through the decision-making process.) Don't buy something you know will tempt you every time you see it in the pantry (unless you can handle temptation!).

Food Selection—by Variety

When you consider how many meals you eat in a week, a month, a year, you begin to realize the burdensome number of eating decisions you have to make. Let's say that every lunch and dinner includes a starch, vegetable, and source of protein, and that you don't want to repeat the same meal twice in one week. That means you will have a total of 42 decisions per week, or 2184 decisions per year to make. And that doesn't even include breakfast. It would be easier if you just ate the same foods each day, but that would definitely get boring. Besides, in order to get well-rounded nutrition, variety is important.

So how do you introduce variety into your meals? Table 24 provides a basic structure for meal planning. It's a mix-and-match approach, in which you can choose a selection from each of the columns as the basis for your meal. I've included some blank rows so you can fill in your favorites.

I'll share with you how it works for dinner, but it works equally well for lunch and breakfast. As I look over the Type of Dish and Cuisine columns, I think I'll make a stir-fry Italian dinner. For my Starch, I'll use pasta (the rotini-shaped variety). The Protein will be halibut. As my Vegetable selections, I'll include zucchini, tomatoes, and onions. All I need to do is stir-fry these ingredients, together with a little olive oil, garlic, basil, and oregano, and I've got dinner.

Food Selection—by the Clock

Because it's breakfast time and the cereal manufacturers have done a good job in advertising their products, cereal seems the right food for breakfast. The egg farmers have done a good job too, since eggs also seem like perfect breakfast food. Yet leftover pizza or a deli sandwich is every bit as acceptable. The Japanese eat fish, rice, and miso soup for breakfast. Don't let the clock determine what your meal should include. There's nothing wrong with having cereal for dinner if that's what you feel like.

My major struggle with the clock is trying to determine what to make for dinner when it's only 8:00 in the morning. How do I know what I'm really going to feel like having at 6:00 that night? Yet, as an ENFJ, I feel it necessary to plan ahead. I sometimes envy Sensors and Perceivers who feel comfortable leaving that decision until they're hungry. Then, whatever they select will probably reflect what they really are in the mood for. Of course, Sensors and Perceivers run a much higher risk of grabbing something that's merely convenient because they haven't left enough time to prepare a dish. An acceptable compromise to me is cooking various meals ahead of time to be packaged and put in the freezer. Then I can make a selection closer to dinner time and defrost it in the microwave oven.

Food Selection—by Consensus

"I'll have what he's having." For many of us who can't decide what to have, having what someone else is having is the easiest

TABLE 24. **Meal Planning**

Type of Dish	Type of Cuisine	Protein	Starch	Vegetable
Casserole	American, Cajun, Tex-Mex	Beef	Rice	Leafy green
Soup	Asian: Chinese, Japanese, Korean, Thai	Poultry	Pasta	Winter squash
Stew	European: Italian, French, German, Spanish, Greek	Fish	Legumes & Dried beans	Summer squash
Entree and side dishes	Middle Eastern: Indian, Persian, Moroccan	Pork	Unusual grains (couscous, bulghur, quinoa)	Yellow, orange, or red (e.g., onions, carrots, tomatoes)
Stir-fry (can be used for all types of cuisine)	Slavic: Russian, Hungarian, Polish	Lamb	Asian noodles	Green (e.g., cabbage, broccoli, celery)
Salad	Mexican	Tofu	Bread	Etc.
		Dairy, Eggs	Potatoes: russet, yams	

decision. The selection could be prompted by wanting to stay in the same price range as others (Thinking preference), or by not wanting to look different (Introverting and Feeling preferences). Group pressure, however subtle, can affect some people. Ordering Chinese food, where everyone shares, can be especially difficult for some. The Feelers believe the nice thing to do is order something everyone else wants even if it really isn't their favorite choice.

Have you ever noticed those who look over other patrons' plates as they are being seated at a restaurant, trying to get an idea of what looks good? They are probably Sensors. For the iNtuitives, the description on the menu may be sufficient to help them imagine what a dish will be like, while Sensors would usually rather see it, even taste it before committing themselves.

The Final Food Selection Decision

If you were to examine your own food selection process, you'd find that many or all of the above-mentioned factors are involved. They are influencers but not determiners. How your personality type deals with them will result in an eating decision. Sensors will probably be swayed by the flavor, Thinkers and Judgers by the numbers (nutrient and price), _S_Ps by impulse and convenience, Judgers by the clock, Extraverts and iNtuitives by variety, and Extraverts and Feelers by consensus. However, all preferences should have their say in the matter. There is no one right answer. Always keep in mind that whatever you choose to eat must fit into your daily nutrient needs.

The Dieter's Decision

The Meal Plans for losing weight I've presented are lifetime eating plans. You get to select the foods you want and eat them when you want. You can be anywhere and find food that works with your Plan. You don't have to panic because you forgot to bring your "special" food with you. Once you find what works for you, you no longer have to make major decisions. Your new healthier way of eating will become a habit. Then you can just allow your body to do its thing, finding its natural weight.

With that said, you still may be enticed by the many diet plans and schemes on the market. Have you seen the plan that promises "you can lose 10 pounds in one week"? That instant gratification will certainly appeal to the _S_Ps. However, even if you were to lose 10 pounds (probably mostly water loss), you wouldn't be able to keep it off.

There are other approaches that offer you a "no-thinking, no-need-to-plan" approach, such as drinking a liquid meal replacement for breakfast and lunch and having a sensible dinner. Perceivers are first in line for this one, appreciating not having to plan ahead. This approach also appeals to Sensors because it's simple. But while it appears that all the nutritional numbers have been worked out for you, a drink in a can cannot contain all the nutrients you'll find in whole foods. More to the point, following this kind of diet plan isn't learning how to eat for a lifetime.

Introverts and Sensors may be willing to try the "one-food plan" such as grapefruit or cabbage soup, not being bothered by its boredom. Yet the only reason they may lose weight is because it's very low in calories. The iNtuitives may try something like this because it seems novel, but they won't stick to it for long. The major problem with this lack of variety is that it is nutritionally inadequate.

The "high/low nutrient plans," such as high-carbohydrate/low-fat and high-protein/low-carbohydrate diets still have the Thinkers scratching their heads. Without there being enough proof yet as to which is the optimum plan, they're still in a wait-and-see mode. Both types of plans have their pros and cons. The Feelers and Extraverts have bought into these plans because their friends have tried them and it's the latest rage. With food manufacturers making foods according to a specific diet plan, you'll find Sensors and Judgers buying. The guesswork and nutrient calculations have been removed and structure has been provided.

It's ironic that dieters spend so much time looking for *the* big secret, when eating normally is all you need to do. It doesn't take anything special to reach a healthy weight. You don't have to be perfect every day. By the end of the week you should have averaged out the days you ate more than your nutrient allowance and those days you ate less.

General Eating Tips

- Don't skip breakfast. By breakfast time, it's been many hours since you had dinner or an evening snack. Your liver can only store so much glycogen for energy. By breakfast, it's time to replenish those glycogen stores.
- You may find that "grazing"—dividing your daily calorie allowance among three meals and two snacks—works best for you.
- Focus your attention on foods you know are nutritious and good for you, instead of constantly thinking about the not-so-healthy foods you think you're missing.
- Concentrate on the *process* of eating healthfully, rather than on the *outcome* of eating healthfully. The results will speak for themselves. When you focus on the outcome, it can cause undue stress when the results aren't as immediate as you would like. *(Sensors, living in the present, will do this naturally, noting accomplishments rather than failures. Perceivers can live with this idea, since the process is more fascinating to them anyway. Judgers and iNtuitives, on the other hand, are more inclined to be focused on future outcomes, with the iNtuitives worrying about whether they can achieve them.)*
- You don't have to be a perfectionist at every meal, trying to make sure that each food fulfills all the healthy guidelines. *(Are you _NT_s and _NF_s listening?)* If you eat a food that is high in fat, sugar, or salt, just balance it with foods that have less of those ingredients—whether at this meal or the next. If you don't get all your servings from each of the food groups in one day, try to make up for it the next.
- Have an arsenal of easy-to-fix, healthy meal ideas for those times when you're too rushed to think about it. *(_N_Js will probably be able to plan for future contingencies this way, whereas _S_Ps will find themselves in the same fix time after time because they're not real planners. Start leaning on your other preferences for help.)*

- Don't consider any food off-limits or forbidden (except for medical reasons).
- Eat without such distractions as television or a book. Focus on what you're doing—eating. You'll enjoy the meal more and run less risk of overeating.
- Keep healthy foods, such as fruits and vegetables, up front in your refrigerator as a reminder. Have them cleaned and ready to eat.

Snacking Isn't Bad for You

Contrary to the opinion of many people, snacking is not bad for you. In fact, it can be very good as long as you consider the snack food part of your daily calorie allowance. Snack foods are not "free" foods.

The major advantage to snacking is that it helps keep your blood sugar at a more consistent level, which, in turn, helps control your hunger level. Consider what you're going to feel like by 6:00 P.M., when you haven't eaten since noon. When you're overly hungry, who knows what you'll put in your mouth? Many of my clients have shared stories about their attack on the refrigerator the minute they walk in the door. It doesn't matter what they eat, as long as they can silence the growls and hunger pains. You may be answering the natural call of hunger, but in most cases, it's not a healthy answer.

If you have an afternoon snack of crackers, pretzels, fruit, or something light but satisfying, you can easily make it until dinner. The same holds true for midmorning snacks. Most important, the decisions about what you eat at the main meal will be more controlled and conscious, rather than merely a reaction to being famished. Remember, the best decisions are proactive, not reactive.

Snack Tips

- Keep healthy snacks visible and convenient. The higher-calorie, higher-fat snacks are best kept in a place that requires some effort to retrieve.

- Many crackers and cookies are now available in bite-size portions. They make you feel as if you're getting more that way.
- Don't eat directly out of the box. Measure out a serving—better yet, measure out half a serving. Just because the food manufacturers have stated a serving size, they don't know how hungry you really are.
- *Healthy carbohydrate snacks:* Seasoned Popcorn (See Recipes, page 343), baked tortilla, or potato chips, fat-free or low-fat crackers and cookies.
- *Healthy fruit snacks:* Fresh fruit, fruit leather, fruit sorbet.
- *Healthy vegetable snacks:* Carrot and celery sticks, flowerettes from cauliflower or broccoli, raw green beans. If you want to add a little interest to the vegetables, try dipping them into salsa or a Dill Dip (See Recipes, page 340.)
- *Healthy cheese snacks:* String cheese, goat cheese on crackers, low-fat cream cheese (Neufchatel) on crackers or bagel, low-fat cottage cheese on bread sprinkled with cinnamon and sugar and broiled.
- *Healthy liquid snacks:* Fruit juice (freshly squeezed, frozen, or bottled), vegetable juice, Fruit Yogurt Shake (See Recipes, page 341), Mocha Shake (See Recipes, page 342.)

Eating Out

Between 1994 and 1995, according to a USDA nationwide food consumption survey, *What We Eat in America,* 57 percent of Americans ate some meals or snacks away from home. This accounted for at least 50 percent of their calorie and fat intake. You may not appreciate how many times you eat out. It's not just limited to sitting down in a restaurant. How about the snack you had at the mall, the quick pick-me-up from the vending machine at work, the hors d'oeuvres at your friend's party, the popcorn at the theater? Each of these eating experiences can be more challenging than eating at home. At home you have more control over the foods available to you, especially if you do the grocery shopping. When you eat away from home, your choices are often more limited. Yet eating out doesn't have to destroy your good intentions. It's just a matter of making good decisions based on everything you are learning in this book. You need to have a plan on how to handle each eating opportunity.

Eating at a full-service restaurant gives you the chance to "have it your way." Ask the waiter how foods are prepared and whether a dish can be prepared by a lower-fat method. At cafeterias, smorgasbords, and buffets, there is a wide variety of foods; while you have little control over the preparation, you have loads of control over the quantity (even if "all you can eat" sounds like too good a deal to pass up!). You could set a limit on the number of dishes you choose and allow yourself only one pass through the line. Fast-food restaurants are now offering more variety, but recently they seem to be scaling back on the healthier choices. Stick to the regular-size options rather than the extra larges (or extra cheese, bacon, or sauce). If you're having a chicken sandwich that's fried, remove some of the breading if you can. Order it without dressing to lower the fat content.

Questions to Ask Yourself

- Do I eat more when I dine out?
- When I order something, do I know whether it's a healthy choice?
- Am I willing to ask the waiter how something is made or request that a change be made to the way a dish is prepared?
- What types of cuisine (Mexican, Chinese, Japanese, French, German, Italian, Middle Eastern, Russian, etc.) do I enjoy the most? Do they tend to be high in fat? Are there lower-fat options?
- For a typical lunch or dinner out, what foods do I think are the largest contributors of fat?
- When I've eaten out and had an appetizer, salad, and bread, have I felt full even before the main course was served? Do I eat everything anyway?
- Do the choices my friends make influence me?
- Do I have dessert because others are having it, or do I truly want it?
- Have I gone to a restaurant before, read their menu, and found nothing that appealed to me? If so, did I still order

a meal hoping it would satisfy me? Would I feel guilty getting up from the table and not ordering at all?

Eating Out Tips

- Enjoy the bread, but go easy on the butter.
- Order dressing, sauces, and gravy on the side. Then dip your fork into the dressing before going for the lettuce leaves; dip your fork into the gravy before stabbing the meat. You'll end up with a lot less of the topping than if you either have the dressing or gravy poured over the top or you take the food and dip it into the sauce.
- Consider ordering an appetizer as your meal, along with a salad. You won't feel forced to eat more than you really want.
- Ask your waiter if you can have your vegetables steamed without butter.
- If something comes fried, ask if it can be broiled instead.
- Ask for a doggy bag before you start your meal. Put half your meal in the container immediately to avoid eating too much and guarantee yourself another meal for the same price. *(You iNtuitives and Thinkers should like this.)*
- Enjoy dessert if you like, but share it with a friend. *(This works for you Thinkers because it is logical, and for you Feelers who feel it's just being considerate.)*
- Order a cup of soup rather than a bowl.
- *Healthy menu choices:* Au jus, baked, barbecued, boiled, broiled, charbroiled, cooked in its own juice, en brochette, garden fresh, grilled, marinated, poached, roasted, smoked, steamed, stir-fried.
- *Not-so-healthy choices:* Au gratin, basted, béarnaise, beurre blanc, breaded and fried, buttered, buttery, casserole, creamed, crispy, escalloped, fried, hash, hollandaise, in butter sauce, in cream sauce, marinated in oil, pan-fried, parmesan, pot pie, prime, sautéed, stewed, stuffed.
- Consider ordering one course at a time to determine when you are reaching a satisfied level. If you're ravenous when you order, you're likely to order more than you really need.

MENU
Appetizers
Crispy Nachos - Corn tortillas smothered in melted Cheddar cheese, served with guacamole and sour cream
Buffalo Style Chicken Wings - Juicy chicken wings smothered in a spicy sauce, served with celery and blue cheese
Fried Mozzarella - Sticks of Mozzarella cheese, battered, fried and served with Marinara sauce
Shrimp Cocktail - Baby shrimp served on a bed of lettuce with our special cocktail sauce
Fresh Fruit Medley - Fresh seasonal fruit served in a pineapple boat
Fried Won Tons - Crispy won tons served with sweet and sour sauce
Soups and Salads
Split Pea Soup - Hearty pea soup just like your mom's, served with sour cream and a warm roll.
Caesar Salad - Fresh-cut romaine lettuce tossed with Romano cheese, croutons, lemon juice and olive oil.
Gazpacho - A refreshing blend of tomatoes, cucumbers, bell peppers, and celery, served chilled
Spinach Salad - Crispy spinach leaves topped with a warm sweet and sour bacon dressing.
New England Clam Chowder - A creamy chowder chock full of clams and fresh vegetables
Fresh Garden Greens - A mix of fresh organic greens served with a raspberry vinaigrette dressing
Entrees
Pastas
Pasta Primavera - Delicate angel hair pasta tossed with grilled fresh vegetables, a touch of olive oil and a sprinkling of Parmesan
Fettuccini Alfredo - Ribbons of fettuccini cloaked in a rich, creamy and cheesy white sauce
Chicken, Beef and Pork
Game Hen - A tender, young bird seasoned with rosemary and served with roasted potatoes and steamed vegetables.
New York Cut Steak - Center cut, premium-aged to perfection. Grilled to your liking. Served with baked potato
Pork Calvados - Tenderloin of pork, roasted with onions, apples and a touch of apple brandy. Served with roasted potatoes.
Veal Parmigiana - A tender veal cutlet, breaded, fried and topped with Marinara sauce and bubbly Mozzarella cheese. Served with buttered spaghetti.
Seafood
Fresh Salmon - Grilled salmon steak topped with sun-dried tomato and basil butter. Served on a bed of rice pilaf.
Fish and Chips - Fresh filet of sole, dipped in a beer batter and fried. Served with English style fried potatoes.
Desserts
Mud Pie - Rich coffee ice cream on a chocolate cookie crust and topped with chocolate sauce and whipped cream
Key Lime Pie - Lime pie on a graham crust, topped with meringue swirls, surrounded by a raspberry sauce
Chocolate Raspberry Cake - Rich dark chocolate cake with raspberry filling, cloaked in dark chocolate.
Fresh Seasonal Fruit - Served in a toasted almond lace basket
Fresh Fruit Sorbets - Assorted flavors

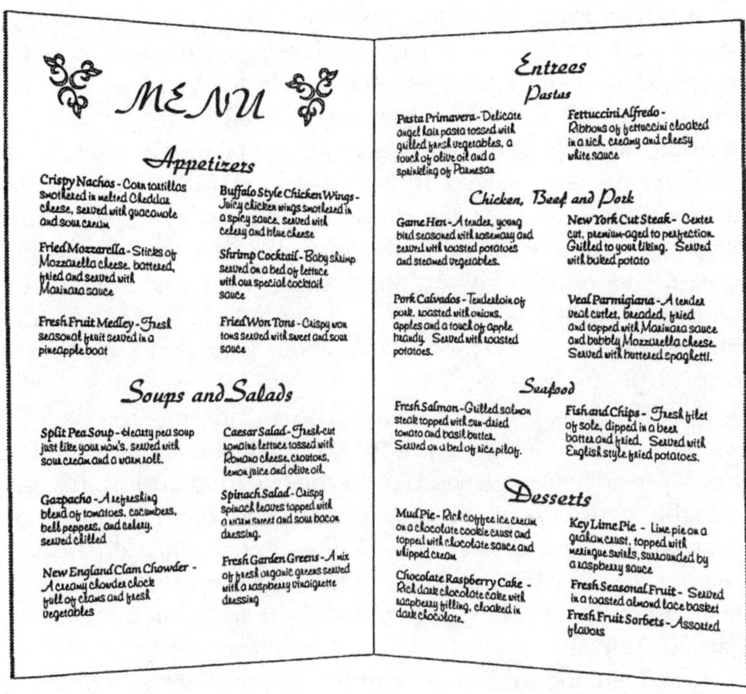

Figure 26. Dinner Menu

- Be adventurous and try new foods, since at home you probably stick with the old standbys.
- When you order, think in terms of the five food groups of the Food Guide Pyramid.

Your Turn—Decision Time

It's time for you to start practicing making some decisions. Call it your final exam. You've learned a great deal so far, and I want to see if you can apply it. So pretend that you've gone out to dinner with some friends. You've been presented with the dinner menu in Figure 26.

What would you order? Use the decision-making process you learned in Chapter 5. The following description is the optimal

Z pattern of decision-making. I want to share some of the things you should consider with each preference. However, to make the decision-making process comfortable for you, you can use your own type's 1–2–3–4 order, if you'd like.

Your **Sensing preference** should be taking a reading of whether you are hungry. It should also provide you with the nutrition facts we discussed earlier, what your Meal Plan is, the flavors you are looking for at the moment, and what you believe to be the amount of fat and other major nutrients in the menu selection (you'll have to use your imagination, since you can't ask the waiter in this case). Think about your past experiences in this type of situation.

Your **iNtuiting preference** should be considering how the various selections on the menu fit into your Meal Plan and whether they'll provide you with foods from the five food groups. It's also probably considering the choices in terms of what might be eaten later, such as dessert. Your iNtuiting preference also notices whether there's a pattern forming here. Are you always choosing beef dishes or avoiding vegetables? Is there something to be learned from that?

Your **Thinking preference** should take the information from the Sensing and iNtuiting preferences and analyze the consequences of the possible selections. Keep in mind the rules of healthy eating. If you eat these foods, will it put you over your nutrient allowances? What is the cost/benefit ratio? From the perspective of the Thinking preference, will you be getting adequate nutrition for the price you're paying for this meal? I appreciate that the Thinking preference is very good at dictating "shoulds," "oughts," and "musts," but don't let it become a dictator. Be thankful that your Feeling preference can balance out these "shoulds" with "wants" and "desires."

Your **Feeling preference** wants to know if you feel comfortable with the choices. Do you think the flavors will bring you pleasure and satisfaction? Will this meal bring enough pleasure for what it is costing from your fat allowance? What influence are your friends going to have on your decision? Will you go along with the crowd?

Don't order until each preference has been heard from. Don't automatically reject anything that is high in fat just because you think that is what you're supposed to do. As you read over the menu, be honest with yourself as to what sounds good and why you think you should order it.

Keep in mind that whether you are an Extravert or Introvert, or a Judger or Perceiver, these preferences are going to influence your decision-making process. As an Extravert, you may be swayed by the others at the table. What are they having? How much are they having? As an Introvert, you will probably be more concerned with your own needs, how hungry you are. You would be more inclined to stick to a plan if you had one.

As a Judger, you have probably accepted the Meal Plan as a workable structure and might even be willing to keep track of the amount of fat and calories you eat. There's a sense of organization to it. The log that accompanies the Meal Plan serves as a partial driving force for you to make choices that fit into it. On the other hand, if you are a Perceiver, you might be less inclined to make selections based on the log. You believe that dining out should be fun, an opportunity to try new things.

If you're struggling with your decision, find others of the opposite type and ask them what they would do. Maybe they can provide another viewpoint you hadn't considered. In the previous chapter, I showed you how each type would use its 1–2–3–4 order to decide whether to eat or not. A similar approach would apply to deciding what to eat. If you need to, refer back to Chapter 5 as a reminder of how your type should handle making decisions. Apply that here.

Answers to Quiz (pages 174–176)

1. b
2. c
3. d
4. b
5. a
6. b
7. b
8. c
9. a
10. d
11. b
12. a
13. d
14. b
15. a
16. a
17. d
18. c

9

Making It a Habit #4: Know When Enough Is Enough

People are very inventive when it comes to making up reasons for eating when they're not hungry. They're just as creative about why they're breaking the rule of eating only until "satisfied":

1. "It smelled so good, I couldn't resist."
2. "It tasted so good, I couldn't stop."
3. "I paid for it, so I'm going to get my money's worth."
4. "I have the clean plate habit."
5. "With all the conversation going on, I really wasn't aware of how much I was eating."
6. "My mother taught me that if I didn't finish my dinner, I couldn't have dessert. Now I eat everything just so I can have dessert."
7. "I know I eat too fast. I'm rarely aware that I've eaten too much until I'm stuffed."
8. "I don't want to have leftovers, because they never taste as good as when the dish is fresh."
9. "I may never get this dish again, so I better eat up now."
10. "As I'm transferring leftovers into a storage container, I sometimes find the container isn't quite big enough. In order not to get another container dirty, I'll just eat the little bit that's left."
11. "I'm eating this dessert to leave a good taste in my mouth."

12. "She was so kind to make this for me. I don't want to hurt her feelings by not finishing it."
13. "Whenever we go for Chinese food, I always seem to eat too much. I'm afraid that if I don't put enough on my plate when the dish is passed to me, there may not be any left if I want more."
14. "I know I shouldn't be eating this, but since I've already blown it, I might as well really enjoy myself."
15. "My mother always told me that I should be grateful for the food we have, considering all the starving children in the world. So I learned to finish everything for them."
16. "The only way I know the meal is over is when I feel stuffed."
17. "If I don't eat it all, it'll be thrown away, which is very wasteful."
18. "I'll just exercise tomorrow to make up for eating too much tonight."
19. "I can't believe the size of the portions they serve."
20. "Nothing you say is going to stop me."
21. "When food is served 'family style,' with the serving dishes on the table, it's so easy to have more than I need."
22. "I'm too embarrassed to ask for a doggie bag, so I just eat everything on my plate."
23. "Give me a buffet or smorgasbord and my eyes have no limit. Only when I've tried one of everything, and had seconds of the really good dishes, is it time to quit."
24. "If someone says, 'Help me finish this,' I feel bad if I don't help them out."
25. "Other people are still eating."

The Personality Element

Let's review these statements again and see the personality preferences at work. It's normally one or two preferences that create habitual responses like these and, in most cases, it's due to the dominant or backup preference. Maybe you've made comments like these, so for each one I have included a "Try this instead" section, a way to use other preferences in your type to get a healthier result. Then you'll have more power to reconsider your decision about eating beyond what your body wants or needs.

1. "It smelled so good, I couldn't resist."
   - *What's going on here?* There are certain smells, like baking or barbecuing, that many people find irresistible. The Sensing preference stores the memories of the pleasure those smells previously brought; the aromas themselves can even stimulate the production of gastric juices, encouraging your appetite.
   - *Try this instead:* You are obviously in the present, which is where you need to be when it comes to eating. But considering that you're already full, you're allowing your external sensors, not your inner barometer, to guide you. Time for some consequential thinking from your Thinking preference. Enjoy the smell, but move on. Eating now would only mean extra calories you don't need. Your iNtuiting preference could come up with ideas for how you can enjoy the food later. What about buying it now, having it wrapped up tightly so roaming fingers can't get in, and save it for when you're really hungry and can appreciate it more?
2. "It tasted so good, I couldn't stop."
   - *What's going on here?* While this person is very much in tune with his Sensing preference ("It tasted so good"), his iNtuiting preference is pushing him to eat more. The thought that the pleasure of this great taste can continue is a "future" thought, not one in the here-and-now.
   - *Try this instead:* Let your Sensing preference take a fullness reading. Be honest with yourself through your Feeling preference and listen to your Thinking preference when it tells you where "more" is going to lead you. Use your iNtuiting preference in a more positive manner to determine how you might put away any extra food for later.
3. "I paid for it, so I'm going to get my money's worth."
   - *What's going on here?* On the surface, this appears very logical. One shouldn't pay hard-earned money on a

meal and then waste it. Yet there is a Feeling component to this statement that is silently saying, "It's mine, and you aren't going to take it away. The only way I can make sure of that is to eat it."

- *Try this instead:* Use your Thinking and iNtuiting preferences to extend your logical economic perspective. Consider taking the extra food home in a doggie bag and having another meal from it. Now that's getting your money's worth and more.

4. "I have the clean plate habit."
   - *What's going on here?* The Sensing preference was trained by the Feeling preference as you were growing up. Your parents might have made you feel guilty about not eating everything on your plate, or you might have been forced to sit at the table until everything was eaten. Your parents probably meant well by thinking it would help you grow up healthy. Now a plate with food left on it brings back those memories, continuing to promote the habit even when you're full.
   - *Try this instead:* I'm sure you'll get tired of my saying this, but you must use your Thinking preference to consider the consequences of overeating—namely, the extra calories that are going to be put away into storage. Your iNtuiting preference should be working on ways to *avoid* cleaning your plate. Try serving only as much food as will fit on half a plate (and no piling on!). Then, midway through the meal, take a fullness reading. Not hungry anymore? Then remove the plate from the table. Return with a glass of water, cup of coffee, or cup of tea, and slowly sip it if the urge comes over you to bring the plate back.
5. "With all the conversation going on, I really wasn't aware of how much I was eating."
   - *What's going on here?* The Extravert's energy is focused on the socializing, so it's not surprising that the conversation was almost more important than the food. Also, eating with others normally extends the length of a meal, giving time to eat more.
   - *Try this instead:* Use your Sensing preference to focus

on your fullness level. If you're a Judger, try to provide some structure to the meal by taking a fullness reading every so often throughout the meal.

6. "My mother taught me that if I didn't finish my dinner, I couldn't have dessert. Now I eat everything just so I can have dessert."
   - *What's going on here?* Though this *sounds* like consequential thinking ("If you eat your dinner, you get dessert") it's really more a case of personal values set by the Feeling preference. It is saying "You've earned your dessert by eating all your dinner. You've been good." The Sensing preference maintains a history of past experiences and continues to dredge them up as a way of justifying your actions.
   - *Try this instead:* You can use your Thinking preference to explain the illogic of that statement, since the rule is *Don't eat past "satisfied."* Of course, it means your Sensing preference needs to concentrate on your fullness level. You could use your iNtuiting and Judging preferences to plan ahead. If you really want a particular dessert, plan ahead by adjusting the amount of food you eat during the meal. (Be careful that this doesn't become an everyday habit, though, or you'll be getting your calories from less nutritious foods.)
7. "I know I eat too fast. I'm rarely aware that I've eaten too much until I'm stuffed."
   - *What's going on here?* The Extravert probably eats so fast because the food actually gets in the way of talking. The iNtuitive might eat fast just so he or she can move on to other things.
   - *Try this instead:* This is definitely a job for your Sensing preference, which has to stay aware of your actions. Meanwhile, your Thinking preference can be telling you where your usual gobble-it-up habit is going to lead you. If you're a Judger, you might consider providing some structure by putting your fork down between bites to slow down the process.
8. "I don't want to have leftovers, because they never taste as good as when the dish is fresh."

- *What's going on here?* This person is using her Feeling preference to pass judgment on leftovers. Her Sensing preference remembers the pot roast from last week that was reheated and became so tough it was impossible to eat. Then there was that chocolate pudding that started separating after a day or so in the refrigerator.
- *Try this instead:* The iNtuiting preference can look at your track record of leftovers and realize there is a pattern there. Maybe every time you make pasta, you make a big pot of it instead of just the required number of servings. Think about what you can change. For example, when you make a recipe, try halving it. Couples whose children no longer live at home are especially vulnerable to cooking too much until they rethink their approach. If you have children who live away from home, you can always send leftovers home with them. They'll love you for it—and so will your body.

9. "I may never get this dish again, so I better eat up now."
   - *What's going on here?* Just as this gets the iNtuitive to eat something when she isn't hungry, it also keeps her eating beyond being "satisfied." Of course, the ridiculous part is the idea that anyone can "fill up" for a lifetime in just one sitting. Is she going to remember the taste any more strongly because she stuffed herself?
   - *Try this instead:* Apply your Thinking preference to explain how illogical it is to believe you can fill up for a lifetime at one sitting. Let your Sensing preference really savor the flavors, putting your full and undivided attention on the food to lock the pleasurable experience away in your memory. At the same time, don't lose awareness of when your body has had enough. Your Feeling preference should tell you that it is being unkind to yourself to overdo it.
10. "As I'm transferring leftovers into a storage container, I sometimes find the container isn't quite big enough. In order not to get another container dirty, I'll just eat the little bit that's left."
    - *What's going on here?* The Sensing preference is seemingly being practical and realistic—why clean another

dish for the sake of a couple of bites? Of course, the problem is that you're eating more than your body really wants or needs.

- *Try this instead:* The Thinking preference can explain to you the pros and cons of having a dirty container versus eating extra calories your body doesn't need. Cleaning the container may mean a little extra effort, but not as much effort as it would take for you to burn off the unnecessary calories.

11. "I'm eating this dessert to leave a good taste in my mouth."
    - *What's going on here?* What an excuse to have dessert! You'd think that if this person really enjoyed the meal, that in itself would leave the good taste. Yet if you grew up in a family where a meal wasn't over until you had dessert, it's understandable why you have the habit. Obviously, Sensing is a strong preference here, but it is the Feeling preference that's putting a value judgment on the need for something sweet and disguising it as a logical statement.
    - *Try this instead:* Let your iNtuiting preference come up with some options for you. You could just brush your teeth, which would solve the problem with a lot fewer calories! (That is something the Thinking preference could see.) A breath mint would also do the trick. If you want chocolate cake, be honest with yourself, but try to determine how you can fit it into your daily calorie or fat allowance. Something else must be eliminated (preferably not the nutritious foods). Just be careful not to do this on a regular basis.
12. "She was so kind to make this for me. I don't want to hurt her feelings by not finishing it."
    - *What's going on here?* Wanting to please others is often at the root of the Feeler's weight and eating problems. A Thinker might not eat any if she felt it didn't fit into her diet. At best, she might figure that one or two bites should logically show that she appreciated her friend's efforts. Yet the Feeler believes that leaving anything on the plate shows a lack of gratitude and enjoyment.
    - *Try this instead:* You need to call up the efforts of your

iNtuiting preference to consider ways to handle this situation that will still allow the Feeling preference to be heard. Ask your friend if she wouldn't mind your taking the food home with you to enjoy later when you're hungrier. Tell her that that way, you get to prolong the enjoyment. Ask for the recipe from her so that she really knows you liked it but are too full right now to finish it.

13. "Whenever we go for Chinese food, I always seem to eat too much. I'm afraid if I don't put enough on my plate when the dish is passed to me, there may not be any left if I want more."
    - *What's going on here?* Chinese dining, where everyone shares the dishes, is plan-ahead eating, something the iNtuiting and Judging preferences are good at. As you eye the dishes, you worry that you'll miss out on something if you wait or if you don't take enough on the first pass. There's a bit of a selfish and protective attitude coming from the Feeling preference.
    - *Try this instead:* You could use your Thinking preference to assure yourself that if you want more of a certain dish, you can always order it. (Of course, the Thinking preference will also be considering the cost of ordering another dish.) Perceivers will appreciate the variety of the Chinese meal, but it can also be their undoing. Just let your Thinking preference guide you in sampling, rather than overindulging in, each dish. Judgers will be eyeballing how much space each dish will take up on their plate to determine how much they can take from each dish. Don't forget to keep your Sensing preference alert for how much *your body* needs, versus how much *your plate* looks as if it needs.
14. "I know I shouldn't be eating this, but since I've already blown it, I might as well really enjoy myself."
    - *What's going on here?* Once guilt has set in, you figure you might as well "really enjoy yourself." There is an unspoken hope from the Feeling preference that burying yourself in the food now will take away the guilt for the time being. It may; but it doesn't last long.

- *Try this instead:* If you allow your Thinking preference a chance here, it can put you straight with some rational thinking. Whatever it is you've already eaten, you've stamped as "forbidden fruit" with your Feeling preference. Inevitably you are going to feel guilty. One rule you should take away from this book is that all foods are allowed (unless you are medically advised otherwise). If you can accept that, then logically you should see that you didn't blow anything. You allowed yourself an indulgence. Keep in mind, though, that you don't have to eat the whole thing to get pleasure from it.

15. "My mother always told me that I should be grateful for the food we have, considering all the starving children in the world. So I learned to finish everything for them."
    - *What's going on here?* Talk about the royal guilt trip parents put their children through, using their Feeling preference. Well-meaning parents say these things as a way of coaxing their children into eating what they believe is a healthy meal. But, it sets up a habit that's very hard to break. It's "the clean-plate" habit with emotional baggage.
    - *Try this instead:* See suggestions in #4. Also, appreciate that you're using your Sensing preference to keep dredging up the past. It's time to change the tape recording you hear in your head. Your Thinking preference can logically explain to you that eating more food than you really need is no way to make up for what starving children don't have. Give to children's charities instead.
16. "The only way I know the meal is over is when I feel stuffed."
    - *What's going on here?* Always open to more experiences, the Perceiving preference allows eating to continue until the stomach is so distended and uncomfortable that it becomes blatantly obvious the meal must come to an end. The iNtuiting preference doesn't help, since its attention is somewhere besides the present.
    - *Try this instead:* By now you can probably answer this one yourself. Your Sensing preference must keep you

grounded in the present so you can focus on your level of fullness. Keep all distractions to a minimum so you can begin to learn what "satisfied" feels like.

17. "If I don't eat it all, it'll be thrown away, which is very wasteful."
    - *What's going on here?* For the Thinker, this is consequential thinking and logical analysis at work. Being wasteful is seen in terms of dollars and cents. The Feeler might say the same thing but assign a personal value to it. This preference will see the emotional effect of wastefulness in terms of hunger in the world or destruction to the environment (for having produced something that won't be eaten).
    - *Try this instead:* This one's easy. Let your iNtuiting preference figure out how to make another meal from these leftovers. You might even be imagining another way to present it so it seems like something different.
18. "I'll just exercise tomorrow to make up for eating too much tonight."
    - *What's going on here?* This is put-off-until-tomorrow-what-you-would-rather-not-do-today thinking (very typical of Perceivers and often iNtuitives). From the Thinking preference's perspective, it sounds like a logical and good idea to use exercise as a balancing mechanism for overeating (not on a regular basis, though). The problem is that when tomorrow comes, something will come up that makes exercise impossible to do (the Perceiver at work again). "Whoops. Oh well, then, maybe the day after."
    - *Try this instead:* The Sensing preference is there to help you to take fullness readings along the way. If you did this diligently, you wouldn't have to be finding a way to burn off what your body didn't need in the first place. Your Feeling preference would be happier as well, since then it can feel it's in control.
19. "I can't believe the size of the portions they serve."
    - *What's going on here?* Blame is being laid elsewhere by the Feeling preference. "The reason I overate is because they served portions that were too large." It's as if all

control has been taken away from you (though, in fact, you are the only one in control of what you eat).

- *Try this instead:* Use your Thinking preference to compare the amount you would normally eat with the amount served. Okay, so it's too much. Now what? Put your iNtuiting preference to work. You could ask for a doggie bag before you even start eating and leave only the amount on your plate that you think will be enough.

20. "Nothing you say is going to stop me."
    - *What's going on here?* This person is grappling for control through her Feeling preference, and to prove it, will even sabotage herself. There is no concern for her level of fullness because the objective is to do the opposite of what has been asked of her.
    - *Try this instead:* Time to call in your Thinking preference and analyze who is being hurt by your actions. Did you check with your Sensing preference to see how full you are? Someone has advised you that he thinks you've had enough. Instead of becoming possessive of what you're eating, take a moment to use your Feeling preference to appreciate that someone cares about you.
21. "When food is served 'family style,' with the serving dishes on the table, it's so easy to have more than I need."
    - *What's going on here?* "Family style" means everything is sitting right there on the table for you to see and activate your Sensing preference. If you're enjoying the flavors, the Perceiving and Feeling preferences support you in having more. This same type of problem occurs when you leave a cookie jar out on the counter or store food in transparent containers.
    - *Try this instead:* This method of serving is just asking for trouble. Your Thinking preference, with the help of your iNtuiting preference, will tell you that the most logical thing to do is serve your food from the stove and then sit down. Why put temptation in your path?
22. "I'm too embarrassed to ask for a doggie bag, so I just eat everything on my plate."
    - *What's going on here?* Your Feeling preference just assigned a value to asking for a doggie bag: it's embar-

rassing. It's worried what other people will think. If you ask for a doggie bag, does it look to others as though you're so financially strapped or cheap you can't afford to just leave it and let the waiter take the extra away?

- *Try this instead:* I know it's hard to use logic when you're dealing with your feelings. However, let your Thinking preference have a shot at this. It just doesn't make any sense to sabotage your efforts at a healthy lifestyle because you're concerned about what other people will think. Who's getting hurt here? Who are these people that they should have such power over you? If you're really too embarrassed to ask for a doggie bag, let the waiter take away your half-eaten plate of food. The cost of the uneaten food is far less than the cost to your body of eating it.

23. "Give me a buffet or smorgasbord, and my eyes have no limit. Only when I've tried one of everything and had seconds of the really good dishes is it time to quit."
    - *What's going on here?* This is obviously a statement by your Sensing preference. The variety part comes from the Perceiving and Extraverting preferences. The Feeling preference is thinking, "I can have all I want. No limits to the number of times I can go back to the buffet." The Thinking preference is considering how little is being paid for so much food.
    - *Try this instead:* Buffets and smorgasbords require a strategy that uses your iNtuiting preference. You could make a deal with yourself before you go that you may try a limit of five different dishes. Or you could serve yourself only one tablespoon of as many foods as you want, as long as no food touches another on your plate. The Thinking preference could try to analyze what it thinks are the ingredients of the dishes and what that means in terms of calories and fat. Any dish made with mayonnaise, cream, or butter is obviously going to be high-fat and high-calorie. On the other hand, food served as close to its natural state as possible, such as vegetables and grains, is less likely to take too big a bite out of your daily calorie allowance.

24. "If someone says, 'Help me finish this,' I feel bad if I don't help them out."
    - *What's going on here?* Not wanting to appear insensitive to someone's needs, your Feeling preference does as it's asked. No thought is given to your own personal needs when someone else requires help.
    - *Try this instead:* The Thinking preference can tell you how illogical it is for you to be eating when you're full just so you can make someone else feel better. Once you've accepted this, you can go back to your Feeling preference to find a diplomatic and caring way to tell your friend why you can't eat any more.
25. "Other people are still eating."
    - *What's going on here?* If others are still eating, that serves as a stimulus to the Extravert. Add the Feeling preference, and you've got someone who wouldn't want someone else to feel uncomfortable about eating alone.
    - *Try this instead:* There's no question you must tune into your Sensing preference and know whether you've had enough to eat. Then the iNtuiting preference can offer up a suggestion: once the "satisfied" stage has been reached and people are still eating—have a cup of coffee or tea. Let the cup take the place of the dinner plate right in front of you, so it seems as if you're still eating.

I hope that you can better see now how your personality preferences influence your decisions. When you apply all your preferences, working on those that aren't necessarily as strong, you can make healthy decisions. As I've said before, you're in the driver's seat. The decisions are yours to make. If you continue with your old way of doing things, don't expect different results, but don't admonish yourself for them. The fact that you're sticking with the old agenda means that, deep down, that really is the way you want to be.

How Do You Know When to Stop?

Recognizing when you're hungry is probably easier than recognizing when you have reached the "satisfied" stage. When you're hungry, your stomach may growl or transmit hunger pangs. It sends out red flags alerting you to the need for nourishment. The "satisfied" stage doesn't have the same red flag system. There are no bells and whistles going off in your body saying, "Don't send anymore down here. I've had exactly the right amount."

Is It Time to Stop When the Plate Is Empty?

There are a couple of problems with waiting until the plate is empty to say you're full. In one case, when you serve yourself, you have to fill your plate with what you think will be the exact amount to satisfy your hunger. Can you really size up your hunger so well as to know it will take one cup of pasta and ½ cup of vegetables and four ounces of meat to fill the void? When you're hungry, your eyes can be bigger than your stomach, so you may serve yourself more than you really need. Or might there be other reasons for putting the amount you do on a plate? My clients have mentioned the following factors as determining their portion size:

- "How much I like the food."
- "Whether or not it's a whole portion of something—like a potato or a muffin."
- "The size of the plate."
- "How much fat is in the food. I tend to be more liberal with low-fat foods."
- "What kind of day I've had."
- "Whether these are leftovers and I don't want to see them again."
- "Whether I want to have leftovers."
- "How much of the plate is showing."
- "What the label on the package says is a serving size."

Now suppose someone else is serving you. How do they know what the right amount is? Think about when you dine out. Customers would feel cheated being served a three-ounce steak and paying $16 for it. In order for restaurants to command the prices they do, they have to pretty much fill the plate. (That is, unless they're one of those exclusive restaurants that present a huge plate with a morsel of meat in the center, artistically set off with a drizzle of sauce and a sprig of herb, and then charge you $25 or more).

I would say that an empty plate is a poor sign of when enough is enough, even though that's what most people use as a guideline.

Serving Sizes

When the new food labeling went into effect in 1994, the Food and Drug Administration and United States Department of Agriculture required food manufacturers to list realistic serving sizes, not sizes that would make the nutrition numbers look good. Also, because serving sizes became standardized for similar foods, you could now compare one product against another. So do take advantage of that information.

But how well can you really judge the size of a serving? For some of you, especially the _S_Js, actual measuring is probably fine. On the other hand, _S_Ps would be happier with something more visual. So consider the list in Table 25 the next time you eat something:

TABLE 25. Serving-Size Visuals

One Serving	Looks Like
Meat (3 ounces)	Deck of cards
Ice cream, rice, pasta, or cereal (½ cup)	Tennis ball
Apple	Softball
Broccoli	Light bulb
Cheese (1 ounce)	4 dice
Jam or margarine (1 teaspoon)	4 quarters

If you've gone through the decision-making process and decided you don't want to measure or even consider the serving-size visuals, I recommend you serve your meals on a smaller plate (and no food touching or piled on another!). At least you run less risk of overeating that way.

Is There Something Physiological That Lets You Know When to Stop?

This might be easier to answer if you understood what happens to the food after it passes your lips. The process of digestion starts in the mouth. Chewing the food breaks it into smaller pieces. Once swallowed, the food moves down to the stomach, where it mixes with gastric juices. The composition of the food determines how long it remains in the stomach. The more protein, fat, and fiber, the longer it stays.

When the first bit of food leaves the stomach and enters the small intestine (about 20 minutes from when it is eaten—if the meal doesn't contain a great deal of fat), a special chemical is released. It slows down the emptying of the stomach, which in turn causes the stomach to enlarge. This distention, or stretching, of the muscles of the stomach serves as a message to the brain announcing that the "food has arrived, so you can now start sending out some fullness signals." I cannot emphasize enough how important it is that you eat slowly. If you eat all your meal in less than about 20 minutes, your brain hasn't yet received any messages to say you could have stopped six bites ago. You will inevitably eat more than your body really needs. If you eat slowly, and really focus on the sensations in your body, you will realize—within this 20-minute time-frame—that the sensation of hunger is gone. It's been replaced by the sense that you are no longer empty. Unfortunately, some people don't know how to recognize that no-longer-empty feeling. For them, only the Thanksgiving-stuffed stage says it's time to stop.

Remember, eat slowly. Then, within 20 minutes of starting to eat, put your fork down and take a fullness reading. (See the Fullness Gauge in Figure 27.) Think about what the levels of fullness would feel like to you. What are the sensations of "slightly full"? "very full"? "topping the tank"? Now compare those feelings with the sense of being "satisfied"—which, in a way, means experiencing no sensations associated with either fullness *or* hunger.

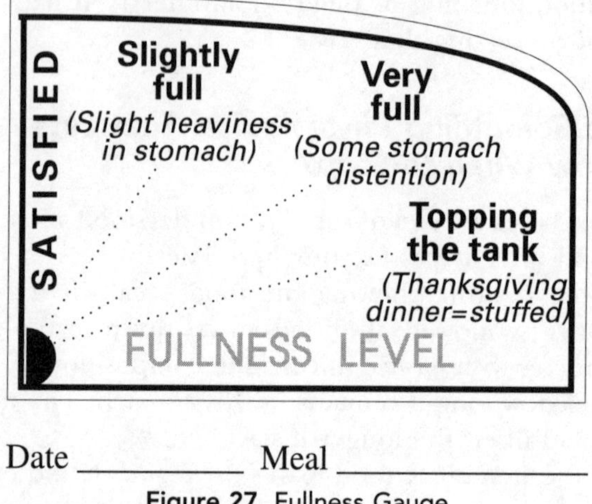

Date __________ Meal ______________

Figure 27. Fullness Gauge

Does Stopping Have Something to Do with Taste?

For some people that "satisfied" level comes when there's no more appeal to the food. However, this often has more to do with satiation of flavor or temperature than with a physical fullness. The taste receptors in your tongue and cheeks simply get bored. Even highly intense flavors can "short-out" your taste buds, not so much from boredom as fatigue; the taste receptors become too overwhelmed to taste anymore. (If you've ever tried hot chili peppers or tabasco sauce, you'll know what I'm talking about.)

Since taste is such an important component of eating, once your taste buds are no longer able to react to the presence of food, there is a sense of "I've had enough." Think about how little food it takes to satisfy you when you have a cold. With smell and taste so intricately entwined, your sense of taste diminishes when your nose is blocked, as does the quantity of food you eat.

Now think about a meal that has a variety of flavors, from salty to sweet, and a variety of temperatures and textures. Your taste buds aren't likely to get bored. On the contrary, they cry out for more. At this point, your radar should be up, trying its hardest to determine if you have reached "satisfied." Otherwise, you'll be at the Thanksgiving-stuffed stage before you know it.

Is the Time to Stop When You Have Eaten Your Required Number of Servings?

Many people appreciate being told what a normal serving size is, along with how many servings they should eat. Meal Plans give them a framework within which to work (which is especially appreciated by Judgers). At least it is a starting point and a way of avoiding overdoing it. Having determined your Meal Plan in the last chapter, you can assume that, give or take a couple of calories, your body needs that amount of food daily. If so, then let your body determine how that food should be distributed throughout the day. Just because your Meal Plan specifies a certain number of servings doesn't mean that's what your body needs or wants. With that kind of thinking, you could go beyond "satisfied."

The Meal Plan cards in Tables 26–30 are *recommendations* for distributing your food choices throughout the day according to the different calorie levels. If you don't want a snack, you can skip it and join that serving up with another meal. Just remember that these are simply suggestions. Only when you are in the process of eating will you know if there is too much or not enough. I've included a blank chart (Table 31), so you can do your own planning, if you'd like.

TABLE 26. Suggested Food Choice Distribution for Meal Plan A

Meal Plan A	Breakfast	Snack	Lunch	Snack	Dinner	Snack
Grains	1	1	1		1	1
Vegetables			1		2	
Fruit	1			1		
Dairy	½		½		½	½
Meat	1 oz		2 oz		2 oz	
Extras: 50 calories from Fat and Sugar						

TABLE 27. Suggested Food Choice Distribution for Meal Plan B

Meal Plan B	Breakfast	Snack	Lunch	Snack	Dinner	Snack
Grains	1	1	2	1	1	1
Vegetables			2		2	
Fruit	1			1		1
Dairy	½		½		½	½
Meat	1 oz		2 oz		3 oz	
Extras: 100 calories from Fat and Sugar						

TABLE 28. Suggested Food Choice Distribution for Meal Plan C

Meal Plan C	Breakfast	Snack	Lunch	Snack	Dinner	Snack
Grains	2	1	2	1	2	1
Vegetables		1	2		2	
Fruit	1			1		1
Dairy	1		½		1	½
Meat	1 oz		3 oz		3 oz	
Extras: 150 calories from Fat and Sugar						

TABLE 29. Suggested Food Choice Distribution for Meal Plan D

Meal Plan D	Breakfast	Snack	Lunch	Snack	Dinner	Snack
Grains	2	2	2	1	2	1
Vegetables		1	3	1	2	
Fruit	1		1	1		1
Dairy	1		½		1	½
Meat	1 oz		3 oz	1 oz	3 oz	
Extras: 200 calories from Fat and Sugar						

TABLE 30. **Suggested Food Choice Distribution for Meal Plan E**

Meal Plan E	Breakfast	Snack	Lunch	Snack	Dinner	Snack
Grains	2	2	2	2	2	1
Vegetables		1	3	2	2	
Fruit	1		1	1		1
Dairy	1		1		1	1
Meat	1 oz		3 oz	1 oz	4 oz	
Extras: 250 calories from Fat and Sugar						

TABLE 31. **Blank Meal Plan**

Meal Plan ___	Breakfast	Snack	Lunch	Snack	Dinner	Snack
Grains						
Vegetables						
Fruit						
Dairy						
Meat						
Extras: _____ calories from Fat and Sugar						

While the Judgers probably are appreciating this structure, I can hear you Perceivers crying out, "Please don't lock me into too tight a schedule." Remember, your personality, not me or anyone else, is going to be your guide in making decisions. View this as a guideline that allows some side excursions if desired. However, all the side excursions count toward your daily allowance for calories, fat, etc.

You Started Eating When You Weren't Hungry

Another major reason for eating past the "satisfied" level is that you started eating when you weren't hungry. If you look at Figure 28, in which the Hunger and Fullness Gauges are lined up side-

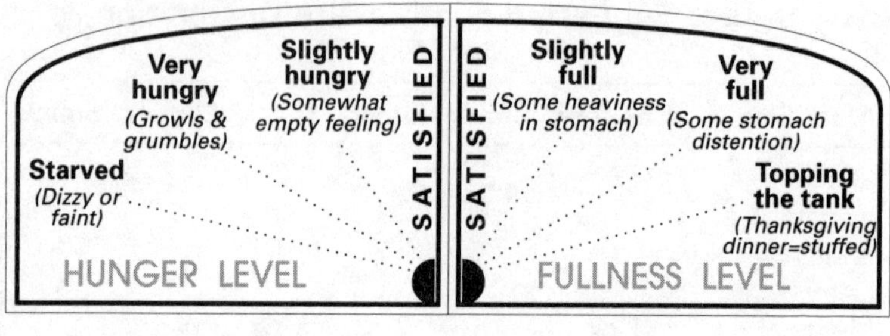

Date __________ Meal ______________

Figure 28. Hunger-Fullness Gauge

by-side, you'll see that the center point for both is "satisfied." What happens when you start eating at the "satisfied" level on the Hunger Gauge? You're inevitably going to go beyond the "satisfied" level on the Fullness Gauge. Only when you start eating below the "satisfied" level on the Hunger Gauge can you possibly stop at the "satisfied" level of Fullness.

In addition, when you start eating when you're not hungry, it is that much more difficult to recognize what fullness really is. There is nothing to compare it to. Then you're more likely to go to the stuffed stage to experience a difference and realize it is time to stop eating.

If you'd like, make some copies of this Hunger-Fullness Gauge to use when you eat. After a week of recording when you started and stopped eating, you'll know if you are really changing your habits, trying not to overeat. (You Judgers should be good at this.) If you decide not to keep a record, at least keep a copy of the gauge with you as a reminder of your goal. Just a glance at it at the beginning and halfway through a meal may be enough for you.

Finding That "Satisfied" Level

You are the only one who can judge what "satisfied" feels like. In order to determine that feeling, you must learn to focus on your body's reaction to what you are eating, putting your undivided attention to the task, being completely in the present without distractions. This is definitely a Sensing job. If only the iNtuitives could hush their brains a little while eating, they too, would be more attentive to the eating process. However, they're often so busy working out ideas and plans for the future, such as considering what they'll be having for dessert, they miss the pleasure of eating right now.

Here are some suggestions my clients have shared with me that might help you find that "satisfied" level:

- Don't eat while watching television or reading a book.
- Don't carry on a conversation with anyone while you're eating. Tell them you'll talk after you finish eating and recognize that you've reached the "satisfied" level.
- Eat with the opposite hand from the one you normally use.
- Eat with a baby spoon or cocktail fork.
- Put your fork down between bites.
- Get up halfway through the meal and take a quick walkabout. Then when you sit down again, see whether your body really wants any more.
- Sit in a different seat at the table. The change of perspective will heighten your awareness.
- Throughout the meal, ask yourself whether the food is still tasting as good as did the first bite.
- When eating something that is high-fat and high-calorie, tell yourself that you can have it again, so there's no need to finish it if you're no longer hungry.
- Imagine that each bite is your last. Are you full yet?

Many of my clients hated giving up watching television or reading while eating. They felt that by doing both activities at the same time, they were being efficient. (Many of these people were _S_Js.) However, they did admit that they didn't get as much pleasure from their food because the distractions made them less aware of the flavors. They also didn't know whether they were full since their attention was focused elsewhere.

The Perceivers found eating with the opposite hand or using a baby spoon fun. The Judgers weren't too excited about this idea, but were willing to give it a try. They both found that it made them have to think more about the eating process. Also, because it was such a struggle, they were more willing to admit to being full when they had reached that level. Why continue to eat beyond "satisfied" when it was such a challenge?

Sitting in a different seat at the table was easy enough for the Extraverts, but the Introverts didn't feel comfortable with it. However, they did admit that doing so made them more aware of their eating, allowing them to more easily recognize when they had had enough. The Extraverts found keeping silent during a meal very difficult. To their way of thinking, why eat with someone if you don't plan to socialize? Having to hold back conversation until the food was gone meant too much silent time. The Introverts were okay with this.

Once you have told yourself that nothing is forbidden and that you can have it whenever you want, you do not have to feel forced to gorge yourself this one time. You'll enjoy the food more because you'll be more willing to take the time to savor the flavor rather than gobble it down in an attempt to make sure you get your fill of it.

Considering each bite to be your last means you are consciously making a decision after each bite whether to continue or stop eating. When my clients had success with it, I knew they had finally learned what it meant to make a conscious decision using their personality. It wasn't just their Sensing preference working. The other preferences were weighing the pros and cons of eating more, what the consequences would be, and the feelings involved.

It's Just a Matter of Making a Decision

If you think making a decision about when to start eating is a big one, the decision about when to stop eating is enormous. If you stop too soon, you'll be hungry within an hour or so. Of course, you could always eat a snack to keep you going till the next meal. What's worse is if you stop too late: you'll be eating more calories than you need, not to mention making yourself uncomfortable. Most people admit that the Thanksgiving-stuffed stage is not pleasant. They also know that getting to that stage on a regular basis leads inevitably to weight gain.

One very important question you must ask yourself to get you out of the habit of eating too much is "How is eating this way going to help me reach the goals I set?" (See Chapter 6.) You mustn't lose track of where you're headed and why. It *is* the reason you bought this book, isn't it?

Appreciate the fact that if you stop at the "satisfied" level, you don't have to make any decisions. It's when you want to eat more than this that you need to bring in the reinforcements (your other preferences), either to talk you out of it or to support you in your actions. The *Z* pattern of decision making can help a lot here. Or apply your 1–2–3–4 order using the Fullness Decision Road Map in Figure 29. (See the Fullness Decision Questions in Table 32 on p. 270.) Be sure you allow each of your preferences its say until you reach a "Don't Eat" response.

It can be very tempting to come up with the decision you want (that is, to continue eating when you're full), and then find information that appears to support your decision. But when you do that you are only fooling and hurting yourself. However, if that is what you want to do, then do it consciously, take responsibility for the results of your actions, and understand the effect your actions will have on your reaching your *life vision.* Don't be like the person in the old antacid commercial who moans, "I can't believe I ate the whole thing," when you made the decision to eat the whole thing!

The *Z* Approach

Sensing Preference Contribution

Let your Sensing preference help you determine if you've reached the "satisfied" stage by "listening to your body talk." Remember, Sensing is the here-and-now preference and is in the best position to tell you what your body needs. Look at the Hunger-Fullness Gauge (Figure 28) and consider what level you've reached. Did you manage to stop at the "satisfied" level, or did you go too far and hit the Slightly full, Very full or Topping-the-tank level?

Allow your Sensing preference to collect details about the

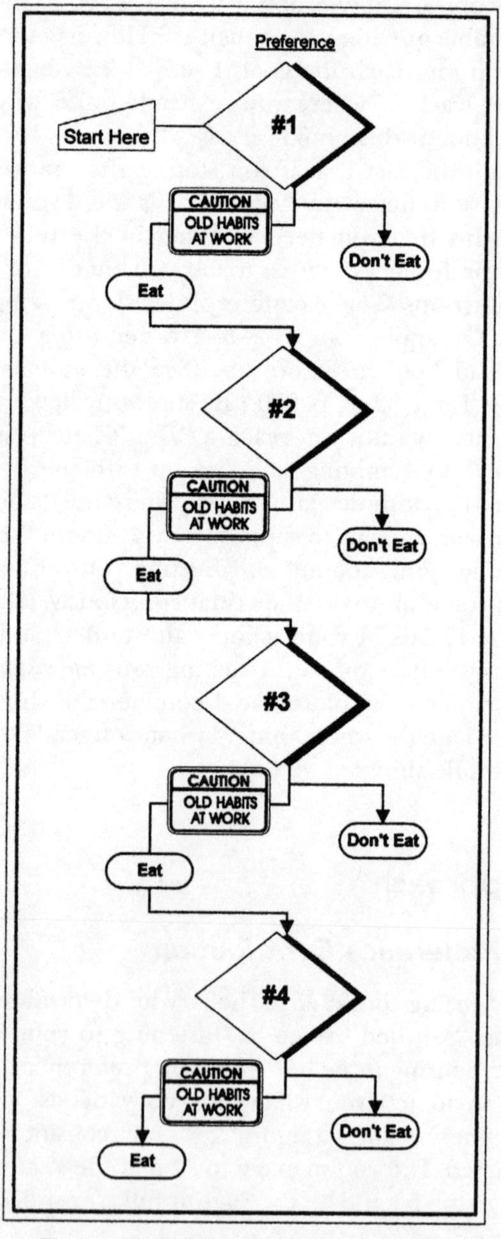

Figure 29. Fullness Decision Road Map

situation, the environment, and your emotions. These will greatly influence your actions and decisions. Try to remember times when you stopped eating at the right moment, and how that felt. Now think of how you felt when you didn't stop in time. All this is information your decision-making processes (Thinking and Feeling) need if you are considering eating when you are full.

iNtuiting Preference Contribution

If you find, through your Sensing preference, that you are full but are going in for more, enlist your iNtuitive preference to help push yourself away from the table. Think about the excuses you're making to eat more than you need. What can you do to eliminate those excuses?

- If you're continuing to eat because you're hoping to be comforted by food, you need to consider some other alternatives. Food should not be used as a pacifier. Take a walk instead of continuing to eat.
- If you're angry with someone, consider writing a letter to that person expressing your feelings instead of burying the anger in food. (And it's probably best not to mail the letter!)
- If you're eating to avoid doing something, find something else to use as an avoidance activity (although you're going to have to face it sometime).
- If you're bored, start a project or hobby, play with a pet, see a movie. Continuing to eat may fill up time in the short term, but eventually you'll have to deal with your problems.
- If you know that you'll be in a meeting or elsewhere that food is unavailable at a time when you're likely to get hungry, you might be tempted to eat more at the present eating opportunity. Yet stockpiling doesn't work. More food often revs up the digestion machine, storing the excess in your fat cells. Not a good thing. Instead of eating more than you need, carry a convenient food source (nutrition bar, bagel, fruit) that you can eat when you do get hungry.

If you found yourself going over the "satisfied" level, then let your iNtuiting preference imagine what it will feel like the next time you eat an amount that gets you right on target. Visualize the sensations and how you'll feel about yourself.

Thinking Preference Contribution

The Thinking preference involves impersonal analysis using generally accepted rules. One important rule is that you **eat only to the "satisfied" stage.** It is only logical, since the calories you're eating beyond that level are not necessary and will go into storage. Think of the consequences if you don't stop. Your Thinking preference knows it can be physically and emotionally damaging to continue.

Your Sensing preference has provided your Thinking preference with the details of the situation. Your iNtuiting preference has come up with alternatives to avoid eating beyond the "satisfied" point. Now let your Thinking preference consider the pros and cons of all this information.

Feeling Preference Contribution

While your Thinking preference is considering the facts of the situation, your Feeling preference is considering the emotions of the situation. The Feeling preference can either be turned outward, worrying about what others are feeling or thinking, or turned inward with concern for yourself. Look over the excuses at the beginning of this chapter and study how the Feeling preference is being used in each case. Is it helping you decide in favor of continuing to eat because of how it will make others feel or because of how it will make you feel?

There's another aspect to look at when the Feeling preference is turned inward. In the guise of wanting to comfort you, it can help you find reasons to support your excuses. Or, because it wants you to succeed, it can make you aware of how you're sabotaging your efforts toward a healthier lifestyle. If you use it in a positive way, your Feeling preference can be your friend.

It's so important that those of you who have a dominant or backup Feeling preference *not* make a decision using your Feeling preference until all your other preferences have been consulted. Then your Feeling preference can allow you to put your stamp of approval on the decision, ensuring that you'll have no regrets about your actions.

Your 1–2–3–4 Order Using the Fullness Decision Road Map

Making a decision when to stop eating isn't all that different from making a decision about not eating when you're not hungry. The major distinction is that in one case, you stop the process of eating and in the other, you never start. Yet you need to consider many of the same questions.

TABLE 32. **Fullness Decision Questions**

Preference	Questions to Consider
Sensing	• Am I still hungry? What sensations of fullness am I experiencing? • Are my eyes bigger than my stomach? • Is it the sight and smell of the food that's making me continue to eat? • What happened the last time I was in this situation? • If I continue to eat, how many extra calories and grams of fat will I be getting that my body doesn't need? • Am I continuing to eat because others are still eating? • What is happening at the moment?
iNtuiting	• If I eat too much, how am I going to feel later? • Is eating beyond "satisfied" going to help me reach my *life vision*? • If I'm enjoying the taste of the food so much, how can I preserve that pleasure? Is eating more of the food the answer? • Am I using food for reasons other than nutrition? Am I eating beyond what my body needs as a way to avoid something? • Am I eating more than I need now because I don't know when I'll be eating again? What planning could I do?
Thinking	• Do I want to overeat because of appetite rather than hunger? • What are the pros and cons of overeating? What do I think is going to happen to these extra calories? • Will this unnecessary amount of food fit into my daily calorie and fat allowance? Will I have to give something up later by overeating now? Is it worth it?

	• Isn't it against the rules to eat when my fullness level registers "satisfied"? • Am I eating this extra food because it's free? • Is it logical to eat when I'm full? Is it as pleasurable?
Feeling	• Am I eating more than my body needs just because "I want it"? • Am I continuing to eat because others are still eating? • Am I eating more than I want because someone gave it to me and I don't want to hurt her feelings? • Am I eating beyond fullness in hopes that the food will finally make me happy, calm, less bored, or unable to begin something I don't want to do? • Don't I care enough about myself to realize what I'm doing to myself? • Am I eating all this food because my mother taught me to "clean my plate"?

10

Making It a Habit #5: Keep It Moving

Many people don't like to exercise. Some got burned out during the "no pain, no gain" era (which, thankfully, no longer exists). Having been made to feel guilty if they didn't suffer while exercising, some pushed themselves so hard that they did hurt themselves and decided to give up. Then there are those who have never given exercise a try and so haven't experienced its benefits. Some people feel they should exercise, but can't seem to figure out how to make it a regular habit.

For every excuse you make, a viable option can be suggested that makes your excuse seem pretty flimsy. Here are some excuses my clients have used in the past to avoid exercising. I have included some suggestions on dealing with the problem.

- **"It's boring."** *Try something new and different. Challenge yourself to learn a new exercise each month. Having an exercise buddy helps.*
- **"I don't have enough time."** *Accumulate physical activity by doing one 10-minute session three times a day. While you ride a stationary bicycle, you can read your mail, a magazine, or watch television. Make fitness a priority.*
- **"I don't like to sweat."** *Exercise in front of a fan or outdoors in the evening when it's cooler.*
- **"The weather is bad."** *Go to the gym, do a mall walk before the stores open, invest in a piece of exercise equipment for your home.*

- **"I'm too tired."** *Give exercise a five-minute try and you'll probably find you've got more energy than you thought. You're probably suffering mental fatigue more than physical fatigue. The fact is, exercise gives you energy because your body becomes stronger and more efficient. Don't get caught in a vicious cycle in which (1) you say you're too tired; (2) you don't exercise; and (3) you become even more tired because you've let yourself become so physically unfit.*
- **"It's too hard."** *Ease up a little, take it slower, and work your way up to speed.*
- **"It's too expensive."** *All you really need is a good pair of athletic shoes.*
- **"There's no place to exercise."** *Join a gym, look into your local YMCA, YWCA, or recreation department.*
- **"I feel self-conscious."** *Exercise with others who are at your same level. Exercise at home where it's private.*
- **"I hate exercise."** *If this is you, at least you're being honest. Yet do you hate dancing, gardening, walking the dog? Maybe it's structured exercise you dislike, and you just need to look for activities that get you moving without too many rules. Think of exercise as playtime. Think about the fun you had as a kid when it wasn't considered "exercise" but "recess."*

The Benefits of Exercise

Eating smart but not exercising is like walking around with only one shoe on. Why are you providing your body with all the nutrients it needs, but not encouraging your body to use those nutrients? If you look at the human body, with all its muscles and bones, you just know we were built to move.

Centuries ago, when we were hunters and gatherers, the term "couch potato" would have had no meaning. Our ancestors had no choice but to rustle up their meals. There were no fast-food restaurants on the corner or ready-to-cook meals to be picked up from the market on the way home. Back then, they were using their bodies to do what they had been designed to do.

I never cease to marvel at the athletes who compete in the Olympic Games. They have exercised their bodies to the point of becoming fine instruments. When they compete, we hear the music their bodies can play. I'm not suggesting that each of us must become an Olympic athlete. However, when you realize what your body is capable of doing, it makes you better appreciate how you are keeping your body from its potential. Exercise not only benefits you physically, it brings mental and emotional benefits as well.

Physical Benefits of Exercise

Exercise helps you to:

- Increase the strength of your heart muscle.
- Decrease your total blood cholesterol while increasing the level of good HDL cholesterol.
- Lower your blood pressure.
- Stabilize your blood sugar level.
- Increase delivery of oxygen to your whole body.
- Increase the action of your intestinal tract, ensuring that everything moves smoothly and swiftly to help you avoid constipation and exposure to carcinogens.
- Lose weight.
- Strengthen your bones; weight-bearing exercise helps your body deposit calcium in the bones.
- Increase your metabolism.
- Maintain lean body mass. (This is especially important for people as they get older. Even if we weigh the same as we did in our youth, we normally have a higher percentage of fat to muscle. Exercise is one way to help maintain lean body mass.)
- Decrease the risk of some chronic diseases, including heart disease, diabetes, hypertension, osteoporosis, and some cancers.
- Increase your flexibility and stamina.
- Burn calories.
- Look better.
- Burn fat.

If you are using exercise as a way of increasing your rate of weight loss on a reducing diet, then consider how the body burns

:avy sack and find your muscles quivering, you know your cles need strengthening.

'ortunately, no matter how out of shape you are or how old are, it's never too late. It may take more time than either would like or expect in order to improve your body, but you do it. In fact, the more slowly you approach the conditioning, more easily your body can adjust and the more likely you to stick with it.

You _S_Ps are probably moaning that you haven't got the ience to wait for results. If you have Thinking in your type, know it's logical for it to take some time, but you still won't happy. Some short-term goal setting is in order for you. For mple, you could say, "By the end of next week, I'll be able do four repetitions of that exercise activity." If you think about long-term goal of 10 repetitions, you may never even get rted. iNtuitives, with your ability to see the possibilities, can content for the time being to look at role models or people know who have made exercise a part of their lives, and agine yourself like that one day. Long-range goal setting is problem for you. It's the occasional I-can-put-that-off-until-morrow syndrome that can get you into trouble. If you're an T_ or _NF_, don't hold out for perfection before you pat urself on the back for making some changes.

As with your other lifestyle habits, you have to decide what's st for you. First and foremost, the right exercise is one that u'll enjoy doing on a regular basis, one that you're willing to today and tomorrow. It doesn't necessarily have to be the me thing all the time. In fact, variety is very important, not nly to avoid boredom, but also to work different sets of muscles. ifferent kinds of activity affect your endurance, flexibility, and rength differently.

Look over the following list and circle those exercises you hink you might enjoy. The Extraverts may have a tendency to o for the group activities, while the Introverts will prefer activities hey can do on their own. The Sensors will go for something hat is tried and true while the iNtuitives might consider the nusual or new. The Thinkers will consider which exercise would pply to their health needs and the Feelers will opt for exercises hey like or that work in harmony with friends and family. Which

fat. Moderate exercise—as compared to intens
more fat. Intense exercise forces the muscles
glycogen (sugar) supplies for energy, whereas n
uses both muscle glycogen and fat from your fa
However, you'll need to exercise longer durin
cise to burn the equivalent number of calorie
intense exercise. Brisk walking is a moderate ex
to jogging, which is more intense. One good thi
ate exercise is that it's easier to maintain on
because there is less risk of injury or burnout.

Mental and Emotional Benefits of Exerc

Exercise helps you to:

- Reduce stress and anxiety and have a genera being; you're less likely to let things get you
- Improve your ability to relax; life becomes m
- Improve your mental outlook and feel you' you have more confidence.
- Sleep better; you wake up refreshed.
- Be more alert and able to concentrate; it clea so you can get the job done better.

Think about why you would personally want to i
physical activity. Whether it's to improve your body o
it has to be your cause, not mine or that of anyone
only way you're going to guarantee yourself full parti
the long term.

The Exercise Trio

The optimum exercise program addresses three aspe
body's health: endurance, flexibility, and strength. You
these every day. If you're huffing and puffing when yo
a flight of stairs, you know your endurance needs i
When you bend over and can't even get close to your
know your flexibility needs improving. When you try t

do you prefer? Check as many as you want, but be sure to include at least one from each category. (Contrary to popular belief, channel surfing television stations is not an exercise—endurance or otherwise!)

Endurance

Aerobic dance
Basketball
Bicycling (outdoor or stationary)
Dancing
Football
Frisbee
Hiking
Jogging or running (outdoors or on a treadmill)
Kick-boxing
Racquetball
Rollerblading
Rowing (outdoor or rowing machine)
Skating
Skiing (cross-country or downhill)
Skipping rope
Softball
Squash
Step aerobics
Step climbing
Swimming
Tennis
Volleyball
Walking (brisk walking or race walking)
Others__________________

Flexibility

Calisthenics
Martial Arts
T'ai chi
Yoga
Others__________________

Strength

Floor exercises (e.g., sit-ups, push-ups)
Free weights
Rubber bands
Weight lifting
Others__________________

The exercise trio work hand-in-hand. When you increase your strength through weight-bearing and resistance activities like weight lifting or push-ups, you can also increase your aerobic activity level. Having flexibility reduces your risk of injury during exercise. The more muscle mass you have, the more efficiently you burn calories.

How Much Is Enough?

Your fitness level and what you're trying to accomplish will help determine the number of minutes you spend exercising. Wanting to *maintain* your level of fitness is one thing. If you are shooting for a marathon, reaching your goal would require much more time.

Some people might think they've had enough exercise when they start to sweat. Others might say it's when they start to hurt (wrong!). While there isn't an exact formula for how much is right, you'll find some guidelines for exercise intensity in the pages that follow.

Let me just remind you of two things. First, it's very important before you start any exercise program to consult your physician, especially if you have a health condition. Take this book with you and ask whether the suggestions here are appropriate for you. Second, before you do any type of exercise, whether it be endurance, weight training or stretching, it's crucial to do a warm-up session, such as walking on a treadmill or riding a stationary bicycle for five minutes and stretching for another five minutes.

Endurance Training Intensity

Another term for endurance activities is *aerobic exercise.* It is called aerobic because the muscles use oxygen to produce the necessary energy. To determine your endurance training intensity, you need to calculate your target heart rate, which is a percentage of your maximum heart rate (MHR). If you're a beginner, it's best to start out at 55–60 percent of your MHR. At the intermediate level, 60–70 percent of your MHR is adequate. If you're a more advanced athlete, you can probably exercise at 70–85 percent of your MHR.

Keeping these percentages in mind, find your age in Table 33 and then locate your target heart rate in the correct column. *(Your maximum heart rate is found by subtracting your age from 220.)*

TABLE 33. **Target Heart Rate**

Age	Maximum Heart Rate (MHR)	55–60% MHR (Beginner or history of heart disease)	60–70% MHR (Intermediate Athlete)	70–85% MHR (Trained Athlete)
20	200	110–120	120–140	140–170
25	195	107–117	117–137	137–166
30	190	105–114	114–133	133–162
35	185	102–111	111–130	130–157
40	180	99–108	108–126	126–153
45	175	96–105	105–123	123–149
50	170	94–102	102–119	119–145
55	165	91–99	99–116	116–140
60	160	88–96	96–112	112–136
65+	150	85–96	93–109	109–132

There are two places on your body where you can easily take a heart rate reading. You can either place your index and middle finger on the side of your neck below your jawbone or on your wrist below the thumb. Feel for the pulse. Count the beats for 20 seconds. Then multiply by three to find out the number of beats per minute. Before you start exercising, take a reading. Then, halfway through your training, take another reading. Make sure you don't go over the range you found in the table.

Strength Training Intensity

A high-intensity resistance program has been shown to be the most effective in improving strength, no matter your age. By strengthening the muscles, you reduce the risk of injury, reduce back pain (often due to weak stomach muscles), improve athletic performance (no matter what the sport), and increase bone density, to just name a few benefits. The major muscle groups to be targeted are those that you use in everyday activities—the shoulders, arms, chest, abdomen, back, hips, and legs. You might even consider getting an anatomy book to see what muscles you'll be working. Then picture those muscles in your mind as you exercise them.

Select weights according to how many repetitions of lifting you can do before fatigue sets in. You should be able to lift the weights about 8 to 12 times before the muscles say, "No more, please." When you can comfortably lift the weights over 20 times, they're too light for strength training or increasing muscle mass, though you'll be improving muscle endurance. At that point, it's time to increase the weight.

Don't forget to breathe while you're lifting weights. Too many people hold their breath during the whole lifting and lowering process, which can affect blood pressure and heart rate. You should inhale before a lift, exhale during the lift, and then inhale when lowering the weight. Work slowly and concentrate on the muscle group you're strengthening. Always remember to work opposing muscle groups, such as your quadriceps (front of thighs) with your hamstrings (back of thighs), or your biceps (front of upper arms) with your triceps (back of upper arms).

Flexibility Training Intensity

Flexibility training is often the most overlooked aspect of exercise. Yet you can reduce many injuries when you are flexible. You should stretch very slowly and only to the point where you feel slight tension. Hold the position for about 20 to 30 seconds. At this point you should be feeling a decrease in tension. Repeat the stretch at least three or four times. Never bounce while stretching; it increases your risk of injury. When you release a stretch, do it as slowly as you started it.

Focus all your attention on the muscle being stretched. Close your eyes and visualize the muscle lengthening. Feel and sense it releasing to a longer position. Feel the release of tension. Enjoy the sense of relaxation that follows. When you keep your eyes closed, you eliminate the tendency to push further than is safe. You are then doing the stretch based on feel rather than what it looks like. Some people believe that unless they see themselves stretching and folding themselves up like a contortionist, they aren't doing an adequate job. If you aren't looking, that is no longer a problem.

You Sensors will probably be best at feeling the stretch because you tend to stay in the present. On the other hand, you iNtuitives probably have your minds off somewhere working on some new idea or visualizing being that contortionist, so you may miss the real experience of the stretch. You will have to be more conscious of what you're doing, both physically and mentally. Because becoming flexible takes some time, you Sensors may question whether you will ever see results. Take a day at a time, focusing on what you have accomplished, not on what you haven't yet achieved.

You can do stretching activities no matter where you are—at your desk, on a plane, in your home. Think about the different muscle groups that need your attention, so your whole body will gain flexibility. What you don't want is stiffness in one set of muscles that opposes the flexibility you gained in another.

Length of Sessions

Before you start an endurance, strength or flexibility activity, do a 5- to 10-minute warm-up. You can't expect your muscles to be ready to respond to a full-intensity workout right after having been still for some time. They need to get acclimated. You can run, walk in place, or ride a stationary bicycle for a few minutes. Include some gentle stretches. End your exercise session with a cool-down session of another 5 to 10 minutes. Just repeat what you did for the warm-up.

- Endurance Activities: If you're a beginner, do the endurance activity of your choice for 20–30 minutes; if you're an intermediate, you might want to tack on another 10 minutes (30–40 minutes); and if you're advanced, tack on an additional 10 minutes (40–50 minutes).
- Strength Activities: Length of sessions should be based on how long it takes you to complete the required number of repetitions.

- Flexibility Activities: The length of your session will depend on the number of stretches and repetitions you decide to do. However, on average, expect to spend 15 minutes if you're stretching to prepare for an endurance or strength-building activity and 30–35 minutes if the session is solely for flexibility training.

Fortunately for those of us who find it difficult to fit exercise into our daily schedules, research has shown that accumulating minutes during the day can add up to a healthful exercise program. If you can get 10 minutes in the morning, 10 minutes at lunch, and 10 minutes before or after dinner for a brisk walk or short bike ride, you'll have easily attained the minimum 30 minutes of physical activity that's recommended. Those of you who want to be more physically fit will take the extra time.

Number of Days Per Week

If you're just trying to maintain your physical fitness level, three to four days a week is sufficient. Exercise every other day to give your muscles a chance to recover. However, if you want to improve, step up the frequency to five days a week. Try aerobic conditioning on three alternate days and strength training on the other days. More than five days a week doesn't give your body a needed rest. Try to do at least a short session of flexibility exercises every day, if possible.

Don't be one of those weekend warriors who, not having had the opportunity to exercise during the week, figures they can make up for it on the weekend. They double the length of their exercise sessions and work at a higher heart rate, feeling that anything short of such an intense workout won't be effective. But all they're doing is increasing their risk of an injury that's only going to set them back further. It's better to sneak in a couple of minutes during the week than to try doing it all on the weekend.

Exercise Tips

- Make it enjoyable. Do exercise activities that you like, not what is popular or what someone else says you should do.
- View exercise as a welcome break, not as drudgery. You may find you are more productive when you get back to work.
- Consider listening to books on tape while you work out.
- Be prepared with an alternate exercise plan in case you get rained out or snowed in.
- Exercise regularly, preferably at the same time each day, so that it becomes a natural part of your routine.
- Exercise right before dinner if you want to control your appetite.
- Exercise first thing in the morning if you're the kind of person who comes up with reasons why you can't exercise during the day.
- Be aware that exercising right before going to bed may make it more difficult to fall asleep.
- Realize that doing some exercise is better than doing none.
- Find an exercise program that suits your schedule.
- Find a friend and join a gym or health club if you enjoy exercising in a group.
- Consider hiring a personal trainer for at least one or two exercise sessions so you can learn what will be a good program for you.
- If you buy nothing else, make sure you purchase a pair of athletic shoes that fit well and are appropriate to your athletic activity.
- Make sure you're able to carry on a conversation with someone while you exercise; if you can, you know you aren't pushing too hard.
- Drink water to replace fluid lost in sweating; you don't really need a sports drink unless you're a competitive athlete.
- Give yourself some extra time to work back up to your previous level of exercise if you haven't exercised for several weeks.
- Focus on the benefits of exercising.
- Be patient; the benefits of exercise may take a number of weeks to show.

- Remember that it's okay to change your exercise routine if what you're doing isn't working.
- Don't punish yourself for missing a day of exercise; there's always tomorrow.

Tips for Getting Physical Activity in Small Ways

- Avoid elevators. Take the stairs whenever possible.
- Park as far away from the shopping mall or store entrance as possible.
- Use a broom instead of a vacuum cleaner to sweep up small jobs.
- Use a portable phone so you can walk around as you talk.
- Don't sit at your desk for more than 30 minutes at a time. Get up, walk around, and then return. (It also helps improve your thinking.)
- Wash and wax your car instead of taking it to the car wash.
- Rake your leaves instead of using a blower.
- Take your pet for a walk instead of sending it outside.
- Try dancing or bowling when you're socializing with friends and family.
- Get up to change the television channel instead of reaching for the remote control.
- Don't use the moving walkways in airports, or if you do, walk.
- Don't telephone co-workers. Go to their offices.
- Hand-chop ingredients for a dish rather than using a food processor.

Some Exercise Myths

- **Myth #1** To build muscle, you need to eat more protein. *(Working a muscle is what builds it. While the body-builders or competitive athletes may have to be concerned about how much protein they're getting, the average American eats more than an adequate amount of protein to support a moderate program of exercise.)*

- **Myth #2** Spot reducing, or exercising specific areas of your body, can help remove fat from those areas (stomach, hips, thighs, and buttocks). *(While exercising those areas will increase the muscle tone and make the area appear firmer, it does not remove the fat from that area only. The increased amount of exercise encourages overall fat loss.)*
- **Myth #3** You can have more energy and improve your fitness performance by taking vitamin and mineral supplements. *(Unless you are a professional athlete, a balanced diet will give you adequate nutrition to maintain a regular exercise program.)*
- **Myth #4** Aerobic exercise, such as jogging or biking, can help prevent the loss of muscle mass. *(Only strength training, in which you contract the muscles against a load, can help to maintain or build muscle.)*
- **Myth #5** "No pain, no gain." *(Listen to your body talk. If it hurts or burns while you're doing the exercise, stop! If you have muscle soreness after a workout, you didn't warm up sufficiently or you worked the muscles too hard or too long.)*
- **Myth #6** Bouncing during stretching helps lengthen the muscle. *(Bouncing can injure the muscles by tearing them and actually shortens the muscle. A proper stretch involves gradual stretching to a muscle's full range until you feel resistance.)*

Advice to the Personality Preferences

Extraverts Should Look For

- Group-oriented or team activities
- A variety of types of exercise equipment
- A gym where there are people with whom you can talk while exercising

Introverts Should Look For

- Individual, or one-on-one, activities
- A type of exercise equipment that feels comfortable, so you can stick with it
- A gym where, if you prefer, you can keep to yourself

Sensors Should Look For

- An activity you can stick with whose results are fairly dependable and can be seen within a reasonable amount of time
- Exercise classes, exercise video tapes, or a personal trainer, since you prefer to be shown how to do an exercise
- Activities that are routine, simple, and realistically geared to your level of ability
- Ways to measure your progress that show how far you've come

iNtuitives Should Look For

- Activities that are different and unusual, since you prefer novelty
- Activities that allow you to easily skip from one to the next and offer a change of pace
- Opportunities to create your own exercise program, tailored to your own needs
- Ways to measure how much further you have to go to reach your goal—without expecting the impossible from yourself

Thinkers Should Look For

- A routine that includes the exercise trio, since you appreciate the logic behind needing all three types of exercise
- An improved ability to do an exercise or sport as your reward—trying not to be too critical of yourself as you go along
- An instructor you can trust and who has credentials

Feelers Should Look For

- Exercise that you yourself enjoy, not just activities whose sole attraction is that a friend does them or likes them
- Feedback and praise for how well you're performing an exercise, since that is what will inspire you to continue
- Any improvement in how you perform or look as reason to feel good about yourself—trying not to be too hard on yourself if you're not progressing as fast as you'd like

- An instructor who's warm, friendly, and seems interested in your personal growth

Judgers Should Look For

- A structured exercise program that lets you know exactly what's expected of you—by counting repetitions of an exercise, taking pulse readings, or exercising for a certain length of time, for example
- A way to track your progress (see the Exercise Log in Table 34)
- The pleasure that comes from knowing that each day's exercise session brings you closer to your goal
- Opportunities to schedule exercise sessions on your calendar to increase your chances that it will be completed

Perceivers Should Look For

- An exercise program that gives you room for flexibility, both in what you do and when you do it
- Activities that are fun, since you are more interested in *what* you're doing than whether it gets you to your goal
- A variety of exercises to do, rather than sticking with the same routine each day
- A way to keep track of your progress that isn't too structured (see the Exercise Log in Table 34—appreciating that you're not the type to keep up the logging process for too long, which is okay)
- Another name for exercise—maybe *physical activity*—that doesn't sound so structured

If you can't seem to make exercise a regular habit, it may be due to the fact that your dominant and backup preferences are busy making up excuses. Try appealing to your #3 and #4 preferences and exercising according to *their* needs.

Making Exercise a Lifestyle Habit

To those of you who have already made exercise one of your lifestyle habits—congratulations! I hope this chapter has given

TABLE 34. **Exercise Log**

Date	Time of Day	FLEXIBILITY EXERCISES Minutes	STRENGTH EXERCISES Pounds*	STRENGTH EXERCISES Minutes	ENDURANCE EXERCISES Type of Exercise	ENDURANCE EXERCISES Minutes

*Write down the number of pounds in your weights.

you some new ideas and strategies. This section is for those of you who are better at coming up with excuses than you are at making exercise a habit. It's time to put your decision-making efforts to work.

If you can't seem to get yourself to exercise, you need to determine *why not.* What preference or part of your personality is getting in your way?

George's son had asked his dad to play ball with him. After a couple of minutes, George became winded and asked for a time-out. He was in poor shape because his Feeling preference had said one too many times, "I don't like to exercise," and so he hadn't. What George needed to do was look to his Thinking preference for the logical reasons why he should exercise and to his Sensing preference for the facts. Because of not exercising, his heart muscle was not as strong as it should have been. It couldn't pump hard enough to eject enough blood with each beat to supply adequate oxygen to his muscles. The less oxygen they got, the harder it was for the muscles to produce enough energy to move. They were sending messages of, "Don't work us so hard. We can't keep up." The end result was that he was not only missing out on playing ball with his son, but also increasing his risk of shortening his life. Using his Feeling preference, he can now see that exercise really means having more fun time with his son.

What if you were about to exercise, but you found yourself making up some reason why you couldn't at that time? (Check out the excuses at the beginning of this chapter.) How are you going to get yourself past that excuse?

If you were exercising and, halfway through, you started making up reasons why you should quit; would you quit? How could you get yourself to continue?

You have some decisions to make.

Questions to Consider for the Exercise Decision Road Map

You'll need to enlist the help of either the *Z* pattern or your personality type's 1–2–3–4 order of decision making (see Table 35 and the Exercise Decision Road Map in Figure 30) to get yourself to a firm and enthusiastic "yes" decision about exercising. Once you've said "Yes!" you don't have to go any further on the Road Map. Just go exercise!

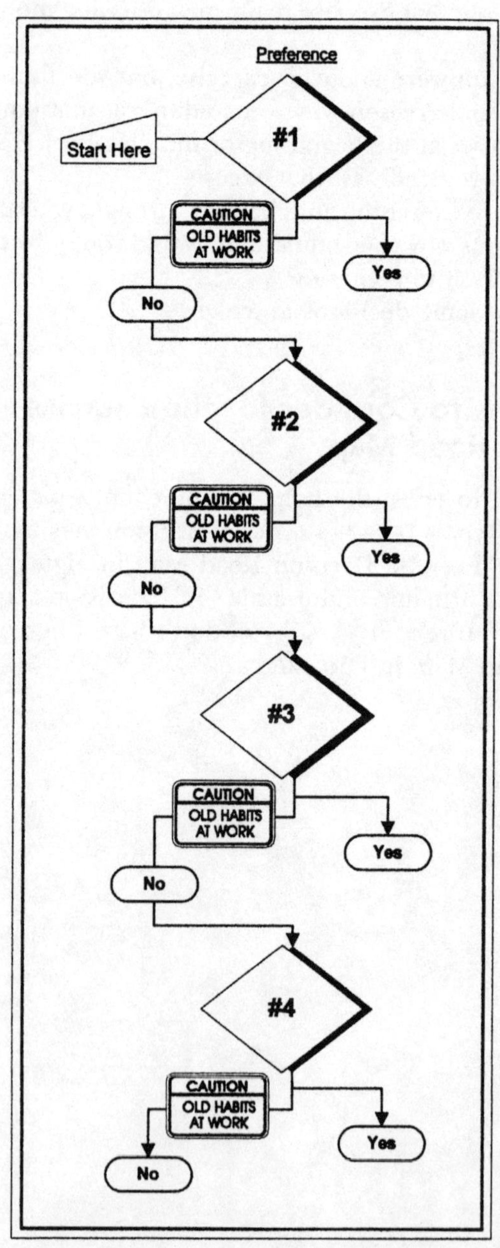

Figure 30. Exercise Decision Road Map

TABLE 35. **Exercise Decision Questions**

Preference	Questions to Consider
Sensing	• Is my being tired stopping me? • Is the weather stopping me? • Is there exercise equipment available? • Am I making up excuses? • Do I wish there were less variety and more routine? • Do I believe I can do these exercises? • Am I losing enthusiasm because I'm not seeing immediate results? • Have I tried doing just 5 minutes to get me going?
iNtuiting	• Am I in my "I'll-do-it-later" mood? • Am I bored with my exercise routine? • Am I still trying to create my own exercise program and am I using that as my excuse for not getting started? • Am I ignoring the possible long-term effects of my not exercising? • Am I developing a pattern of avoidance?
Thinking	• Have I thought about the benefits of exercise? • Am I ignoring the consequences of not exercising? • Do I believe there isn't enough time to do a "decent" session so I am going to avoid it altogether? • Is skipping exercise the logical thing to do?
Feeling	• Am I skipping exercise because my friend can't join me today? • Won't it bother my conscience when I tell my friend I can't exercise today when it's because I really don't want to bother? • Is it that I don't like this activity? • Am I avoiding exercise today because I feel fat or think others will see me as fat? • Do I believe exercise can relieve my boredom, anger, frustration, etc.?

11

Making It a Habit #6: Learn to Relax

When I started writing this book, I thought about putting this chapter first. Many of our poor lifestyle habits are due to stress. Think about the times you grabbed something to eat because you were angry, frustrated, or bored. How about the excuses you make for not exercising? "I'm up against a wall on this project. It has to be done by tomorrow. There's no way I'm going to fit exercise in as well." Quite possibly, if you had stress under control, you might not have some of the unhealthy lifestyle habits you'd like to change.

Stress is a fight-or-flight response, which in an emergency may be a valuable reaction, but can be taxing on the body if experienced too often. Many of us feel as if we're regularly on a battlefield. If it's not a deadline we have to meet at work, it's having to drive our kid's soccer team to an out-of-state game, or dealing with a failing compressor on our refrigerator.

Not all problems can be attributed to people and things outside of ourselves, though. We bring on a great deal of our own stress. You _NT_s tend to be perfectionists, never quite satisfied with the job you've done. You _NF_s tend to be idealists, who feel you have yet to bring meaning to your life or that of others. You _S_Ps, after making a decision on impulse, often fret over whether it was the best decision you could have made. You _S_Js, with your need to serve, often take on more than you can handle.

Sometimes having to act out of character is stressful. Being alone too long can create tension for an Extravert. An Introvert, on the other hand, can find that being in a crowd too long or being forced to express ideas in a group situation produces stress. Perceivers often struggle with the demands of making quick decisions or of having to work in an overly structured environment. By contrast, Judgers are uncomfortable having to work in a disorganized setting or having to respond to last-minute demands.

Some level of stress can help improve performance, efficiency, and motivation. Ask any competitive athlete, public speaker, or air traffic controller. It keeps them on their toes, making them more alert and more focused. There is a point, though, when stress can be harmful. Too much pressure can cause people to make serious mistakes. Knowing what to do to manage stress is paramount to having a completely healthy lifestyle.

What Is Stress?

What does stress mean to you? How do you deal with it? Some people seem better equipped to handle stress. What do they know that would be helpful to the rest of us? When I looked up the definition of *stress* in the *Random House College Dictionary,* I found it interesting to see what was listed first:

> **stress** (stres), *n.* **1.** importance or significance attached to a thing . . . **7.** *Physiol.* any stimulus, as fear or pain, that disturbs or interferes with the normal physiological equilibrium of an organism. **8.** physical, mental, or emotional strain or tension.

I'm sure you can relate to the physiological definition of stress. There's no question that stress disturbs our equilibrium and sense of well-being. However, look again at the first definition. If you didn't attach any significance to an event, it wouldn't cause you any stress. Take the example of the compressor in your refrigerator dying. Instead of fretting about how much it's going to cost you to replace it (do you have an alternative?) or that you'll have to stick around all day until the service repair person comes to fix it, you could take the opposite tack. What if you told yourself that you were very fortunate to get 20 years out of one compressor, that the service repair person can come out today instead of tomorrow or next week, that they have the part in stock, and best of all, that you have time to get some things done at home while you wait? You see, **we can choose the way we want to react to a situation.** (Though at the time, you may not be thinking that way!) It's your decision to get aggravated or not. Don't forget, whenever you have a decision to make, you and your personality are in control. We'll be going into more detail about that a little later.

If I were to add another definition to *stress* it would be "the degree of difficulty one has in adapting to change." Change may be either good or bad, but in both cases, it can be stressful. Getting a promotion can be as stressful in its own way as losing a job. They both reflect change. Think about all the changes that take place in your life and how you've reacted to them. Do you think you handle change well? *It is your mental attitude towards change that determines how stressful you find something, and your mental attitude is very much influenced by your personality type.* The following is a list of stressors that I made up with the help of my clients. See if you have experienced any of these situations and think about what you would add of your own.

Change of employment	Move to another city
Financial problems	Problem with employer
Marriage	Holidays
Birth of a child	Personal achievement
Divorce	Retirement
Death of a loved one	A competitive athletic event
Personal injury or illness	A major exam

Most of these are major changes. Whether planned or not, they can be stressful. We must learn to handle the accompanying stress by calling on our coping skills, which we'll discuss in a little while. When you have consciously made a choice to change, such as improving your lifestyle habits, *undertake the changes in small steps.* Work on each step, achieve success, and then move on to the next. It is self-defeating to make health changes in a way that causes you stress.

Everyday Hassles

While you wouldn't question the idea that *major* crises in your life cause stress, you may be underestimating the stress created by little everyday hassles and your reaction to them. Let's say you're on your way to the grocery store. It's just your luck—the light turns red as you approach the intersection. You start drumming your fingers on the steering wheel. You arrive at the grocery store and can't find a parking space, except one that seems so far from the store you *"could'a"* walked from home! After filling your cart, you find that you've picked the slowest checkout line in the store. You keep watching the line you *"should'a"* chosen, agonizing over the fact that you *"would'a"* been at the cash register already if you had made the right decision.

The main problem here is the feeling that you have little control over the situation. There's an interesting correlation between stress and control. The amount of stress you experience is inversely related to the amount of control you have or believe you have over your circumstances. The more control you feel you have, the less stress you'll encounter, because you're involved in the situation, exploring, learning, and managing its outcome. Adopting a problem-solving attitude helps you get rid of the stress. Action of some sort is the key. Otherwise, you are forced to *react,* and are more likely to feel powerless as a result.

There is another element you should consider—how important the situation is or the circumstances are to you. The value you assign (using your Feeling preference) will determine how much energy you could or should, dedicate to it. While you're brooding about being in the wrong line in the grocery store, the person behind you may be enjoying the extra minutes to thumb through the tabloids and read up on the latest gossip.

Nipping your stress reaction in the bud is the best approach. It means, though, that you have to consciously be watching yourself, Sensing when you are beginning to fume. Using your Feeling preference, ask yourself whether this situation is really worth the time and energy it will take to brood about. Are you going to allow yourself to be controlled by it?

Don't Be a Worrywart

Another potential cause of stress is worry. The worrywart spends a great deal of time anticipating that something bad is going to happen in the near or distant future. (Worrywart iNtuitives can be very good at this, since the future is where they spend their time. Those iNtuitives who are not worrywarts are instead using their energies to come up with alternatives to avoid the possible problems.) Worrying is an indication that you believe you don't have control over the outcome of a situation or event. You may worry, "If I lose my job, I won't be able to pay the bills;" "My father died of heart disease. I may also," "If I don't get this project finished, my boss will get mad at me;" "If I eat this chocolate eclair, I'll get fat." Some of these situations are actually within your control. Stop worrying and take action instead. If you really aren't in a position to do something about it, worrying is truly a waste of time and energy.

Take a moment to think about something that's been worrying you. What scenarios are going through your mind? Did you feel a quickening of your pulse, a butterfly in your stomach, some muscle tension across your shoulders or through your chest? Those feelings are no different than the real fight-or-flight response you would have if the situation actually took place. You have just inflicted unnecessary stress on your body.

What's interesting is that we often "catastrophize" a situation, exaggerating the possibilities and risks way out of proportion, only to find it wasn't necessary. Do you remember when you were a child and your mother told you you were going to be vaccinated? The idea of a needle entering your arm may have given you quite a fright. Even before you found out that the experience wasn't as bad as you had envisioned, you had already done a lot of suffering.

This is what we do to ourselves all the time when we worry. It makes us alert to a problem that needs solving and gets us working on a solution, but that's as far as worry should go. I think the following saying, based on the "Serenity Prayer" by Reinhold Neibuhr, sums it up quite nicely:

> *With serenity, accept the things you cannot change.*
> *With courage, change the things that can be changed.*
> *With wisdom, know the difference.*

There's no point in fighting battles you know you can't win—*accept the things you cannot change.* And if there's a battle you *can* win, worrying about it will get you nowhere; you need to put all your personality preferences to work to come up with a way to handle the situation—*change the things that can be changed.* Take action. Then you can change worry into hope, the belief that you can successfully get through this.

Replay versus Rehearse

How many times have you replayed a negative event in your head, reliving every emotional reaction you had when it first happened? (Sensors are very good at this, as are iNtuitives under stress.) Each time you rerun that scene, you are inflicting stress on your system. Instant replay may be great for a football game, but it doesn't have any benefits, unless you plan to learn from the situation and change your reaction the next time. When you find yourself starting a replay, tell yourself "Stop it. This is getting me nowhere. I don't need to do this to myself."

If you're not willing to drop it, take that same situation and rehearse in your mind what you would do if you had it to do over again. Make it come out favorably for yourself. Take the following scenario as an example. You've had an argument with someone you love. As you relive it in your mind, you feel the tension and frustration all over again. What if you could recreate the scene in your mind? What would it look like? You are both talking calmly with each other, allowing the other person to share his or her feelings and opinions. There is recognition of what each person is saying; there's understanding; there's even empathy. The argument is avoided, and instead of yelling at each other, you give each other a hug. Think about how you would feel. Every time you want to relive the argument, relive it as agreement.

Remember, every time you start the replay, interrupt it with the rehearsal. What I'm asking you to do is stop Sensing and start iNtuiting.

The Warning Signals

We react to stress in many ways—physically, emotionally, behaviorally, and/or mentally. Unmanaged stress can lead to a weakening of the immune system, putting your body at a higher risk for diseases and health problems. What are the warning signals that let you know you are in the first stages of stress?

The Body's Reaction to Stress

Imagine yourself walking alone down a dark alley at night. You hear footsteps behind you. They seem to be in step with yours. As you pick up the pace, you notice that so do the footsteps. You're afraid to look back. There's nowhere to run, no shops are open, no one around to help. You can feel your heart pounding. Your throat has suddenly become dry. Swallowing is difficult. Finally the alley ends, there is a main boulevard and plenty of people to give you a sense you are no longer alone. Now you turn around to see your pursuer. It is an elderly woman holding out the scarf that dropped out of your pocket.

You have just gone through a fight-or-flight reaction followed by relief and joy. The adrenaline is pumping. Your heart rate, blood pressure, rate of breathing, metabolism, and flow of blood to the muscles of your arms and legs have all increased. A ready supply of glycogen for energy has been made available by your liver and muscles. Hormones and chemicals have been produced to make your body ready for action. Once the threat is gone, it may take hours for your body to reabsorb and use up the chemicals that have been activated, which can be exhausting to the body. This same physical reaction occurs when you get the winning Bingo number, burn your finger on the stove, take a math exam, perform in front of an audience, and so on.

Low-level stress can take its toll over time. Headaches, backaches, restlessness, difficulty sleeping, and stomachaches can all be symptoms of how you deal with stress. Your immune system can become depressed. Because these symptoms often develop slowly, you may not realize what is causing them.

Far too many people turn to food as their coping mechanism, often gaining weight because of it—to say nothing of indigestion. They are not feeding their body but their emotions. When a gazelle is faced with a potential threat, such as being stalked by a lion, it knows to forgo eating; the blood and oxygen that would be necessary to digest the food would have to be diverted from the stomach to its legs if it is to escape quickly. It's curious that people don't react the same way. When they are experiencing stress (''a potential threat''), many eat. Yet their body isn't ready to digest the food any more than the gazelle's body. The food is going to sit stagnantly in their stomach until the threat and the body's reaction to the threat has passed.

Emotional Reaction to Stress

You know that you're in the grip of stress when you feel angry, frustrated, anxious, nervous, depressed, tearful, unhappy, edgy. You feel powerless and out of control. As long as you continue to feel this way, you are inflicting the fight-or-flight response on your body. You need a way to deal with these stressors, and it may come down to how you use your type to alter your perception of them and what you believe you can do about them.

On the flip side are the emotional reactions to the positive stresses or good things happening in your life. You're ecstatic, jubilant, euphoric. They're definitely good feelings, but they, too, can drain you.

Behavioral Reaction to Stress

In negative stressful situations, you may turn to food in hopes that it will distract you from your unpleasant feelings and emotions. It worked when you were a child and your mother offered you a cookie after you skinned your knee. As adults, we may still believe the cookie will help. We also reach for food when something good happens. (After all, it's traditional to celebrate good feelings and happy occasions with good food and drink.)

Eating isn't the only way people deal with stress. Smokers may smoke too much. Drinkers may abuse alcohol. People who chew gum may chew it compulsively and with great force. Some people grind their teeth at night, waking up with sore jaws in the morning. We may become insomniacs or sleep excessively. Stress can turn people from Dr. Jekyll into Mr. Hyde. If they normally are soft-spoken, they may find themselves becoming loud and bossy. It's almost as if, by controlling others, they can feel in control of themselves.

The Mind's Reaction to Stress

Stress can affect your concentration, your ability to remember things, and your creativity. Decision making becomes difficult, causing you to doubt yourself. You worry more and don't believe you are in control of your life. Your sense of humor diminishes, and when things get really bad, life can look hopeless. You may blame yourself or others for the problem. Your mind may go over and over the situation, burning an indelible mark on your psyche.

What's interesting is that just the thought of something negative can produce a bodily reaction. Picture yourself in a classroom, and imagine the teacher accidentally scraping her nail on the blackboard. Or visualize yourself inadvertently biting into a piece of aluminum foil, scraping it against your fillings. What was your reaction? (Just writing it sent shivers down my back!) What about when you're tired from a full day's work? You crawl into bed, turn off the lights and close your eyes, only to find all the day's events replaying themselves. Every time you think about something negative, you actually cause your body to react as if it were really happening. It's fight-or-flight all over again.

Stress Is a Habit

Your reaction to some incidents becomes almost second-nature, a reflex you no longer think about. Let's say that the first time someone cuts in front of you while you're driving, you blow your horn and curse under your breath. If you figure that's a satisfactory reaction to this stressful situation, you'll do it again next time it happens. From then on, your reflex reaction will be to blow your horn and be angry. But the habit won't be doing you any good. It will only succeed in aggravating you further. Eventually, just the thought of someone cutting in front of you will get you angry.

Stinkin' Thinkin'

Everyone has certain irrational beliefs that can lead to distorted thinking. Such thinking can, in turn, be stressful because of the negative emotional reaction it causes. Only when you become aware of what these beliefs are and how damaging they can be can you change your negative habitual responses. The following is a list of different negative thinking habits; each is accompanied by an example. Which of these habitual responses sounds most like you?

- **All-or-nothing** thinking: "If I can't eat and exercise perfectly every day, it's not even worth trying."
- **Hearing-the-negative-in-the-positive** thinking: "When Jane told me how thin I looked, she was just trying to be nice. I know it's not true."
- **Generalizing** thinking: "I wasn't able to lose weight on the last diet. There's no reason to assume I can succeed on this one."
- **Catastrophizing** thinking: "If I eat any fat, I just know I'll die of heart disease."
- **Shoulda-coulda-woulda** thinking: "I should have exercised today."
- **Calling-yourself-names** thinking: "Just call me 'Blimp' for short. Goodyear was thinking of using me for the next televised football game!"

- **Jumping-to-conclusions** thinking: "Once you hear what I ate, you're going to think I've been bad."

You need to learn how to take these thoughts, defuse them, and substitute more positive thinking in their place. You have a decision to make.

Your Shadow Side

As you know by now, your personality type consists not only of your dominant and backup preferences, but also of your third and fourth preferences. Throughout this book, I've shown you how each of the preferences plays a part in the decisions you make—whether they're about goal setting, eating, or exercising. I have encouraged you to *consciously* and deliberately use your preferences to take advantage of what they have to offer. Your dominant preference will tend to lead, while your other preferences serve the dominant one. Learning to use all your preferences consciously will open up many more possibilities to you. Yet when you are under extreme stress, are very tired or ill, or are under the influence of alcohol or drugs, not all your thoughts, feelings, and actions may be under your conscious control. What you see then is the result of your fourth, or least-developed preference, acting immaturely and in an unconscious way attempting to take the role of your dominant preference. When that happens, your fourth preference has become your *shadow* preference.

Your dominant preference is like the driver of a car. Now, imagine what would happen if a five-year-old with no driving experience tried to drive the car from the backseat! That's what happens when the fourth preference takes over when you are under stress. You start doing and saying many ineffectual or destructive things that you normally wouldn't.

Experiencing Your Shadow Preference under Stressful Conditions

Let's see what your shadow side is experiencing when you are confronted with an extremely stressful situation. Remember, it's happening unconsciously. The shadow preference becomes an exaggeration, often a negative one, of what that preference would normally do consciously. You become controlled by it. Note that an average amount of stress may not create the profound responses that follow.

- **If you are a dominant Sensor, your shadow preference is iNtuiting.**
  As a dominant Sensor, you normally pay more attention to what is happening in the present. However, when under extreme stress, your shadow preference—iNtuiting—takes over. You look at future possibilities unrealistically, often in a negative way. You may set goals that are too grandiose. You can't seem to see the right road to take. Decision making may be crippled.
- **If you are a dominant iNtuitive, your shadow preference is Sensing.**
  As a dominant iNtuitive, you normally concern yourself with future possibilities. However, when under extreme stress, your shadow preference—Sensing—takes over. Your senses may be heightened to such a degree that you indulge in sensual pleasures uncontrollably (food being high on the list). If continually under stress, obesity and health problems may occur.
- **If you are a dominant Thinker, your shadow preference is Feeling.**
  As a dominant Thinker, you are normally concerned with the logical analysis of a situation. However, when under extreme stress, your shadow preference—Feeling—takes over. You are overcome by strong feelings and emotions with which you feel uncomfortable. You may become enraged or depressed easily. Your emotions may not even relate to the situation. Your normal logical approach to problems is unavailable to you.
- **If you are a dominant Feeler, your shadow preference is Thinking.**
  As a dominant Feeler, you are normally concerned with the emotional aspects of a situation—how others are affected, and how you value the situation. However, when under

extreme stress, your shadow preference—Thinking—takes over. Decisions are based on faulty logic, often an all-or-nothing and overgeneralized thinking. You come to conclusions that are questionable at best. You may start judging yourself mercilessly, finding yourself not thin enough, not good enough, not worthy enough, not competent enough.

Breaking Free of Your Shadow Preference

In order to break the grip of your shadow preference, you first have to realize that it has taken hold of you. Once again, you must become your own best observer. Imagine you are a spectator watching your thoughts, feelings, and actions. You can sense the tension building. You can feel yourself transforming from Dr. Jekyll into Mr. Hyde. You know that if you don't catch it early, the results can be devastating. Before you explode, you need to defuse the bomb. The best way to do that is to exaggerate your dominant preference. It will get you back into character.

- **If you're a dominant Sensor:** Do something that uses your senses. Work in the garden, do needlepoint or woodcarving. Visit a museum. Pay your bills.
- **If you're a dominant iNtuitive:** Plan a trip. Read a book. Set a new goal.
- **If you're a dominant Thinker:** Start analyzing something. What made me act with my shadow preference? What could happen if I had stayed in the throes of my shadow preference? Update your calendar. Organize a project.
- **If you're a dominant Feeler:** Do something nice for someone. Nurture yourself with a bubble bath or walk in the park. Play with a pet.

Stop It Before It Starts

As the saying goes, "An ounce of prevention is worth a pound of cure." It's better to learn to relax *before* stress hits you. That way you don't have to worry about your shadow side. Exercise and recreational activities can be stress reducers because they force us to slow down. They temporarily divert our attention from the stressors in our lives, helping us to maintain some sort of balance. Intense exercise can even produce endorphins or mood-lifting chemicals. However, these activities are not necessarily relaxing, since they can elicit a physiological response that calls on some of the same hormones and chemicals we use in a fight-or-flight response.

However, there are many relaxation techniques that, when practiced on a regular basis, can physically and psychologically alter your stress reaction and improve your overall well-being. They give your body the opportunity to release relaxation chemicals, slow down metabolism and breathing, and decrease muscle tension.

The most effective techniques are deep breathing, meditation, progressive muscle relaxation, and visualization. You will find a description of each over the next several pages. Give one or more of these a try to find which feels most comfortable for you. Improvements in your sleeping, eating, and coping patterns will tell you that what you've selected is working. In the long term, you could be decreasing your risk for many diseases. When you no longer depend on substances such as caffeine, alcohol, or nicotine to get you through the day, you'll know you're doing something right.

Under no circumstances should you view these relaxation techniques as a "must." If you do, they'll become just another stressor in your life. I grant you that, until you've experienced the benefits of these techniques, you might view the process as work. It will take some time to feel comfortable with a method and reap its rewards. When you start, five minutes may be all you can do. That's fine. As you progress, you'll find yourself wanting to extend the time and find yourself saying, "I'm worth it."

You can do these techniques anywhere, any time, for as little as a couple of minutes or as long as you like. Hopefully you'll get to the point where relaxation has become a part of your daily routine every bit as much as eating and sleeping are. Relaxation is a very special "me" time, a time for caring for yourself. You'll know that it's being effective when you feel better, have more energy, and are no longer allowing outside influences to control you.

Getting Ready

No matter what technique you use, there are several things you need to consider.

1. Find a quiet environment where you will be undisturbed. Subdued lighting is best. Set an alarm clock or a timer for 20–30 minutes. That way you can release your mind from worrying that you'll be late for something or not get other things completed.
2. Remove any constraining items (jewelry, glasses, belts, shoes).
3. Get into a comfortable position, whether it's sitting in a lounge chair or lying flat on a bed or the floor. If you choose to lie flat, place a rolled towel under your neck to elevate your chin. Also, place a pillow or several blankets under your knees to ensure that the small of your back is against the flat surface. Do not cross your arms or legs.
4. Try to empty your mind of all thoughts. However, if you find your mind wandering as you perform the techniques, just *gently* disregard the thoughts and go back to your relaxation method. Don't get anxious because you think you're not doing it right. It can take quite some time before you're able to empty your mind of thoughts. The main reason you're likely to struggle with this is because you're not truly living in the moment. You're probably thinking about the past or the future.
5. Breathe slowly, easily, and naturally. Many people get frustrated that they can't seem to keep thoughts from invading their mind when meditating. Focusing on your breathing will help. When you sense that your mind is wandering, gently bring your focus back to your breathing.
6. Closing your eyes usually helps keep you focused and less distracted by your environment.
7. If you find yourself falling asleep while doing these techniques, find an earlier time when you aren't tired. The idea is not to make up for a poor night's sleep. It's to intentionally generate relaxation chemistry.
8. After you finish a relaxation session, remain seated or lying

down quietly for a few minutes, allowing your senses to come back to your environment gradually.

9. These techniques take practice. No matter which one you find most favorable, do it regularly and consistently. It's no different from learning to play an instrument. In this case, the instrument is your body. Try to set aside the same time each day, and appreciate that this is your special time, a time that shouldn't be interrupted or neglected.

Deep Breathing

Most people don't appreciate how shallowly they normally breathe. They never totally fill their lungs to their capacity, nor exhale fully. Shallow breathing means you are not getting the optimum amount of oxygen into your lungs when you inhale. Without sufficient oxygen to your lungs, your blood has less to take to your cells. The less oxygen to the cells, the less energy they can produce. It's like slowly starving your cells of what they need. That's why we yawn when fatigued. The brain, feeling starved for oxygen, stimulates the yawning reflex, which forces you to inhale more deeply, gather up more oxygen and rejuvenate the brain. In addition, exhaling shallowly means that you are not ridding your body of all its waste products.

When you are under stress, your breathing may be shallow, even though it is a time when you need oxygen the most. Learning to breathe deeply is not only valuable as a relaxation technique to deal with feelings of anxiety, depression, irritability, muscle fatigue, and tension; it is essential for a healthy body.

The best position to do deep breathing is lying down. Close your eyes and relax, resting the palm of one hand gently on your stomach and the other on your chest. Let the tension drain out of you into the floor. Breathe normally through your nose. Now focus on the movement of your stomach with each inhale and exhale. As you inhale, feel your abdomen rise. As you exhale, your abdomen should lower. Try to concentrate the energy of your breaths into your stomach. Your chest should hardly move, just your abdomen. It may be easier for you to count slowly 1–2–3–4 as you inhale, pause for two counts and then exhale on a 1–2–3–4 count. Once you have a comfortable rhythm established breathing in and out through your nose, try inhaling through your nose and exhaling through your mouth. Remember to breathe very, very slowly and deeply but without any strain. With each inhalation, visualize the fresh oxygen traveling throughout your body from your lungs to the tips of your toes and fingers and to your brain, nourishing each and every cell. On each exhalation, visualize the waste products being expelled from your body. Continue for at least 15 minutes.

Take note of the sensations you are experiencing. The more you practice this technique, the more quickly you'll reach the relaxation state. Remember, deep breathing is always at your disposal when you sense yourself getting tense. Wherever you are, just close your eyes, take a few deep breaths, and feel the tension drifting away.

Meditation

Meditation is basically focusing your attention on a word, a vision, a sound, or even an imaginary energy force, so that other internal or external signals won't be able to intrude on your consciousness. You become one with the object of your meditation. Consider meditation a time to rest your mind. Stay in the moment. The best experiences will come when you relax your body and breathe slowly and gently.

Mantra Meditation

The mantra is a word or syllable that you repeat silently during meditation. You can choose a word that has meaning for you, but many meditators prefer the *om* sound. It produces a vibration that resonates throughout your body. Say it slowly and draw it out. Focus your mind on the sound and the vibrations. Create a rhythm of repetition that is comfortable for you. If you find thoughts or other stimuli intruding, redirect your focus to the word or syllable. Don't judge yourself or become impatient. Just gently bring your attention back to your mantra. It's often helpful to say it aloud if you find your mind wandering. If you are mechanically repeating the mantra without attention to it or its effect on your body, consider changing your mantra. The idea is to stay focused and in the present. Continue to do this for about 15 minutes, keeping your breathing slow and relaxed and taking care that there is no tension anywhere.

Vision Meditation

In vision meditation, you focus your attention on an object. The best position for it is sitting in a comfortable chair or sitting cross-legged on a cushion placed on the floor. A candle, an object that has special meaning to you, a flower, or a picture of a landscape scene all work well. Concentrate on the object before you. Just look. Notice all its details. Don't think about it, just experience it. This will be difficult at first because your mind is going to want to say something, however simple (for example, "What a beautiful flower"). If you're looking at the landscape picture, don't try to imagine yourself there and what you'd be doing. Just look at it and allow it to affect you. If you've chosen a candle, gaze at it until you feel you can no longer look at it. Then close your eyes and continue to experience the impression it has left on your retina. When you no longer have a sense of the candle, gaze at it again. Have a sense of all tension draining out of you as the object captures your attention.

Sound Meditation

In other forms of meditation, the idea is to block out sounds and sights so that you can concentrate on a word or vision. This form of meditative experience is different. Close your eyes and focus your attention on all the sounds around you. Don't try to figure out what they are or what's causing them or see a picture in your mind of what they are. Don't think of where you've heard that sound before. Just listen. Stay in the present. I find that being in the woods or out in nature somewhere is the best place to do sound meditation. The beauty of the birds chirping, the wind rustling through leaves, the scurrying of small animals through the underbrush—all make for a fulfilling experience. Remember to breathe slowly and gently, relaxing all the muscles of your body.

Energy Meditation

Whether sitting or lying down, close your eyes and breathe slowly, deeply, and gently. Now imagine a warm light shining down on the top of your head. You are being bathed in a warm glow. The energy from this light enters your head and starts to flow downward. You can feel its warmth running down over your face, your nose, your ears, then your neck and onto your shoulders. As the energy passes through your body, it drains away the tension and replaces it with relaxation and warmth. It radiates from your shoulders through your arms all the way to the very tips of your fingers. Let this energy travel very slowly so that it can touch every cell on its way. Now the warm energy slowly continues through your body, over your chest and back, your stomach, hips, thighs, calves, ankles, and down all the way to the very tips of your toes. All tension is dissipating and there is an overall warmth caressing your body.

Make sure you allow your imagination to work slowly and thoroughly. Don't skip any part of your body. If thoughts enter your mind, gently wash them away with the warm light.

Hand Meditation

Studies have shown that touch has a very healing quality. Babies grow up stronger and healthier when touched a great deal. Someone's hand on your shoulder or on your hand can be comforting. Of course, we don't always have someone around, so we can learn to do it to ourselves through hand meditation. It is easy, convenient, and doesn't take a great deal of time.

Sitting or lying down with your eyes closed, breathe slowly, deeply, and gently. Bring your hands together and allow your fingers to explore each other in a motion like washing your hands. Now slowly stroke the top of your left hand with the fingers from your right hand, starting at the wrist and ending at the tip of the fingers. Repeat this at least five times. When completed, reverse hands. Now stroke the palms the same way, remembering to do it very, very slowly. The stroke should be almost sensual and caressing. Next, surround the thumb of your left hand with the fingertips of your right hand. Starting at the base of the thumb, stroke all the way to its tip. Continue with the remaining fingers on your left hand. Repeat this at least five times very, very slowly. Then switch hands. Concentrate on the sensation in your hands. When thoughts start to enter your mind, gently remind yourself to focus on your fingers and the sensations in your body.

Progressive Muscle Relaxation

I'd like you to try a little experiment. Stop for a minute and just relax. Now, how do you feel? I'll bet that, even though you may think you relaxed, you probably still have some tension in your muscles, your breathing is somewhat irregular (rather than slow and smooth), and your brow is slightly furrowed. You are probably not completely relaxed.

Progressive relaxation is a technique you can use to get rid of the residual tension that commanding yourself to relax cannot accomplish. It is achieved by tensing a muscle group and then releasing it. The contrast between tensing and releasing is relaxation. It is called progressive relaxation because you'll be working muscle groups from your head down over your entire body. You basically contract the muscles, hold the tension for several seconds, and then relax those muscles, feeling the tension drain away.

To get the best results, you need to be sitting or lying comfortably and breathe slowly and gently. How you breathe during this exercise is important. Each time you do a contraction-relaxation repetition:

1. Inhale before you start the contraction.
2. Exhale while you tense the muscles.
3. Inhale while you hold the contraction.
4. Exhale during the release of the muscles.
5. Do one more deep inhalation and exhalation before starting another repetition, taking time to note the sense of relaxation in the muscles.

Don't hurry the process or force any muscle beyond just a slight tension. This should not cause you pain or discomfort. Being in a darkened room and closing your eyes during this procedure helps focus your attention on the particular muscle group and avoid any visual interruption of your concentration.

Start with your head. Inhale deeply. Then, as you exhale, raise your *eyebrows* as far up as you can, scrunching your *forehead.* Inhale as you hold it. Do you feel the muscle tension? Now exhale as you slowly release the contraction. Do one more deep inhalation and exhalation. Can you feel the difference? Try it again. Does your forehead feel more relaxed now than before you started? Do it a third time. Next comes the *exaggerated smile.* Imagine yourself saying "oh," "ah" and "ee," making the sounds (though you don't have to vocalize them) by exaggerating your mouth movement. While you say "oh," feel the muscles tense as your mouth forms the shape of an "o." Then open your mouth wide as it forms the "ah" sound. Lastly, feel the corners of your mouth pull upward while simultaneously pulling up on your neck muscles to form the "ee" sound. Hold it. Slowly release. Do this two more times. (This is also a great exercise to strengthen facial muscles and retard sagging.)

Let's move onto your *neck.* To achieve relaxation in your neck muscles, you will be working the muscles in the front and back of the neck. Bend your head forward as if you are going to touch your chin to your chest. At the same time, push your neck backwards. Tighten the muscles. Concentrate on the tension as you tighten the muscles. Now relax. Let the muscle go. Notice the difference between the state of relaxation and tension. Repeat two more times. Enjoy the feeling of deep relaxation and let that relaxation continue before going on to the next set of muscles.

Don't forget about your breathing, inhaling and exhaling at the right moments.

Now to your *shoulders.* Slowly raise your shoulders toward your ears and slightly back in a half-circular motion. You should feel it between your shoulder blades. Hold it. Slowly release by making a half-circular motion in the opposite direction to return to your starting posture. Repeat two more times. Now do it in reverse by raising your shoulders toward your ears and rotating them slightly forward in a half-circular motion. You may feel this in your pectoral or chest muscles. Hold and then slowly release, rotating in the opposite direction to return to your original posture. Again, enjoy the deep relaxation of the muscles before moving on.

Your arms will be done in two steps. First, you'll work on the *upper arm.* Pull your elbow into your body and down, but without moving your lower arm. Hold that tension and then relax. Repeat two more times. This next contraction will focus on your *forearms.* Rest the inside of your arms on a flat surface. Moving your hands at the wrist, raise just your hands and bend them back towards the top of your arms. Hold and slowly release. Repeat two more times.

Make a fist with each *hand.* Hold that tension, hard. Release. Repeat two more times.

Progressive relaxation of the lower part of your body produces the most obvious degree of relaxation because you are working with your body's large muscle groups. Tense the muscles in your *stomach* as if you were going to get hit in the abdomen. Make it hard. Release and repeat two more times. Squeeze your *buttocks* together. It should actually make you feel like you are rising off your chair or bed. Hold and slowly release. Repeat two more times.

You work your legs as you did your arms, first on the *upper leg,* followed by the lower leg and foot. To work the muscles in your thighs, tighten the muscles in the front and back of your leg as much as possible. Hold and slowly release. Repeat two more times. For the muscles in your *lower leg,* bend your feet at the ankle, pulling your toes up and raising them toward the top of your shins. Hold and slowly release. Repeat two more times. Lastly, to relax the muscles in your *feet,* point your toes as if you were a ballet dancer. Hold and slowly release. Repeat two more times.

Now that you have progressively relaxed your whole body, remain still and breathe deeply, enjoying total relaxation. If you find a muscle group that still seems slightly tense, repeat the exercise on that muscle group. The more you practice this, the more responsive your muscles will be. This method is especially useful for people who have trouble falling asleep at night or who find they have sporadic muscle twitches.

Visualization

As we discussed earlier, when you relive bad experiences in your mind, you inflict on your body the same fight-or-flight response you had originally. In a sense, your thoughts become your reality. Logically, then, if all your thoughts were positive ones, your body should be in a healthier state.

Visualizing is somewhat like daydreaming, just a little more structured. As in the *Uncle Remus Stories* by Joel Chandler Harris in which Brer Rabbit had his ''laffin' place,'' I want you to use visualizing as a way of reaching your ''laffin' place'' or happy spot. It's a place of your own creation, so by definition, it is a perfect place. Nothing negative or unhappy can happen here.

Let me share with you my ''laffin' place'' to give you an idea of how this works. As I close my eyes, I breathe deeply and slowly and relax into my chair. My ''laffin' place'' is a sparkling white beach on an island where warm trade winds blow. The breezes caress my face and body. The water looks aqua blue and so crystal clear, I can see right to the bottom. The sun shines overhead, its warmth penetrating into my very core, relaxing all my muscles. The waves lap up onto the beach in rhythmic procession. As each wave retreats into the ocean, it takes one more layer of stress and tension from my body. I'm strolling along the beach, my feet sinking into the warm sand with each step. I take a moment to wriggle my toes in the sand. Next I notice the yellow hibiscus flowers, the red ginger plants, the leathery green foliage, the white jasmine with its fragrant perfume. There are yellow-breasted finches and hummingbirds. Their sounds are sweet and melodic, in rhythm with the lapping water. I listen to hear their conversations. I decide to sit down on the beach to enjoy every moment. No thoughts, just the sheer joy of the experience.

Before I know it, 20 minutes have passed, the alarm has gone off and it is time to return to reality. Yet I return refreshed.

Select somewhere or something special to you. It doesn't have to be a nature scene. It could be making bread, painting a picture, playing golf, or gardening, anything that is personally satisfying to you. See it in all its details and experience the emotions. Feel as if you are really there and it is really happening to you. After visiting your ''laffin' place'' a number of times, you should be able to conjure up the image any time you feel tension beginning to well up. Just that momentary thought can quickly change your mood.

Other Methods

Communing with Nature

Just look at the concrete jungles and sterile environments within which we work. We've lost touch with nature. That's sad, because there is probably nothing more relaxing than enjoying the beauty of trees and flowers or watching the antics of squirrels and birds. It's especially nice in spring, when the trees' new growth is a fresh, bright green, or when the buds on a bush start to burst through their jackets. The smell of pine needles or flowers in bloom can produce a heady feeling. Try taking a stroll or sitting on a park bench to take in nature's bounty. Maybe go to the zoo and watch the animals. Take your pet for a walk. If you don't have one, walk your friend's pet. Don't think . . . just be. This may be very hard for you iNtuitives and Introverts, who will struggle to keep your brains still. One moment you'll be very good about just looking. Then, before you know it, you'll find that your mind has wandered to a thought. Communing with nature is a very here-and-now experience, something you Sensors and Extraverts should easily relate to.

Humor

Have you had your laugh today? Laughter can truly be the best medicine. At least, it was for Norman Cousins, a journalist who contracted a supposedly incurable connective tissue disease. He wasn't going to go out without a fight, so he fought back with laughter. He watched old *Candid Camera* films and the Marx Brothers movies, read cartoons and funny stories. He also took very large doses of vitamin C. At the time, doctors didn't appreciate that laughter stimulates the release of endorphins, morphine-like chemicals that have painkilling capabilities. Endorphins have also been found to stimulate the immune system. Laughter can also help strengthen the heart muscle.

Think about how you feel after you've had a good laugh. If you're like most people, you feel better. So what tickles your funny bone? Try a dose of it every day. Here are some ideas I have heard over the years. They may seem childish, but then, how often do children get stressed?

1. Put on a clown's nose and watch the reactions. You'll have made light of the stressful situation, and the laughter you cause in others can be infectious.
2. Pop popcorn without putting the lid on the popcorn maker. (Okay, so you'll have some cleanup, but think of the fun you'll have.)
3. Use alphabet soup to make up a short sentence.
4. Tape a line on your clothes with a sign that says "I've had it up to here!"
5. Use chopsticks to eat Jell-O®.
6. Try juggling marshmallows. Afterwards, have a marshmallow fight with someone.

Relaxation Tips

- Share your worries and concerns with someone else, especially someone with an opposite personality type. He or she will have a different perspective that may help a lot.
- Consider what you're watching on television or what you are reading. Sometimes the news can be stressful. Even television dramas can be depressing. The newspapers tend to fill their front pages with wars, deaths, and mayhem. Maybe turn to the cartoon section instead. Remember, you can choose what you are exposed to.
- Write your stressful thoughts down on paper. Sometimes removing them from your brain and putting them on paper makes you look at them differently. Then tell yourself that the stressful thoughts are no longer going to control you and throw the paper in the waste basket. Let your emotions go with the paper.
- Get the facts about the situation that's bothering you. It may be that you are allowing your imagination to get the better of you because you don't have all the information you need.

- It's okay to say "no" occasionally when someone asks you to do something.
- Planning ahead will often help eliminate anxiety. Practice "what if" situations, rehearsing what you would do in a stressful situation. See yourself handling the situation with ease.
- Learning to manage your time better will give you less reason to get stressed because of time constraints. Living in the moment also helps, since you are *dealing* with the situation, not fretting about the possibility of it occurring or its potential outcome.
- Be careful about what you think or say. It could become your reality. When you say something like "He's going to kill me when he sees what I've done," appreciate that those words are being accompanied by a mental picture. The incident may never come to pass, but you have just inflicted a fight-or-flight response on yourself. Better to make positive statements or affirmations, such as "I am capable" or "I am at peace." You'll be surprised how convincing you can be.
- Keep asking yourself what are the possibilities in the situation. How can you make a lemonade out of what you think is a lemon?
- Avoid hassles. For example, if you find yourself regularly rushing off to work in the morning with little time for breakfast, make something the night before that you can either eat at home or take with you. Try getting up fifteen minutes earlier in the morning to have time to address the inevitable morning mishaps. If you don't like driving in rush-hour traffic, consider a carpool or public transportation. Maybe you can arrange to work a different shift.
- Simplify your life.
- Have a backup plan for those "just in case" situations.
- Do a minirelaxation session whenever you feel tension beginning to erupt. Anything you learned in this chapter can be done for as short a time as several minutes and still provide some benefits.
- When you're feeling stressed, try writing your thoughts and feelings in a journal. Explain the situation and what you're

experiencing. At the end of the week, look over your journal and see if there is a common thread. That's what you will need to pay attention to.

- Get the unpleasant jobs done early in the day, so the rest of the day you can be free from anxiety.
- Develop a hobby you enjoy and look forward to doing. You deserve some "me" time.
- When you're under stress, put your Thinking preference to work to analyze the situation. Let your Sensing preference gather the facts for your Thinking preference. What's the problem that is causing you stress? What is keeping you from seeing the solution? Put your Feeling preference to bed temporarily. Allow your Thinking preference to sort everything out and show you that the catastrophe you fear is quite unlikely to happen and that your reaction is blown out of proportion. Let your iNtuiting preference come up with alternatives to help change the situation or at least view the possibilities of the situation differently. Put these possible solutions through your Thinking preference to analyze their pros and cons. Now you can let your Feeling preference put its stamp of approval on your plan for dealing with the situation.

12

Making It a Habit #7: Make It Last

Do you plan to *change* or do you plan to *grow* from what you have learned in this book? There is a major difference between change and growth. How you view these two concepts may determine whether you will achieve success in establishing healthy lifestyle habits for the long term. Growth involves developing and using all your personality preferences. Maturity does not inevitably come with change; it does come with growth. That is what is going to "make it last."

While growth always entails change, change does not always bring about growth. We think of growth in positive terms, whereas change can go either way. In addition, change doesn't have to be permanent. You can change right back. On the other hand, with growth, you are transforming and becoming someone different. It's like the caterpillar that has transformed itself into a butterfly. It hasn't just changed; it can never go back to being a caterpillar. It has *grown* into being a butterfly.

Most people who have tried to improve their lifestyle habits and found themselves back where they started were only *changing* their habits, not *growing* permanent new ones. They superimposed rules on themselves that they never really bought into or that worked with their personality. The effort may have been for a short-lived purpose (for example, losing weight for a class reunion) or because someone else wanted it for them. Once the pressures for changing were lifted, the old habits kicked back in.

Growth means adding and integrating new ideas, thoughts, facts, and skills. When we "go on a diet," we are not integrating anything. Once we have achieved our goal, we'll "go off the diet" just as quickly. That is change, not growth. What I'm asking you to do is grow from all you've learned in this book. Let your less-favorite preferences develop and become assets to your growth process. Take a proactive stand and allow your preferences to determine what additions you want to make and how you hope to transform yourself. Think again about your *life vision,* for that is what you will be transforming into.

Mind Trails

There are billions of cells in the brain that are capable of communicating with each other. Once a pathway of communication has been established, it is there forever. Some of those pathways are our memories. The more we call upon certain memories, the more indelibly etched they become in our mind, the ruts of those pathways becoming figuratively deeper. That is what has happened with your habits. They are pathways in your brain that have been used over and over again so that you may sometimes feel you can't climb out of their ruts.

Fortunately, you have billions of cells that you haven't even tapped into and that are just ready and waiting for you to write new habits on. With the help of this book and conscious effort on your part, you can be blazing new mind trails. These trails can become just as established as your old unhealthy habits. In fact, the more you use your new habits and the less you use your old habits, the more likely it is that the new habits will become your natural response and require no thought. If you don't make an effort to continually use your new habits but allow yourself to fall back into your old unhealthy habits, your brain will never make the connection that the new habits are the ones to use. And so you will just be making deeper ruts in the unhealthy habit trails.

It Won't Happen Overnight

If you could have your way (at least you _S_Ps, anyway), you'd probably like to wave a magic wand and have the transformation and the growth take place in an instant. But life doesn't work that way. The caterpillar must weave a cocoon and hibernate for a time before emerging as a butterfly. A human baby takes nine months before making its appearance in the world. An elephant takes 22 months. Why should we expect to transform overnight into a person who believes in and is driven by healthy lifestyle habits?

Growth takes time. There will be an interval of transformation followed by an interval of constancy, a plateau that we must live through before embarking on another cycle of transformation and constancy. Most people view these plateaus with agony, often feeling defeated. Yet, reaching a plateau provides you with the opportunity to refocus your attention on another aspect of your growth and allows what you have already achieved to become fully integrated. As I shared with you in the previous chapter, you shouldn't try to change all your habits at once. First of all, the task is too overwhelming. Second, if you work on one or two things at a time, you can switch to something else when you reach the inevitable plateau. Since growth refers to transforming the total you, it really doesn't matter if you work on various habits in a piecemeal fashion, as long as you are continually moving forward. That may be a little easier for you iNtuitives than for you Sensors. iNtuitives don't mind working randomly on numerous new things, whereas Sensors prefer to do things in a step-by-step sequential order. Sensors may prefer to work on one objective at a time, allowing that objective its possible plateau, and then picking up with that objective once again when you feel you're ready to move ahead.

You never stop growing (and I don't mean from side to side!). The transition you are making will bring an end to many old habits. Then there will be stages of learning, periods of integrating what you are learning, and the new beginnings of healthier habits, when you adjust to your new approach. You don't have to give up everything about yourself to grow. Think about all the valuable experiences and learning you've already stored away.

You needn't regret giving up an old unhealthy habit for something new. Just know that you are growing in the process. It shows that you realize something in your old way of doing things isn't working and you need to find something that does. Hopefully this book has set you on the path of growth, providing you with a variety of facts and skills, so that you can discover what works for you. Then, over time, you can integrate your new learning by experimenting with it. Now is the time when you can view things through a new filter and see the opportunities that lie in store. If it feels comfortable, consider it your new beginning. As the saying goes, "This is the first day of the rest of your life."

Keeping an Eye on Yourself

This journey of growth is your personal journey, directed and guided by you. Someone else may see things you're doing that are unhealthy. However, until *you* see and take on the changes as your own personal *cause,* nothing is going to be altered. It's going to take a watchful eye on your part to discover what unhealthy lifestyle habits you have. Once you see your trouble spots and accept that they're problems, you can select the knowledge and skills necessary to fix them.

Self-awareness may be easier for the Sensors than for the iNtuitives since it requires you to stay in the present. The iNtuitives are too often considering how they can be different "one of these days" and can easily lose sight of where they are right now. However, it's necessary to be fully aware of both your present condition and the transformation you'd like to see happen. That is why Sensors need to work on their iNtuiting skills and iNtuitives need to work on their Sensing skills.

Monitor by Measuring

No matter what habits you're trying to improve, taking some pertinent measurements lets you know that you are on track. For example, if you want to lower your blood cholesterol, a periodic blood cholesterol test can reassure you that your new healthy way of eating or the exercise program you've started is accomplishing the task.

If you are trying to lose weight, *occasionally* stepping on the scale is okay. But if you insist on taking a daily measurement, you'll only be fooling yourself. Since it takes a decrease of 3500 calories (through less calorie intake and more energy expenditure) to lose one pound, it's impossible to accomplish that feat in one day. (Don't believe those supermarket tabloids and magazines telling you that you can lose five pounds in one day!) So why tease or torment yourself every day, expecting the good fairy to miraculously change the numbers on the scale for you? It may only prove demotivating. If you've been good about exercising and eating healthfully, you are replacing fat with muscle, which is going to weigh more. Unless you have a body-composition analysis performed that shows you the change in your body's percentage of fat, you're going to believe that the extra pounds on the scale mean your new habits aren't working. Actually, I believe that just looking at yourself naked in the mirror will tell you much of what you need to know. Weighing yourself once a week is more than enough.

Keeping records can be very enlightening and encouraging. In Chapter 10, I provided you with an exercise log. If you fill it out diligently, you'll be able to monitor your progress. You'll see how your exercise repetitions, amount of weights being lifted, and length of exercise time have increased. It's easy to lose track of your accomplishments when all you notice is what you're doing today and ignore where it all began. I firmly believe that we're never too old for gold stars. So stick some on your log and reward yourself with something special.

Don't forget about the Meal Plans in Chapter 8. You can be monitoring your progress on them as well. If you're into computers, you might consider buying some nutrition software that helps you keep track of what you're eating, analyzes your diet, records how much you're exercising, and even graphs the results.

Set Limits

It's very easy for the pounds to start creeping on as we get older. If you have had success losing weight, you also know how pounds seem to be attracted to a newly reduced body. Avoiding weight gain (unless you start out underweight) should definitely be part of the game plan to reach your *life vision.* Monitoring is a valuable tool for the process, as is setting limits. If you're maintaining your weight within two to three pounds, congratulations. Keep up the good work. (The fluctuation is probably due to water retention.)

However, if you gain more than three pounds, you have something to think about. Those pounds represent additional fat, not just additional water. (One exception could be menstruating women, who retain a great deal of water at that time of the month.) Now it's time to become concerned and consider what you are doing that can be contributing to the problem (unless it's related to a health problem). Have you stopped using the decision-making process? Are you no longer trying to stay consciously aware of what you are doing? Without any limits, it's too easy to go beyond a three-pound gain and promise yourself "one of these days I'll have to get serious and do something." The next time you look, it's a 10-pound gain.

Once your weight has increased that much, it is very hard to take it off. At this point, your Feeling preference will be telling you what a failure you are and that this whole weight game is hopeless. You can never win. Your Sensing preference will be reinforcing your negative view of yourself by pointing out how big you've gotten. (If it were in the right frame of mind, it could remind you of how good you looked at your healthy weight and how history could repeat itself in a positive way.) Your Thinking preference will be logically pointing out to you why you've failed (but it, too, could use logic to show you how to get back on track). Your iNtuiting preference will still be hopeful that one day things will get better. It's a matter of how you want to use your preferences.

The point I want to make here is that setting yourself a limit (a value you assign) can save you a lot of heartache and work later. This limit can apply to your weight, the amount you eat, what you are choosing to eat, and so on. It tells you when to put on the brakes, when the red lights should start flashing, and when your conscious awareness needs to kick in again.

Select Targets

Targets give you something to shoot for. For example, when you decide to do pushups, you should decide how many are reasonable for you. Let's say your target is 25 pushups. That target gives you something to aim for. You may be more willing to put up with a little discomfort knowing the end is not far away (that is, unless you set too callenging a target). As you're doing your 25 pushups, you realize by the sixteenth pushup you may not make it to 25. Do you quit at 16? Can you do maybe 3 more pushups? By having set 25 as your target, you may be willing to push yourself to come close to that target.

Without a target, you may quit at the first sign of difficulty. However, at the moment when you're wondering if you can go beyond 16, you could reset your target of 25 to 20. It now looks achievable. If you're honest with yourself, you might have set your target too high and, in turn, set yourself up for failure. So there is no harm in resetting the target when you begin to assess what you are capable of. Better to change the target than to give up completely.

Rewards and Accolades

What would satisfy you as a reward for a job well done or progressing nicely? When people used to lose weight through abstinence from their favorite foods, their reward tended to be those foods. However, you now know that the best approach to healthy lifestyle eating habits is to eat everything you like but in moderation. So you no longer have to look to food as the reward. That would just be sabotaging your great efforts.

What else would measure up to reward status for you? Receiving praise for making progress toward your goals may be sufficient reward. People noticing the results of your efforts makes the accomplishment that much sweeter. Of course, a new outfit or a trip somewhere wouldn't be too bad either.

Why don't you try this idea? Cut up a sheet of 8½-inch x 11-inch paper into 12 approximately equal-size pieces. On each slip, write a reward for accomplishing a task. Fold the pieces of paper in half and put them in a jar. When it comes time to reward yourself, close your eyes and pull out a suggestion.

What's Standing in Your Way?

Trying to change too many things about yourself at one time can stop the growth process. Appreciate that to change one habit, you may have to change other habits at the same time. Therefore, setting out to change too many habits at one time may set up an avalanche of changes that cannot be easily integrated into your daily life. For example, you may have the unhealthy habit of skipping breakfast because you don't have the time to make something for yourself before running off to work. Not only are you asking your body to run on the few reserves you have left from dinner the night before, you've increased the chances that you'll grab something at work that is less than healthy. Once you decide that eating breakfast is a healthy thing to do, your habit of leaving yourself just enough time to get dressed and out the door will have to change. You may have to create a new habit of planning ahead—making breakfast the night before (something that may be challenging for you Perceivers). Adding exercise to this new morning ritual may be too much at first. If you are used to getting up at the last minute, the addition of both exercise *and* breakfast before you head off to work may set you up for failure. It may be better to include only breakfast in your morning ritual and save exercise for after work. Become comfortable with that routine before considering exercise in the morning.

As long as you are reacting to situations rather than being proactive, you are not growing. Reacting means staying afloat, using whatever skills you presently have to maintain your current position. This is not growth. It's not even change. To accomplish growth and change, you must be proactive. Learning new knowledge and skills, as well as making choices, is at the root of proaction. When you think of the two words, *re-action* and *pro-action,* you can appreciate the difference. *Re-action* means responding or acting against some force, typically in a similar fashion as before. However, if what you did before didn't work, why do it again? *Pro-action,* on the other hand, means acting in a forward or advancing direction, which should produce different and potentially better results.

Doggedly staying in your comfort zone, with its old habits, can pose a threat to growth. Most people don't like making mistakes. When you venture outside your comfort zone by trying new ways of doing things, you're bound to stumble occasionally. But the best learning comes from trying new things and making mistakes. This testing and experimenting stage enables you to see what works and what doesn't. If you did everything perfectly, it means either that you're a genius or that you're not stretching yourself beyond your present capabilities. However, I'm not suggesting that you stretch too far at each stage of learning because you first need to be successful to want to continue the process.

That brings us to self-esteem. **Without good self-esteem and a belief in your ability to grow, you won't be able to grow.** You may feel that your unhealthy habits are evidence of how weak and incapable you are of altering your ways. Yet this thinking is like the dog chasing its tail. Until you're willing to see yourself differently, you'll continue to "chase your tail," acting in the same way that makes you believe you aren't capable of change. What will make you believe in yourself?

1. Feeling that you are in control helps. Accepting change as your personal responsibility makes you feel less like a victim. Every time you find yourself pointing a finger away from yourself and at someone or something else, realize that you're trying to take the burden of accountability off yourself.
2. Trying something new, something with a low risk of failure, and seeing your accomplishment, can increase your belief that you are capable. Failure because of lack of effort should not be construed as personal failure but the result of lack of motivation and commitment. If this is happening, it's time to go back to the drawing board and think about why you set off on this journey in the first place.
3. Breaking the task into small steps—multiplying your opportunities to succeed—is another way to increase your belief in yourself. Success with one step or task can promote success with others.
4. Enlisting the help of someone else who can provide feedback, especially positive feedback, can also be beneficial.

Your dominant personality preference can stand in your way. Your dominant preference is accustomed to doing things in a certain way and isn't always happy to let your less-favored preferences take over. Intentionally staying in the present, where you can watch your dominant preference at work, will help you to make changes. You must consciously work at developing your other personality preferences, since that really is at the heart of growth. Use the Decision Road Maps frequently to keep you on track.

Just a Lot of Talk?

Do you really want to change, or are you just a lot of talk? Unless you are truly motivated to grow, you will just find yourself making temporary changes. It will look good on the surface, but deep down you'll know the truth: "I really don't want to change." For instance, if you don't like to exercise but are jogging because your friend is, or you were told that it would be good for you, your attempts will be short-lived.

How much commitment to growth do you have? At the time you make the decision to change a habit, you could probably rate your commitment a "10" on a scale of 1 to 10 (10 being the greatest amount of commitment). However, your resolve to change may diminish over time. If you're a Sensor and your efforts are not producing immediate results, you will be disappointed. If you're an iNtuitive, and your efforts are not up to your expectations, you will be disappointed. You need to reassess the approach you're using to change a habit. It may not be as appropriate as you thought or as fitting to your personality type as you would like. Also, the original reason to change may no longer exist, and might need to be reassessed.

It's important to reassess your level of motivation and commitment, being sure you really want to grow. In the movie *Star Wars—The Empire Strikes Back,* Yoda, the Jedi Master, is teaching Luke Skywalker what it takes to become a Jedi warrior. Yoda challenges Luke to raise his spacecraft from the marshy waters into which it crashed. Luke says, "All right. I'll give it a try." To this Yoda replies, "No! Try not. Do, or do not. There is no 'try'." I pose the same directive to you. You must not *try* to transform your lifestyle habits, for *trying* simply means you are not fully invested in the process and are willing to accept failure. You must *do,* for only by *doing* will you exert all your efforts until you succeed.

Relapses Are the Result of Decisions You Make

To experience a lapse means you've reverted back to your old habits. It doesn't mean you're a failure. It may be that you didn't learn the lessons of a healthy lifestyle well enough. Or maybe you encountered a situation that had previously triggered unhealthy responses, and you fell back into your old habits without thinking. Maybe someone pressured you into repeating a bad habit, and you didn't feel strong enough to resist the pressure. I believe that relapses are due to poor decision making or even to the absence of decision making and are great opportunities from which to learn and grow.

Much as we would like to blame others, the environment, the situation, or even our own weakness for causing us to revert to our unhealthy habits, the lapse or relapse doesn't just happen. It is essential that you appreciate, no matter what the circumstances, that lapses or relapses are products of the decisions you make. Sometimes you may not think so because the decisions are being made out of conscious awareness using previous habitual responses. When you realize you are falling back into your old habits, it's time to reassess your decision-making process. You're probably ignoring valuable input from some of the preferences. If so, it's time to reread Chapter 5, Breaking Habits—Making Habits.

Lapses are understandable when you begin your journey to your *life vision.* You're in the learning stages, and to expect perfection is only setting yourself up for defeat. (Are you _NT_s and _NF_s listening?) Staying in the present will help you avoid lapses because it forces you to address what's going on at the moment and make decisions accordingly. If you experience a succession of relapses, it means you are not staying aware of your actions, nor employing the skills you have learned nor accepting that it is your personal responsibility to grow. When you find this happening, it may be wise to reread Chapter 1, Know Where You're Headed and Why, and reassess your goals. Your life vision should be like the proverbial carrot that lures you on and encourages you to make the necessary decisions.

Many of the decisions you must make may be difficult and stressful, and you may find yourself avoiding them. Yet that is just acting like the ostrich with its head in the sand. You cannot grow from avoiding difficult situations.

Like most people, you may have a tendency to rationalize or justify an unhealthy action or behavior. You'll pull out all the stops with your Thinking preference, making the reasons for the behavior sound very logical, or use your Feeling preference to undervalue the significance of an unhealthy behavior so that you can continue it without guilt. Whatever you do is based on a decision, however poorly made. Remember, every decision you make should be one you feel comfortable with and can easily support. If you don't feel comfortable with the decision, you need to go over the process and decide again.

When you have a craving for something, it's just a warning sign that you must concentrate more on the decision-making process. The more you try to ignore a craving, the stronger it will get. If you don't address it early on, its power will grip you. Then your decision to satisfy the craving won't consider the input from all your preferences. If you give into a craving, it should be because, after collecting the facts about the situation, analyzing those facts, considering the alternatives and the effect on you and others, you still believe the craving should be satisfied. You needn't chastise yourself since a consciously made decision, done with all your preferences, should not be considered a lapse. Take note, though, that continually satisfying your cravings by twisting the decision-making process into affirming your cravings is a lapse, because your decisions are not being made with the intent of moving forward toward your *life vision.* If you're feeling guilty or regretting your decision, then your craving is a lapse.

If you find your decisions are too often based on "shoulds," don't be surprised if you tend to lapse more frequently. For many people, "shoulds" mean deprivation, which, in turn, eventually ends up in overindulgence. It also implies that someone or something outside of yourself is imposing the rules, rules that you may not have bought into. It's better to make your decisions on the basis of "wants" because then there is self-fulfillment. Of course, self-fulfillment must take your *life vision* into account so it doesn't end up as pure pleasure-seeking.

There are situations that are outside your decision-making control. For example, you may be on medication that stimulates your appetite. However, what you end up eating is your decision. You may be restricted by your doctor to bedrest, meaning exercise may be out of the question. However, before you make the final judgment, ask your doctor. A leisurely stroll may be allowed.

Being prepared will help you to avoid lapses. We all pretty much know what situations are going to make us act in our old ways with our unhealthy habits. Taking a little time before you encounter that situation to plan what you'll do is time well spent. For Introverts, who like to rehearse and think things over before experiencing something, preplanning is no problem. Judgers are also very good at planning. It's the Extraverts, Sensors, and Perceivers I worry about. The Extraverts can be influenced by other people and follow their lead. The Sensors, who live in the here-and-now, will tend to be reactive rather than proactive and have a greater tendency to fall into their old traps. This is especially true for _S_Ps, whose tendency toward instant gratification may outweigh the potentially negative effect of relapsing. You'll need to look to some of your other preferences to help you out. Again, think in terms of the Decision Road Maps.

A Little Reminder

While you more naturally allow your dominant and backup preferences to be heard, remembering to use the complete 1–2–3–4 decision-making approach guarantees your less-favored preferences a chance to have their say. A clever trick to be sure you tap into all your preferences is to use your fingers as a reminder. Hiding your hand in your pocket or under the table, as you go through using your 1–2–3–4 order, first lift your pointer finger as you consider your dominant or #1 preference's contribution, then lift your middle finger to represent your backup or #2 preference's contribution, then your ring finger for #3, and lastly

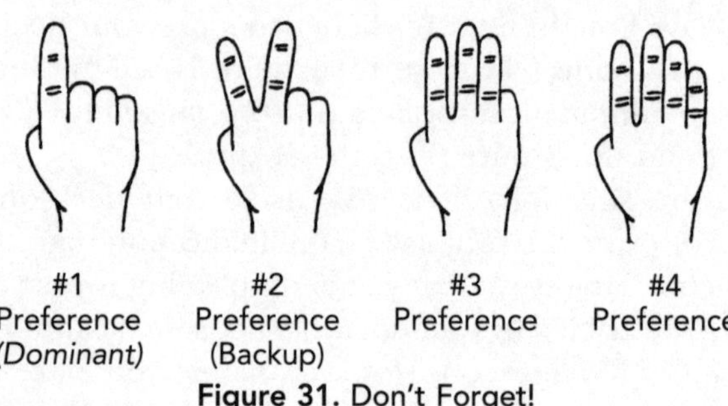

Figure 31. Don't Forget!

your pinky finger for #4. When you end up with all your fingers extended, you know you've considered the input from all four of the preferences. (See Figure 31.)

A Little Support May Be of Value

Extraverts have no qualms about making a public announcement about their plans, and may even ask others for help to keep them on track. That's not to say that Introverts won't ask for help. However, they may need to take some private time to decide what they want to do, start doing it and then, once they're sure about the approach, share it with a few special individuals.

Enlisting the help of others is not only for moral support, but for possible constructive suggestions. If someone else has been through what you're going through, why not take advantage of what they've learned? There is no question that experience is your best teacher, but it doesn't hurt to head off in the right direction. Isn't that why you are reading this book? You may find that having company on your path to a healthier lifestyle makes the journey more enjoyable.

Consider finding others whose dominant personality preference is the same as your backup or less-favored preferences. They can provide you with the support your less-favored preferences need in order to grow. They view life from a different perspective because of their different personality type. We each have something very valuable to offer. The older we get, the wiser we get. That's because our less-favored preferences have had the opportunity to develop, which provides a more expanded view of life.

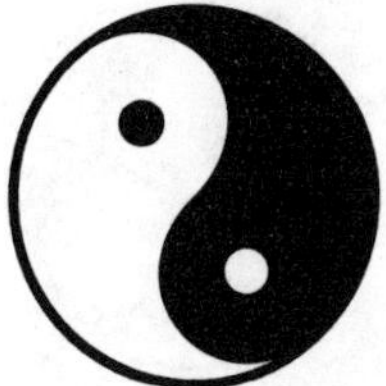

Figure 32. The Symbol for Yin and Yang

Until that happens, seek out those people who can enrich your less favored preferences.

For example, if you're an ESTP, ESFP, ISFJ, or ISTJ, your dominant Sensing is trying to convince you that what you're doing isn't working: "Look, I don't see any change." A dominant iNtuitive can encourage you to keep on your path to your *life vision* by saying, "Tomorrow you'll see a difference" and suggesting ways for you to get there. A dominant Feeler can tell you how proud she is of what you're doing and that you should feel the same way. A dominant Thinker can explain to you logically how the healthy eating and exercising you are doing is going to produce results—if not today, then soon. Others can help bring a more balanced approach to your growth process. What's great about having others involved in this process is that they don't bring the negativity about your goals that you might personally experience. What better cheering section could you ask for?

The Balancing of Type

One of the basic concepts in the Chinese Tao is the concept of yin and yang—achieving balance. Life isn't a matter of either/or, right/wrong, good/bad, black/white, win/lose, all/nothing. It is a dynamic interaction of opposites. That is the reason for the yin/yang symbol. (See Figure 32.) Something or someone isn't all good (the white portion of the symbol). Some bad exists within it (the black dot). In like manner, something or someone isn't all bad (the black portion). Some good exists within it (the white dot).

When you think of this yin/yang concept as applied to person-

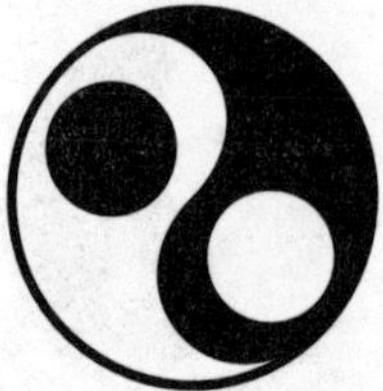

Figure 33. The Symbol for Yin and Yang, adapted to show an increased balance of opposites

ality types, you can better appreciate the contribution of all the preferences. You may be a dominant Sensor (say, the white portion), but you have some balance from the iNtuitive preference (the black dot). You may have a backup preference of Thinking (say, the black portion), but have the balance from the Feeling preference (the white dot).

What you need to do to keep your life in balance is to grow your less-favored preferences so they may more fully contribute to the decision-making process and, in turn, improve your lifestyle habits. Only when Sensing and iNtuiting, Thinking and Feeling, Extraverting and Introverting, and Judging and Perceiving are more in balance will you be able to reach your *life vision.* (See Figure 33.) It will take some conscious effort on your part, but I know you'll find the results are worth it.

Success Comes to Those Who Believe

In *The Empire Strikes Back,* Luke learns another very good lesson from Yoda. Through his concentration and use of the Force, Yoda is able to lift the spacecraft from the water. Luke exclaims, "I don't believe it." And, as Yoda so succinctly puts it, "That is why you fail."

Only when you believe you can alter your lifestyle habits, will you succeed. Your *life vision* is yours for the taking. Yes, it will take some time and effort on your part. Yet anything worth having is cherished that much more when earned. You can't look to someone else to do this for you. You've made the first big step by wanting to learn how. As an ENFJ and nurturer, I hope I've been able to give you the knowledge to make it possible.

RECIPES

The recipes that follow are designed to be delicious, healthy and, especially, easy to make. They are organized into six categories: Appetizers and Beverages, Desserts and Sweets, Main Dishes, Soups, Salads, and Vegetables. Each recipe contains nutrition information in the form you see on food package labels. Not only do you learn about the amount of nutrients in a serving, you also learn the *% Daily Value* for those nutrients. This gives you an idea of how much of your nutrition allowance is used up when eating a serving from a particular recipe.

I have tried to keep the sodium content fairly low. Those of you who are not salt-sensitive, feel free to add more salt to taste. The *Nutrition Facts* for each recipe will reflect the salt content based on the stated ingredients. So, if you add salt, keep in mind that one teaspoon of salt contains a little less than 2400 mg of sodium, the recommended daily maximum based on the guidelines of the American Heart Association.

In a number of recipes, I have made suggestions for "optional" ingredients. These ingredients were not included in the nutritional analysis of the recipe.

Olive and canola oils were used in many of the recipes because of their high monounsaturated fat content. If you choose to use safflower, corn, or some other vegetable oil instead, the *Total Fat* content won't be affected, but the nutritional analysis for the *Saturated Fat* content may change.

Fat-lowering tip: If you want to lower the fat content of a recipe, use about 2 tablespoons of broth instead of sautéing in oil. As you continue to sauté, you may need to add a little more liquid to keep the food from sticking to the pot.

Cabbage Bundles

1 tablespoon toasted sesame seeds
½ pound ground turkey breast
1 tablespoon canola oil
1 cup cooked brown rice
1 tablespoon light soy sauce
½ teaspoon Chinese Five Spices
1 teaspoon sugar
½ teaspoon salt
4 tablespoons sherry wine or chicken broth
Napa cabbage or Savoy cabbage leaves
Cilantro sprigs (optional)

NUTRITION FACTS	
Servings per Recipe 4	
Amount Per Serving	
Calories 210	Calories from Fat 50
	% Daily Value*
Total Fat 6g	**8%**
Saturated Fat 1g	**2%**
Cholesterol 50mg	**17%**
Sodium 510mg	**21%**
Total Carbohydrates 16g	**5%**
Dietary Fiber 1g	**6%**
Sugars 3g	
Protein 21g	
Vitamin A 7% •	Vitamin C 18%
Calcium 3% •	Iron 8%

In a frying pan over medium-high heat, toast the sesame seeds for 5 minutes or until golden brown, shaking pan continuously. Remove sesame seeds to a small dish.

Using the same frying pan, brown the ground turkey in the oil. Add the rice, sesame seeds, soy sauce, Chinese Five Spices, sugar, salt, and wine or broth. Simmer over low heat, stirring occasionally for about 5 minutes.

While the turkey mixture is simmering, clean the cabbage leaves, shaking off the excess water. If using the Napa cabbage, cut off the firm ends, reserving for a vegetable stir-fry (if desired). If the leaves are quite large, cut in half.

To Serve: Place two cabbage leaves on a plate. Mound about two tablespoons of the turkey mixture in the center of the leaves. Garnish with sprigs of cilantro, if desired.

To Eat: Wrap cabbage leaf around turkey mixture to make a packet.

Dill Dip

NUTRITION FACTS	
Servings per Recipe 8	
Amount Per Serving	
Calories 70	Calories from Fat 50
	% Daily Value*
Total Fat 6g	**8%**
Saturated Fat 1g	**4%**
Cholesterol 4mg	**1%**
Sodium 60mg	**3%**
Total Carbohydrates 6g	**2%**
Dietary Fiber 0g	**0%**
Sugars 2g	
Protein 2g	
Vitamin A 1% •	Vitamin C 1%
Calcium 5% •	Iron 0%

1 cup plain nonfat yogurt
¼ cup mayonnaise
1 teaspoon dill weed
2 teaspoons vinegar or lemon juice

Mix all the ingredients together and refrigerate for at least 1 hour.

Serving Suggestion: Serve with fresh cut-up vegetables, grilled fish or chicken, veggie burger, steamed artichokes.

Fruit Yogurt Shake

3 ounces fruit-flavored nonfat light yogurt
½ cup nonfat milk
½ banana* or *½ cup fresh fruit
½ cup crushed ice

NUTRITION FACTS			
Servings per Recipe 1			
Amount Per Serving			
Calories 120		Calories from Fat 0	
		% Daily Value*	
Total Fat 0g		**0%**	
Saturated Fat 0g		**0%**	
Cholesterol 2mg		**1%**	
Sodium 110mg		**4%**	
Total Carbohydrates 22g		**7%**	
Dietary Fiber 1g		**3%**	
Sugars 15g			
Protein 7g			
Vitamin A	15%	Vitamin C	7%
Calcium	28%	Iron	1%

Place all the ingredients in a blender and blend until smooth.

Mocha Shake

NUTRITION FACTS			
Servings per Recipe 1			
Amount Per Serving			
Calories 100		Calories from Fat 0	
			% Daily Value*
Total Fat 0g			**0%**
Saturated Fat 0g			**0%**
Cholesterol 2mg			**1%**
Sodium 75mg			**3%**
Total Carbohydrates 18g			**6%**
Dietary Fiber 1g			**2%**
Sugars 16g			
Protein 5g			
Vitamin A	15%	• Vitamin C	2%
Calcium	16%	• Iron	2%

¼ cup strong coffee
½ cup nonfat milk
1 tablespoon fat-free chocolate syrup
½ cup crushed ice

Place all the ingredients in a blender and blend until smooth.

Seasoned Popcorn

Popcorn, air-popped
Vegetable-oil spray

Choice of Seasonings:
Ground thyme
Poultry spice
Dill weed
Ground caraway
Butter flakes
Seasoned butter flakes (cheese, dill)
Cinnamon and sugar

NUTRITION FACTS	
Servings per Recipe 4	
Amount Per Serving	
Calories 60	Calories from Fat 6
	% Daily Value*
Total Fat 1g	**1%**
Saturated Fat 0g	**0%**
Cholesterol 0mg	**0%**
Sodium 0mg	**0%**
Total Carbohydrates 12g	**4%**
Dietary Fiber 2g	**10%**
Sugars 0g	
Protein 2g	
Vitamin A 1% • Vitamin C 0%	
Calcium 0% • Iron 2%	

Preheat the oven to 350°.

Air-pop your popcorn. Place the popcorn in a single layer on a cookie sheet. Spray with the vegetable oil spray and then sprinkle with one or more of the seasonings and salt (optional).

Cook in oven for 5–8 minutes.

Note: The *Nutrition Facts* are for the popcorn seasoned with thyme, poultry spice, dill weed, or ground caraway. If you add butter flakes or seasoned butter flakes, the *Sodium* will be 180mg and 8% DV. If you add cinnamon and sugar, the *Total Carbohydrate* will be 25g and 8% DV, the *Sugars* will be 12g.

Tofu Tuna Triangles

½ package (16 ounces) soft tofu
1 can (6½ ounces) tuna (canned in water)
1 tablespoon fresh dill weed, chopped or *½ teaspoon dried dill weed*
¼ cup sweet gherkin pickles, chopped
¼ teaspoon garlic salt
2 tablespoons low-fat mayonnaise
4 whole wheat fat-free flour tortillas

Makes 24 triangles.

NUTRITION FACTS	
Servings per Recipe 6	
Amount Per Serving	
Calories 140	Calories from Fat 48
	% Daily Value*
Total Fat 5g	**8%**
Saturated Fat 1g	**5%**
Cholesterol 6mg	**2%**
Sodium 400mg	**17%**
Total Carbohydrates 11g	**4%**
Dietary Fiber 6g	**24%**
Sugars 0g	
Protein 12g	
Vitamin A 2% •	Vitamin C 1%
Calcium 3% •	Iron 4%

In a colander, drain the tofu for at least 1 hour. Mash with a fork or a potato masher. Let stand for 30 minutes. Drain any excess liquid. Drain the can of tuna fish and flake with a fork into fine pieces. Mix together with the tofu. Add all the remaining ingredients except the tortilla and mix well.

Cut each tortilla into 6 triangles. Place a teaspoonful of the tuna mixture at the broad end of the triangle. Roll up and place on a serving dish. Continue the process with the remaining triangles. Refrigerate for about one hour.

Bugs Bunny Soup

1 pound ground turkey breast meat
1 cup chopped onion
Vegetable-oil spray
2 tablespoons peanut butter
6 cups chicken broth
3 cups coarsely grated carrots
½ teaspoon curry powder (more if desired)
1 teaspoon sugar
4 tablespoons margarine
¼ cup flour
1½ cups nonfat milk
½ cup nonfat plain yogurt
Paprika

NUTRITION FACTS			
Servings per Recipe 6			
Amount Per Serving			
Calories 235		Calories from Fat 85	
			% Daily Value*
Total Fat 9g			**14%**
Saturated Fat 2g			**10%**
Cholesterol 37mg			**12%**
Sodium 760mg			**32%**
Total Carbohydrates 15g			**5%**
Dietary Fiber 2g			**8%**
Sugars 7g			
Protein 23g			
Vitamin A	252% •	Vitamin C	9%
Calcium	12% •	Iron	9%

Spray a soup pot with the vegetable-oil spray. Over medium-high heat, brown the turkey meat and onion for about 5 minutes until the meat is no longer pink and the onion is somewhat translucent. Take a little of the broth and add to the peanut butter to make a soupy mixture. Add this mixture, the remaining broth, carrots, curry powder, and sugar to the pot. Bring to a boil, then cover and simmer for about 1 hour.

Melt the margarine in a small saucepan over medium-high heat. With a wire whip, blend in the flour until smooth. Slowly add the milk, stirring constantly until smooth and thickened. Stir this mixture into the carrot soup, continuing to cook for another 20 minutes.

To Serve: Spoon into bowls and top with a dollop of plain yogurt and a sprinkling of paprika.

Pork and Tofu Soup

3 quarts low-sodium chicken broth
1 pound pork tenderloin
1 pound firm tofu
½ pound fresh spinach leaves
½ pound Napa or Savoy cabbage
1 cup fresh cilantro sprigs
1 pound fresh udon (Japanese noodles) or spaghetti
2 cloves garlic, minced
1 teaspoon grated fresh ginger
2 tablespoons light soy sauce
1 cup canned or frozen white corn (drained)
1 cup sliced fresh mushrooms
Sesame oil (optional)

NUTRITION FACTS	
Servings per Recipe 8	
Amount Per Serving	
Calories 280	Calories from Fat 67
	% Daily Value*
Total Fat 7g	**10%**
Saturated Fat 2g	**8%**
Cholesterol 50mg	**17%**
Sodium 385mg	**16%**
Total Carbohydrates 24g	**8%**
Dietary Fiber 3g	**13%**
Sugars 4g	
Protein 29g	
Vitamin A 53% •	Vitamin C 33%
Calcium 11% •	Iron 19%

Cut the pork tenderloin into 1-inch x 2-inch x ¼-inch thick slices. Then cut the tofu into 1-inch cubes. Next, clean the spinach leaves, cabbage, and cilantro and shake dry. Remove the stems of the spinach and cilantro, keeping the cilantro leaves separate from the other vegetables. If the spinach leaves are quite large, cut in half. Cut the cabbage into thin shreds.

In a big soup or pasta pot, cook the udon or spaghetti until just tender and still chewy.

In an 8-quart soup pot, combine all of the ingredients except the udon or pasta and ¼ cup of the cilantro leaves. Bring the mixture to a boil, then simmer until the pork is cooked, approximately 15 minutes. Add the udon or pasta until warmed through.

Serving Suggestion: Serve in deep bowls and top with fresh cilantro leaves. Drizzle a small amount of sesame oil on top, if desired.

Scallops and Leek Chowder

NUTRITION FACTS	
Servings per Recipe 6	
Amount Per Serving	
Calories 340	Calories from Fat 78
	% Daily Value*
Total Fat 9g	**13%**
Saturated Fat 3g	**13%**
Cholesterol 48mg	**16%**
Sodium 740mg	**31%**
Total Carbohydrates 34g	**11%**
Dietary Fiber 4g	**16%**
Sugars 6g	
Protein 31g	
Vitamin A 13% •	Vitamin C 26%
Calcium 16% •	Iron 14%

2 pounds leeks
1 pound red-skinned potatoes
½ pound ham steak
1 pound small scallops
1 tablespoon olive oil
¼ cup flour
3 quarts low-sodium chicken broth
1 teaspoon dill weed
2 cups nonfat milk

Remove and discard the green tops and root ends from the leeks. Slice lengthwise and rinse well; then slice crosswise. Scrub the potatoes and cut into ½-inch cubes. Cut the ham steak into ½-inch cubes and the scallops into 1-inch pieces, if too large.

In an 8-quart soup pot, brown the ham cubes in the olive oil. Add the leeks and sauté until limp, about 5–10 minutes. Sprinkle the flour over the ham and leeks and stir until well coated. Stir in the broth, dill, and potatoes. Bring to a boil and then simmer until the potatoes are tender, about 15–20 minutes.

Add the milk and scallops, stirring frequently over low heat until scallops are cooked, about 8–10 minutes. Be sure not to overcook scallops, or they will become tough.

To Serve: Spoon into deep bowls and sprinkle with fresh chopped parsley.

Tomato Bean Bisque

- *1 pound tomatoes (skinned and cubed)*
- *2 onions, thinly sliced*
- *2 cloves garlic, minced*
- *1 tablespoon olive oil*
- *1 quart regular-strength chicken broth*
- *½ pound fresh green beans (cut in 1-inch pieces)*
- *½ cup chopped fresh basil leaves*
- *French bread (4 ½-inch-thick slices, toasted)*
- *¼ pound part-skim-milk mozzarella cheese, grated*

NUTRITION FACTS	
Servings per Recipe 4	
Amount Per Serving	
Calories 290	Calories from Fat 96
	% Daily Value*
Total Fat 11g	**16%**
Saturated Fat 4g	**20%**
Cholesterol 16mg	**5%**
Sodium 1080mg	**45%**
Total Carbohydrates 32g	**11%**
Dietary Fiber 5g	**20%**
Sugars 7g	
Protein 17g	
Vitamin A 35%	Vitamin C 60%
Calcium 27%	Iron 14%

In a 4- or 5-quart pot, bring about 3 quarts of water to a boil. Drop the tomatoes into the water for about 1 minute. Lift out and drain. Run under cold water, pull off the skin, and cut out the core. Cut tomatoes into cubes.

In an 8-quart soup pot, over medium-high heat, sauté the onions and garlic in the olive oil until translucent, about 5–10 minutes. Add the tomatoes, broth, beans, and basil. Bring to a boil and then simmer until the beans are cooked but still bright green and crisp.

Meanwhile, toast the French bread slices.

To Serve: Spoon the soup into oven-safe soup bowls. Top the soup with a slice of French bread and then sprinkle with grated mozzarella cheese. Place bowls on a cookie sheet and place under the broiler of your oven. Broil until the cheese is melted and golden brown, about 5 minutes.

Asian Slaw

2 tablespoons sesame seeds
4 cups thinly shredded cabbage
⅓ cup seasoned rice vinegar
1 tablespoon canola oil
4 tablespoons simple sugar syrup *
¼ teaspoon fresh grated ginger
¼ cup chopped cilantro (optional)

* **Simple sugar syrup:**
1 cup sugar
1 cup water

NUTRITION FACTS		
Servings per Recipe 6		
Amount Per Serving		
Calories 110	Calories from Fat 36	
		% Daily Value*
Total Fat 4g		**6%**
Saturated Fat 0g		**0%**
Cholesterol 0mg		**0%**
Sodium 150mg		**6%**
Total Carbohydrates 18g		**6%**
Dietary Fiber 1g		**6%**
Sugars 12g		
Protein 1g		
Vitamin A 1%	•	Vitamin C 25%
Calcium 4%	•	Iron 2%

In a frying pan over medium-high heat, toast the sesame seeds until golden, about five minutes. Remove and cool.

Combine with remaining ingredients and chill for about 1 hour.

Simple sugar syrup: In a small saucepan, boil the sugar and water over high heat until syrup thickens slightly. Allow to cool undisturbed. Use 4 tablespoons for this recipe and store the remainder in a cool place. (Great for iced tea!)

Chinese Green Bean Salad

1 pound green beans, washed and ends removed

Dressing:
½ cup rice or sherry vinegar
4 tablespoons canola oil
2 tablespoons oyster sauce
2 tablespoons teriyaki sauce
¼ cup sugar
1 tablespoon sesame seeds (optional)

NUTRITION FACTS	
Servings per Recipe 6	
Amount Per Serving	
Calories 130	Calories from Fat 63
	% Daily Value*
Total Fat 7g	**11%**
Saturated Fat 1g	**3%**
Cholesterol 0mg	**0%**
Sodium 340mg	**14%**
Total Carbohydrates 17g	**6%**
Dietary Fiber 2g	**10%**
Sugars 10g	
Protein 2g	
Vitamin A 10% •	Vitamin C 12%
Calcium 4% •	Iron 7%

Choose one of the following methods to cook the green beans:

1. *To microwave*—Place beans in a 2-quart baking dish and cover. Microwave on high for 5 minutes or until tender but still crisp and bright green.
2. *To boil*—Bring 4 quarts of water to a boil, add green beans, and bring the water back up to a boil. Continue to cook for about 5 minutes, until the beans are tender but still crisp and bright green.

Plunge the green beans into cold water for about 5 minutes to cool them quickly. Drain well.

Mix the remaining ingredients for the dressing.

Arrange the green beans lengthwise in a shallow serving dish. Pour the dressing over them, sprinkle with sesame seeds if desired, and refrigerate for at least one hour.

Dilled Cottage Cheese Salad

1 cup green beans* or *1 cup asparagus
2 cups low-fat 1 percent cottage cheese
1½ teaspoons dried dill weed
¼ teaspoon onion salt (optional)
1 teaspoon dill or balsamic vinegar
Red-leaf lettuce
French bread, sliced and toasted

NUTRITION FACTS	
Servings per Recipe 4	
Amount Per Serving	
Calories 170	Calories from Fat 18
	% Daily Value*
Total Fat 2g	**3%**
Saturated Fat 1g	**5%**
Cholesterol 5mg	**2%**
Sodium 630mg	**26%**
Total Carbohydrates 19g	**6%**
Dietary Fiber 2g	**8%**
Sugars 4g	
Protein 17g	
Vitamin A 12% •	Vitamin C 10%
Calcium 11% •	Iron 8%

Wash, trim and cut the beans or asparagus into 1-inch pieces. Combine with all the remaining ingredients except the lettuce. Place a mound of the salad in the middle of a lettuce leaf. Serve with toasted French bread slices.

Marinated Vegetables

½ cup green beans, ends removed and sliced diagonally into 1½-inch pieces
½ cup zucchini, julienne cut
½ cup cherry tomatoes, halved
½ cup small baby carrots or regular carrots, cut into ¼-inch slices
½ cup cauliflower, cut into small flowerettes
½ cup broccoli, cut into small flowerettes
½ cup pea pods (snow peas or sugar snap peas)
½ cup yellow bell peppers, seeded and cut into 1-inch pieces

Dressing:
¾ cup olive oil
¼ balsamic vinegar
1 teaspoon sugar
1 teaspoon dried tarragon
1 teaspoon onion salt

NUTRITION FACTS	
Servings per Recipe 8	
Amount Per Serving	
Calories 70	Calories from Fat 45
	% Daily Value*
Total Fat 5g	**8%**
Saturated Fat 1g	**5%**
Cholesterol 0mg	**0%**
Sodium 300mg	**13%**
Total Carbohydrates 7g	**2%**
Dietary Fiber 2g	**7%**
Sugars 5g	
Protein 1g	
Vitamin A 58% •	Vitamin C 63%
Calcium 2% •	Iron 4%

Combine all the vegetables in a deep bowl. In another bowl, whisk the salad dressing ingredients together. Pour over the vegetables and toss. Transfer the vegetables and dressing into a flat shallow container and refrigerate for at least 3 to 4 hours or overnight, stirring occasionally. Drain before serving.

Mediterranean Rice Salad

1 purple onion, chopped
Vegetable-oil spray
1 small eggplant (about 1 pound), diced with skin
2 tablespoons water
3½ cups zucchini, cut into ¼-inch slices
½ pound mushrooms, sliced
¼ teaspoon each dried oregano and thyme leaves or *1 teaspoon chopped fresh oregano and thyme*
1 can (8 ounces) ripe olives, drained and sliced
2 cups cooked short-grain rice
¼ cup balsamic vinegar
¼ cup olive oil
1 cup cherry tomatoes, halved
¾ pound bay shrimp
2 lemons, thinly sliced
Salt to taste
Red-leaf lettuce

NUTRITION FACTS	
Servings per Recipe 10	
Amount Per Serving	
Calories 230	Calories from Fat 73
	% Daily Value*
Total Fat 8g	**13%**
Saturated Fat 1g	**6%**
Cholesterol 0mg	**0%**
Sodium 353mg	**15%**
Total Carbohydrates 32g	**11%**
Dietary Fiber 3g	**13%**
Sugars 4g	
Protein 8g	
Vitamin A 12% •	Vitamin C 19%
Calcium 5% •	Iron 15%

Spray a deep frying pan with the vegetable-oil spray and sauté the onions over medium-high heat until almost translucent. Add the eggplant and water and continue cooking until the eggplant is tender. Remove to a bowl. Again spray the frying pan with vegetable-oil spray and sauté the zucchini over high heat, browning the slices on both sides until tender-crisp. Be careful not to overcook. Add the zucchini to the bowl containing the onions and eggplant. One more time, spray the frying pan with the vegetable-oil spray and sauté the mushrooms until tender. Add them to the bowl, along with the oregano, thyme, olives, rice, vinegar, and oil. Chill the mixture for about 1½ hours.

Before serving, stir in the tomatoes.

To Serve: Line each salad bowl with red lettuce leaves and mound the rice mixture. Top with the shrimp and garnish with the lemon slices.

Sweet Pasta Salad

6 cups cooked pasta (macaroni, rotini, penne, etc.)
2 crisp apples (peeled and grated)
¼ cup raisins
¼ chopped nuts (walnuts, pecans, or almonds)
4 cups zucchini (grated)

Dressing:
¼ cup olive oil
2 tablespoons apple cider vinegar
1 teaspoon grated orange rind
2 tablespoons honey
1 teaspoon cinnamon
¼ cup orange juice
¼ teaspoon salt

NUTRITION FACTS	
Servings per Recipe 8	
Amount Per Serving	
Calories 260	Calories from Fat 90
	% Daily Value*
Total Fat 10g	**15%**
Saturated Fat 1g	**6%**
Cholesterol 0mg	**0%**
Sodium 76mg	**3%**
Total Carbohydrates 40g	**13%**
Dietary Fiber 4g	**15%**
Sugars 15g	
Protein 6g	
Vitamin A 5% •	Vitamin C 18%
Calcium 3% •	Iron 11%

Dressing: Whisk all the ingredients together.

In a deep bowl, combine all the ingredients, including the dressing. Toss well to incorporate the dressing. Refrigerate for at least 2 hours.

Three-Bean Casserole

1 cup chopped onion
¼ pound low-fat turkey bacon, cut into 1-inch pieces
½ pound ground turkey breast meat
Vegetable-oil spray
2 cans (15½ ounces each) lima beans, drained
1 can (15½ ounces) kidney beans, drained
1 can (16 ounces) baked beans
½ cup catsup
1 cup brown sugar
1 teaspoon prepared mustard
1 teaspoon salt (optional)

NUTRITION FACTS	
Servings per Recipe 10	
Amount Per Serving	
Calories 300	Calories from Fat 30
	% Daily Value*
Total Fat 3g	**5%**
Saturated Fat 1g	**2%**
Cholesterol 27mg	**9%**
Sodium 870mg	**36%**
Total Carbohydrates 54g	**18%**
Dietary Fiber 8g	**33%**
Sugars 28g	
Protein 17g	
Vitamin A 7% •	Vitamin C 21%
Calcium 9% •	Iron 17%

Preheat oven to 375°.

Spray a large frying pan with the vegetable oil. Over medium-high heat, sauté the onions, bacon, and ground turkey until cooked. Drain any accumulated fat. Combine the meat mixture with the beans and remaining ingredients in a casserole dish. Cover and bake for 1 hour and 15 minutes.

Serving Suggestion: Accompany casserole with a crisp garden salad.

Chinese Wraps

1 pound pork tenderloin, cut into thin slices
4 tablespoons light soy sauce
½ teaspoon grated ginger
1 tablespoon olive oil
Vegetable-oil spray
1 onion, cut into strips
1 cup bean sprouts
1 cup carrots, julienne cut
2 tablespoons water
½ cup water chestnuts, sliced
½ cup bamboo shoots, strips
1 teaspoon sesame oil (optional)
6 fat-free flour tortillas
½ cup plum sauce
2 cups cooked basmati or jasmine rice
½ cup fresh cilantro, chopped

NUTRITION FACTS	
Servings per Recipe 6	
Amount Per Serving	
Calories 395	Calories from Fat 55
	% Daily Value*
Total Fat 6g	**9%**
Saturated Fat 2g	**8%**
Cholesterol 60mg	**20%**
Sodium 645mg	**27%**
Total Carbohydrates 54g	**18%**
Dietary Fiber 8g	**33%**
Sugars 10g	
Protein 27g	
Vitamin A 106% •	Vitamin C 10%
Calcium 5% •	Iron 10%

Pork: Marinate the pork tenderloin in 2 tablespoons of the soy sauce, along with the ginger. Let stand for 20 minutes. Heat the olive oil in a large frying pan or wok over medium-high heat and cook the pork slices. Set aside.

Vegetables: Spray a large frying pan or wok with the vegetable-oil spray. Over medium-high heat, sauté the onion, bean sprouts, and carrots, adding the water to steam the vegetables. When the bean sprouts are limp and the carrots tender, add the water chestnuts, bamboo shoots, remaining 2 tablespoons of soy sauce, and sesame oil (optional). Cook for another 2–3 minutes. Remove from burner.

Assembling wraps: Spread the plum sauce over the center of the 6 flour tortillas. Spoon about ⅓ cup of cooked rice on each tortilla, arranging it down the center of the tortilla. Divide the vegetable mixture over the rice, followed by the pork and cilantro. Tightly roll the tortilla over the mixture, tucking the ends in to make a pocket.

Serve with extra plum sauce, if desired.

Curry Chicken

1 onion, chopped
2 apples, peeled and diced
2 carrots, diced
3 skinless chicken breasts (cut lengthwise and then cut crosswise into 1/4-inch thick slices)
Vegetable-oil spray
2 tablespoons margarine
2 tablespoons flour
1 cup chicken broth
1 cup nonfat milk
1 teaspoon curry (adjust as desired)
1 teaspoon coconut extract
1 teaspoon salt (optional)
1 tablespoon light soy sauce
1/2 teaspoon grated fresh ginger root
3 cups cooked basmati or jasmine rice

NUTRITION FACTS			
Servings per Recipe 6			
Amount Per Serving			
Calories 375		Calories from Fat 70	
			% Daily Value*
Total Fat 7g			**11%**
Saturated Fat 2g			**9%**
Cholesterol 75mg			**25%**
Sodium 360mg			**15%**
Total Carbohydrates 41g			**14%**
Dietary Fiber 3g			**11%**
Sugars 10g			
Protein 32g			
Vitamin A	151%	Vitamin C	9%
Calcium	8%	Iron	8%

Spray a large frying pan with vegetable-oil spray. Then, over medium-high heat, sauté the onion, apples, and carrots until the onions are translucent and the carrots tender. If necessary, add a small amount of water to keep the mixture from sticking. Set aside in warm dish.

Again, spray the frying pan with vegetable-oil spray. Sauté the chicken pieces until browned and cooked through. Add to dish with apple mixture.

Sauce: In a saucepan over medium heat, make a roux by melting the margarine and adding the flour until well incorporated.

Slowly add the broth and milk, stirring constantly. Add the remaining ingredients and continue to cook until thickened.

Stir the sauce into the chicken mixture and serve over rice.

Donatella

1 pound extra lean ground beef
2 onions, chopped
2 cloves garlic, crushed
1 can (10¾ ounces) tomato soup, condensed
½ pound mushrooms, sliced
1 can (9.3 ounces) niblet corn, drained
6 cups cooked pasta (macaroni, rotini, penne, etc.)
½ teaspoon dried basil
½ teaspoon dried oregano
½ cup grated Parmesan cheese

NUTRITION FACTS	
Servings per Recipe 8	
Amount Per Serving	
Calories 320	Calories from Fat 65
	% Daily Value*
Total Fat 7g	**11%**
Saturated Fat 3g	**14%**
Cholesterol 55mg	**18%**
Sodium 495mg	**21%**
Total Carbohydrates 54g	**18%**
Dietary Fiber 3g	**11%**
Sugars 4g	
Protein 25g	
Vitamin A 8% •	Vitamin C 42%
Calcium 10% •	Iron 25%

Preheat oven to 350°.

In an 8-quart oven-proof pot, sauté the ground beef and onions together until the meat is browned, adding a little water if necessary to keep it from sticking to the pan. Stir in the remaining ingredients. With the back of the spoon, smooth out the top surface of the mixture.

Place the pot, uncovered, in the oven and bake for 1 hour or until bubbly.

Fettuccine with Eggplant and Pesto

1 cup firmly packed fresh basil leaves, plus whole basil leaves for garnish
½ cup freshly grated Romano or Parmesan cheese
Vegetable-oil spray
1 eggplant, cut into 1-inch cubes (leave skin on)
1 large purple onion, chopped
3 cloves garlic, minced
1½ cups chicken stock or broth
3 tablespoons olive oil
1 pound dried fettuccine
¼ cup toasted pine nuts
Salt to taste (optional)

NUTRITION FACTS	
Servings per Recipe 6	
Amount Per Serving	
Calories 370	Calories from Fat 140
	% Daily Value*
Total Fat 15g	**23%**
Saturated Fat 3g	**14%**
Cholesterol 19mg	**6%**
Sodium 335mg	**14%**
Total Carbohydrates 46g	**15%**
Dietary Fiber 1g	**7%**
Sugars 4g	
Protein 14g	
Vitamin A 4% •	Vitamin C 5%
Calcium 11% •	Iron 11%

Put the basil leaves, cheese, and olive oil in a food processor and process until smooth. Then set aside.

In a large frying pan coated with vegetable-oil spray, sauté the eggplant until browned. Set aside. Add more vegetable-oil spray and sauté the onion and garlic until tender and translucent. Return the eggplant to the frying pan. Add the stock and simmer uncovered, until the stock is reduced by one-fourth, about 8–10 minutes.

While the eggplant mixture simmers, fill an 8-quart pot about three-fourths full of water. Bring to a boil and add the fettuccine. Cook according to package directions, usually about 10–12 minutes. Drain.

Combine the fettuccine, eggplant mixture, and basil mixture in a large serving bowl. Toss well, salting to taste.

To Serve: Garnish with basil leaves and top with pine nuts.

Garden Sandwich

NUTRITION FACTS	
Servings per Recipe 4	
Amount Per Serving	
Calories 335	Calories from Fat 160
	% Daily Value*
Total Fat 17g	**27%**
Saturated Fat 3g	**14%**
Cholesterol 0mg	**0%**
Sodium 565mg	**23%**
Total Carbohydrates 41g	**14%**
Dietary Fiber 9g	**37%**
Sugars 7g	
Protein 9g	
Vitamin A 22% •	Vitamin C 43%
Calcium 8% •	Iron 20%

1 to 2 large tomatoes
8 mushrooms
1 cucumber
2 avocados
1 purple onion
Alfalfa sprouts
Fresh basil leaves (several per sandwich)
8 slices multi-grain bread
Fat-free Italian vinaigrette

Cut the vegetables into ¼-inch slices. Assemble the sandwiches, evenly dividing the ingredients. Slice the sandwiches in half or thirds and serve with the Italian vinaigrette in a dish for dipping, if desired.

Halibut Paprikash

NUTRITION FACTS
Servings per Recipe 4

Amount Per Serving	
Calories 385	Calories from Fat 60
	% Daily Value*
Total Fat 7g	**10%**
Saturated Fat 1g	**5%**
Cholesterol 75mg	**25%**
Sodium 410mg	**17%**
Total Carbohydrates 44g	**15%**
Dietary Fiber 3g	**12%**
Sugars 7g	
Protein 36g	

Vitamin A	32%	•	Vitamin C	6%
Calcium	19%	•	Iron	21%

4 halibut steaks (4 ounces each)
1 cup chopped onions
½ teaspoon minced garlic
1 teaspoon olive oil
1½ cups chicken broth
2 tablespoons flour
1½ tablespoons paprika
1 cup plain nonfat yogurt
3 cups cooked egg noodles

Place the halibut steaks in a broiler pan. Broil on both sides until the fish flakes with a fork, approximately 5–8 minutes per side. Do not overcook.

Meanwhile, in a frying pan over medium-high heat, sauté the onions and garlic in the olive oil. Continue cooking until the onions are translucent. Add the chicken broth. Stir the flour and paprika into the yogurt and then stir the yogurt mixture into the onions. Continue to cook over low heat until the sauce is thickened.

To Serve: Place the warm noodles on a serving dish. Top with the halibut steak and cover the fish and noodles with the sauce.

Lemon Rosemary Beef

1 clove garlic
1 pound flank steak, trimmed of fat
Salt to taste

Sauce:
1 tablespoon butter
½ pound mushrooms, sliced
1 clove garlic, crushed
½ cup sherry wine
1 tablespoon flour
½ cup beef stock
¼ cup lemon juice
1 teaspoon grated lemon rind
1 teaspoon dried rosemary or 2 teaspoons chopped fresh rosemary
Salt to taste

NUTRITION FACTS	
Servings per Recipe 4	
Amount Per Serving	
Calories 295	Calories from Fat 110
	% Daily Value*
Total Fat 12g	**19%**
Saturated Fat 6g	**29%**
Cholesterol 55mg	**18%**
Sodium 340mg	**14%**
Total Carbohydrates 9g	**3%**
Dietary Fiber 1g	**3%**
Sugars 3g	
Protein 29g	
Vitamin A 6% •	Vitamin C 16%
Calcium 2% •	Iron 16%

Meat: Peel the clove of garlic. Cut it in half and rub both sides of the flank steak with the cut sides. Salt the meat, if desired. Broil the meat to your liking. As the meat is cooking, make the sauce.

Sauce: In a frying pan, melt the butter on medium-high heat and add the sliced mushrooms and crushed garlic. Sauté the mushrooms until tender and slightly browned. Add the sherry wine to deglaze the pan. Mix the flour, beef stock, lemon juice, lemon rind, and rosemary together. Add to the frying pan and continue to cook over medium heat until the sauce has thickened. Salt to taste.

To Serve: Cut the flank steak on an angle into thin slices. Fan out the pieces on a serving platter and top with the sauce.

New Orleans Style Red Beans and Rice

NUTRITION FACTS	
Servings per Recipe 4	
Amount Per Serving	
Calories 370	Calories from Fat 118
	% Daily Value*
Total Fat 13g	**20%**
Saturated Fat 3g	**16%**
Cholesterol 55mg	**18%**
Sodium 1540mg	**64%**
Total Carbohydrates 47g	**16%**
Dietary Fiber 5g	**18%**
Sugars 6g	
Protein 21g	
Vitamin A 24% •	Vitamin C 62%
Calcium 4% •	Iron 23%

---

2 cups cooked brown rice
1 onion, chopped
1 tablespoon olive oil
2 stalks celery, thinly sliced
1 green pepper, seeded and chopped
2 cups beef broth
1 cup cooked red beans, drained
12 ounces low-fat smoked turkey sausage, cut into 2-ounce portions
Vegetable-oil spray

Prepare the brown rice according to package directions.

In a deep saucepan, sauté the onion in the olive oil until translucent. Add the celery and green pepper, continuing to sauté until slightly tender. Add the beef broth, then the rice and beans. Cover pot and cook over low heat for 1 hour, stirring occasionally. If it seems to be getting too dry, add more water. The finished dish should have a creamy, gravy consistency.

Grill the sausage or brown in a frying pan that has been sprayed with a vegetable-oil spray.

To Serve: Spoon the bean and rice mixture onto a plate and place the sausage on top.

Nut Crusted Chicken in Raspberry Vinaigrette

NUTRITION FACTS		
Servings per Recipe 6		
Amount Per Serving		
Calories 360	Calories from Fat 165	
		% Daily Value*
Total Fat 18g		**28%**
Saturated Fat 3g		**16%**
Cholesterol 130mg		**44%**
Sodium 400mg		**17%**
Total Carbohydrates 10g		**3%**
Dietary Fiber 2g		**9%**
Sugars 6g		
Protein 39g		
Vitamin A 5%	•	Vitamin C 6%
Calcium 4%	•	Iron 11%

---

1 egg
½ cup chopped pistachio nuts
6 chicken breasts, skinned
2 tablespoons olive oil
Salt to taste

Vinaigrette:
2 tablespoons olive oil
½ cup fresh or frozen raspberries
2 tablespoons sugar
1 tablespoon red wine vinegar
¼ cup bacon bits

Chicken: In a bowl, whisk the egg. Put the chopped pistachios in a flat shallow dish. Dip each chicken breast in the egg and then coat one side with the nuts. Sprinkle with salt, if desired. Heat the oil in a large frying pan over medium-high heat. Place each breast nut-side up in the frying pan and cook, browning the bottom side. Then turn and brown the nut side, watching carefully not to burn the nuts. If necessary, lower the heat.

Vinaigrette: In a small pot, heat together all the ingredients. Keep warm.

To Serve: Top each chicken breast with the vinaigrette.

Todo Tofu Tortilla

1 ripe avocado, thinly sliced
2 teaspoons lemon juice
1 cup thinly shredded cabbage
½ cup shredded cheddar cheese
6 fat-free whole wheat flour tortillas
1 can (15½ ounces) fat-free refried beans
1 package (10½ ounces) soft low-fat tofu
Vegetable-oil spray
1 cup salsa

NUTRITION FACTS	
Servings per Recipe 6	
Amount Per Serving	
Calories 210	Calories from Fat 58
	% Daily Value*
Total Fat 6g	**10%**
Saturated Fat 1g	**5%**
Cholesterol 0mg	**0%**
Sodium 860mg	**36%**
Total Carbohydrates 28g	**9%**
Dietary Fiber 13g	**51%**
Sugars 2g	
Protein 14g	
Vitamin A 19% •	Vitamin C 17%
Calcium 14% •	Iron 16%

Prepare and Set Aside: Thinly slice the avocado. Sprinkle the lemon juice over the avocado slices and cover tightly. Thinly shred the cabbage and place in a bowl. Shred the cheddar cheese and place in another bowl. Warm the tortillas in a 200° oven.

As you heat the refried beans in a sauce pot or in the microwave oven, prepare the tofu.

The Tofu: Drain the tofu. Cut it lengthwise into 6 equal slices. Then cut each slice in half lengthwise. In a frying pan sprayed with vegetable-oil spray, brown the tofu slices on both sides.

To Serve: Spread about 3 tablespoons of refried beans on each tortilla and top with the avocado, cabbage, tofu, salsa, and cheese. Roll up tightly.

Fruity Jasmine Rice

NUTRITION FACTS	
Servings per Recipe 8	
Amount Per Serving	
Calories 355	Calories from Fat 28
	% Daily Value*
Total Fat 3g	**5%**
Saturated Fat 1g	**3%**
Cholesterol 2mg	**1%**
Sodium 399mg	**17%**
Total Carbohydrates 72g	**24%**
Dietary Fiber 4g	**14%**
Sugars 5g	
Protein 8g	
Vitamin A 8% •	Vitamin C 3%
Calcium 2% •	Iron 6%

1 purple onion, chopped
1 tablespoon canola oil
1 cup cooked yellow split peas
3 cups cooked jasmine or other fragrant rice
½ cup chopped mixed dried fruit (combination of any of the following: apricots, prunes, raisins, cranberries, apples, etc.)
1 teaspoon ground cinnamon
1½ cups chicken stock or broth
Salt to taste

In a frying pan over medium-high heat, sauté the onion in the oil until soft and translucent. Place onions in a medium-sized saucepan, along with the remaining ingredients. Bring to a boil, then lower the heat and simmer, uncovered, stirring frequently. Continue cooking until the rice has a creamy consistency, approximately 30 minutes. Salt to taste.

Grilled Vegetables

NUTRITION FACTS	
Servings per Recipe 4	
Amount Per Serving	
Calories 190	Calories from Fat 70
	% Daily Value*
Total Fat 8g	**12%**
Saturated Fat 1g	**6%**
Cholesterol 0mg	**0%**
Sodium 160mg	**7%**
Total Carbohydrates 27g	**9%**
Dietary Fiber 3g	**11%**
Sugars 3g	
Protein 5g	
Vitamin A 8% •	Vitamin C 117%
Calcium 5% •	Iron 9%

3 Japanese eggplants **or** ***1 Mediterranean eggplant***
1 red bell pepper
1 green bell pepper
2 zucchini
2 tablespoons olive oil
Bulb of garlic
Foccacia bread
Salt to taste

Prepare and Set Aside: Wash the vegetables. Trim the ends of the eggplants and zucchini and cut lengthwise into ¼-inch-thick slices. Remove the stems and seeds from the peppers. Quarter the peppers. Brush both sides of the vegetable pieces with the olive oil and grill on both sides until tender and browned, approximately 5–8 minutes per side.

Garlic: Put the whole bulb of garlic with skin in a pot. Cover with water. Bring to a boil, then simmer until the cloves are tender.

To Serve: Place the bulb of garlic in the center of a platter, arranging the vegetable slices around it. Serve with warmed foccacia bread.

To Eat: Pull off a clove of garlic from the bulb and pop it out of its skin by pinching it at its base. Spread the softened garlic over bread and then top with the vegetable slices. Salt, if desired.

Hungarian Sauerkraut

NUTRITION FACTS	
Servings per Recipe 6	
Amount Per Serving	
Calories 110	Calories from Fat 24
	% Daily Value*
Total Fat 3g	**4%**
Saturated Fat 1g	**2%**
Cholesterol 0mg	**0%**
Sodium 180mg	**8%**
Total Carbohydrates 21g	**7%**
Dietary Fiber 2g	**6%**
Sugars 6g	
Protein 2g	
Vitamin A 0% •	Vitamin C 10%
Calcium 2% •	Iron 3%

2 tablespoons olive oil
1 onion, chopped
2 tablespoons caraway seeds
1 small head of cabbage, shredded
3 russet potatoes, peeled and grated
2 tablespoons sugar
½ cup water
1 teaspoon salt
1 tablespoon apple cider vinegar

In a deep frying pan, brown the onion and caraway seeds in the olive oil. Add the cabbage, potatoes, and sugar and continue to sauté until the cabbage and potatoes are slightly limp and starting to brown. Add the water and salt, then cover and cook over medium-low heat for 30 minutes, stirring occasionally. Remove cover, add vinegar, and continue to cook until all liquid has been absorbed, approximately 10 minutes.

Minty Carrots

NUTRITION FACTS	
Servings per Recipe 6	
Amount Per Serving	
Calories 70	Calories from Fat 19
	% Daily Value*
Total Fat 2g	**3%**
Saturated Fat 1g	**2%**
Cholesterol 0mg	**0%**
Sodium 66mg	**3%**
Total Carbohydrates 12g	**4%**
Dietary Fiber 3g	**14%**
Sugars 8g	
Protein 1g	
Vitamin A 647% •	Vitamin C 20%
Calcium 4% •	Iron 6%

1½ pounds carrots
1 tablespoon chopped fresh mint
1 tablespoon margarine
1 teaspoon flour
1 tablespoon water

Peel carrots and cut diagonally into ¼-inch slices. Place in a pot with about ¼ inch of water and the chopped mint. Bring water to a boil, lower heat, cover and steam until tender, about 10 minutes. Add more water if necessary. Remove carrots with slotted spoon to a plate.

Make a soupy flour paste by mixing the flour with 1 tablespoon of water.

Add the remaining ingredients to the liquid in the pot, including the flour paste. (If all the water was absorbed by the carrots, add ¼ cup of water to the pot.) Cook over medium heat until slightly thickened. Return carrots to pot and toss to coat.

To Serve: Spoon onto plate and garnish with fresh mint sprigs.

Orange Yam Bake

NUTRITION FACTS			
Servings per Recipe 6			
Amount Per Serving			
Calories 295		Calories from Fat 100	
		% Daily Value*	
Total Fat 11g		**18%**	
Saturated Fat 2g		**10%**	
Cholesterol 0mg		**0%**	
Sodium 132mg		**5%**	
Total Carbohydrates 50g		**17%**	
Dietary Fiber 5g		**18%**	
Sugars 27g			
Protein 2g			
Vitamin A	141%	Vitamin C	73%
Calcium	5%	Iron	7%

2 pounds (approximately 2 medium-size) yams (scrubbed and ends removed)
2 oranges
¼ cup honey
2 tablespoons margarine (melted)
¼ cup chopped macadamia nuts

Preheat oven to 350°.

Cut the yams into ½-inch slices. Wash the skins of the oranges and then cut them into ¼-inch slices.

In a flat, shallow pan, alternate and slightly overlap the yam slices with the orange slices.

Mix the melted margarine and honey together. Drizzle over the yams and oranges.

Cover with aluminum foil and bake for 45 minutes. Uncover the yams and sprinkle with the macadamia nuts. Continue to bake for another 15 minutes or until the yams are tender.

Potato Spinach Cups

2 pounds russet potatoes, peeled and cut into large chunks
1 tablespoon olive oil
1 onion, chopped
1 clove garlic, crushed
1 package (12 ounces) frozen chopped spinach, thawed
¼ teaspoon nutmeg
¼ cup nonfat milk
¼ cup bacon bits
Salt to taste
Vegetable-oil spray
½ cup grated Parmesan cheese

NUTRITION FACTS			
Servings per Recipe 6			
Amount Per Serving			
Calories 230		Calories from Fat 50	
			% Daily Value*
Total Fat 6g			**9%**
Saturated Fat 2g			**9%**
Cholesterol 5mg			**2%**
Sodium 297mg			**12%**
Total Carbohydrates 37g			**12%**
Dietary Fiber 5g			**21%**
Sugars 4g			
Protein 9g			
Vitamin A	92%	Vitamin C	33%
Calcium	21%	Iron	9%

Preheat oven to 375°.

Potatoes: Either boil in a big pot of water or microwave until tender. Drain. Mash the potatoes with a ricer, electric mixer, potato masher, or a fork. (Don't use a food processor because it will give your potatoes a gluey texture.)

Spinach and Onions: In a large frying pan, heat the olive oil. Sauté the onion with the garlic. Add the spinach and continue to cook until the spinach is heated.

Mix the potatoes and spinach with the nutmeg, milk, bacon bits, and salt, if desired. Spoon into custard cups that have been sprayed with a vegetable-oil spray. Sprinkle with the Parmesan cheese. Bake in an oven until the cheese has browned, about 15 minutes.

Thai Sweet Squash Stew

8 cups hubbard or similar winter squash (rind removed and squash cut into 1-inch cubes)
6 cups chicken broth
4 cups yams (cut into 1-inch cubes)
3 cups zucchini (cut into ½-inch slices)
4 ounces bean threads ("Saifun")
2 teaspoons coconut extract
½ cup evaporated nonfat milk
Cilantro sprigs

NUTRITION FACTS	
Servings per Recipe 8	
Amount Per Serving	
Calories 250	Calories from Fat 20
	% Daily Value*
Total Fat 2g	**3%**
Saturated Fat 1g	**3%**
Cholesterol 0mg	**0%**
Sodium 620mg	**26%**
Total Carbohydrates 51g	**17%**
Dietary Fiber 11g	**42%**
Sugars 7g	
Protein 10g	
Vitamin A 196% •	Vitamin C 45%
Calcium 10% •	Iron 11%

Place hubbard squash and broth in a deep soup pot. Bring to a boil, then lower heat and simmer until squash is almost tender. Add the yams and zucchini, continuing to cook until they are tender, approximately 20–25 minutes.

While the stew is cooking, place the bean threads in a bowl and cover with hot water. Let sit for 10 minutes. Drain completely. Once yams and zucchini are tender, add the bean threads, extract, and milk. Continue to cook for another 10 minutes.

To Serve: Spoon into soup bowls and garnish with cilantro sprigs.

Thyme Tomatoes on Toast

French bread, cut into ½-inch-thick slices
3 large tomatoes, cut into ¼-inch-thick slices
2 tablespoons margarine
2 tablespoons flour
¾ cup chicken stock or broth
½ cup nonfat milk
¼ teaspoon thyme
Salt
1 cup chopped mushrooms (about ½ pound fresh mushrooms)

NUTRITION FACTS	
Servings per Recipe 6	
Amount Per Serving	
Calories 140	Calories from Fat 45
	% Daily Value*
Total Fat 5g	**8%**
Saturated Fat 1g	**5%**
Cholesterol 0mg	**0%**
Sodium 316mg	**13%**
Total Carbohydrates 20g	**7%**
Dietary Fiber 2g	**6%**
Sugars 3g	
Protein 5g	
Vitamin A 20% •	Vitamin C 21%
Calcium 5% •	Iron 7%

Preheat oven to 325°.

Cover the bottom of a 9-inch x 13-inch baking pan with the French bread slices. Top each bread slice with a tomato slice. Set aside.

In a small saucepan over medium heat, melt the margarine. Add the flour, whisking until the flour is well incorporated into the margarine. Remove the pot from the flame. Whisk in the chicken stock, milk, and thyme. Salt to taste. Decrease heat to low and return pot to the flame, continuing to stir until the mixture has thickened into a creamy sauce consistency.

Pour over the tomato and French bread slices. Sprinkle chopped mushrooms on top. Bake for 20 minutes.

Almond Jewels

NUTRITION FACTS	
Servings per Recipe 4	
Amount Per Serving	
Calories 190	Calories from Fat 2
	% Daily Value*
Total Fat 0g	**0%**
Saturated Fat 0g	**17%**
Cholesterol 2mg	**44%**
Sodium 110mg	**42%**
Total Carbohydrates 39g	**7%**
Dietary Fiber 0g	**36%**
Sugars 37g	
Protein 6g	
Vitamin A 35% •	Vitamin C 2%
Calcium 6% •	Iron 30%

1 package unflavored gelatin
2 tablespoons water
2 cups nonfat milk
½ cup sugar
1 teaspoon almond extract
1 can (11 ounces) mandarin orange segments, natural style
Mint sprigs (optional)

Dissolve the gelatin in the water and set aside. Combine the milk and sugar in a saucepan. Heat to boiling. Add the dissolved gelatin and continue to stir until totally incorporated into the milk mixture. Stir in the almond extract.

Pour into an 8-inch x 8-inch pan and refrigerate until gelled.

To Serve: Cut the almond gel into 1-inch cubes. Serve in glass dishes, spooning the mandarin orange segments and some of their juice over the cubes. Decorate with mint sprigs, if desired.

Brown Rice Pudding

2 cups cooked brown rice
2½ cups nonfat milk
½ cup sugar
½ cup dried apricots (diced)
2 tablespoons pine nuts
¼ teaspoon cinnamon
1 teaspoon vanilla extract
½ cup canned apricot halves, juice packed (drained)

NUTRITION FACTS	
Servings per Recipe 6	
Amount Per Serving	
Calories 225	Calories from Fat 22
	% Daily Value*
Total Fat 2g	**4%**
Saturated Fat 1g	**2%**
Cholesterol 2mg	**1%**
Sodium 55mg	**2%**
Total Carbohydrates 47g	**16%**
Dietary Fiber 1g	**6%**
Sugars 25g	
Protein 6g	
Vitamin A 35% •	Vitamin C 4%
Calcium 14% •	Iron 7%

In a deep saucepan, combine rice, milk, sugar, dried apricots, pine nuts, and cinnamon. Simmer, stirring frequently, until most of the milk has been absorbed and the consistency is creamy. This should take about 15–20 minutes.

Remove from the heat and stir in the vanilla extract.

To Serve: Place in dessert bowls and top with one canned apricot half, cut-side down.

Chocolate Clouds

NUTRITION FACTS	
Servings per Recipe 6	
Amount Per Serving	
Calories 170	Calories from Fat 0
	% Daily Value*
Total Fat 0g	**0%**
Saturated Fat 0g	**0%**
Cholesterol 0mg	**0%**
Sodium 50mg	**2%**
Total Carbohydrates 39g	**13%**
Dietary Fiber 1g	**3%**
Sugars 36g	
Protein 3g	
Vitamin A 0% •	Vitamin C 0%
Calcium 1% •	Iron 2%

4 egg whites (at room temperature)
¼ teaspoon cream of tartar
⅔ cup sugar
½ cup fat-free chocolate syrup
6 maraschino cherries

Preheat oven to 400°.

With an electric mixer on high, beat the egg whites until foamy. Add the cream of tartar and beat a little longer until soft peaks form. Add the sugar gradually, one tablespoon at a time, continuing to beat until all the sugar has been absorbed and stiff peaks have formed. To check that you have beaten the whites sufficiently, run a spatula across the bottom of the bowl, creating a valley in the middle. The sides of your valley shouldn't budge.

Fill a jelly roll pan or large shallow pan with boiling water, 1 inch deep. With a large spoon, drop 6 large mounds of egg whites into the water. Do not allow them to touch. Bake, uncovered, for 5–10 minutes until meringues are golden.

To Serve: Lift each meringue from the water with a slotted spoon and place in individual dessert dishes. Drizzle each meringue with chocolate syrup. Top with a maraschino cherry.

Date Oatmeal Bars

Filling:
2 cups finely cut pitted dates
½ cup brown sugar (firmly packed)
1 tablespoon flour
1 cup water
1 tablespoon vanilla extract

Crust:
1 cup all-purpose flour
1 tablespoon baking soda
¾ cup brown sugar (firmly packed)
2 cups rolled oats
¾ cup melted margarine
Vegetable-oil spray

NUTRITION FACTS	
Servings per Recipe 36	
Amount Per Serving	
Calories 120	Calories from Fat 37
	% Daily Value*
Total Fat 4g	**6%**
Saturated Fat 1g	**4%**
Cholesterol 0mg	**0%**
Sodium 160mg	**7%**
Total Carbohydrates 21g	**7%**
Dietary Fiber 1g	**5%**
Sugars 13g	
Protein 1g	
Vitamin A 10% •	Vitamin C 0%
Calcium 1% •	Iron 3%

Preheat oven to 375°.

Filling: Combine the dates, brown sugar, and flour in a small saucepan. Add the water and bring to a boil. Then simmer for about 10–15 minutes or until thickened. Add the vanilla extract. Set aside to cool.

Crust: Combine the flour, baking soda, brown sugar, and oats in a deep bowl. Gradually add the melted margarine, stirring to incorporate into flour mixture. Spread evenly ½ of the oatmeal mixture in the bottom of a 13-inch x 9-inch x 1-inch baking pan that has been lightly greased with vegetable-oil spray. Top oatmeal layer with date mixture. Then sprinkle remaining oatmeal mixture on top of the date layer. Pat lightly with a spoon.

Bake for about 20 minutes. Cool in pan. Cut into 2-inch x 1½-inch squares.

Meringue Cookies

NUTRITION FACTS	
Servings per Recipe 18	
Amount Per Serving	
Calories 50	Calories from Fat 0
	% Daily Value*
Total Fat 0g	**0%**
Saturated Fat 0g	**0%**
Cholesterol 0mg	**0%**
Sodium 12mg	**1%**
Total Carbohydrates 11g	**4%**
Dietary Fiber 0g	**0%**
Sugars 11g	
Protein 1g	
Vitamin A 0% •	Vitamin C 0%
Calcium 0% •	Iron 0%

4 egg whites (at room temperature)
½ teaspoon lemon juice
1 cup sugar
1 teaspoon vanilla extract

Options:
½ cup chocolate chips or
½ cup diced dried apricots or
½ cup raisins or
3 tablespoons of each of the above

Preheat oven to 200°.

Line 2 lightly greased cookie sheets with parchment paper or brown paper.

With an electric mixer on high, beat the egg whites until foamy. Add the lemon juice and beat a little longer until soft peaks form. Add the sugar gradually, one tablespoon at a time, continuing to beat until all the sugar has been absorbed and stiff peaks have formed. To check that you have beaten the whites sufficiently, run a spatula across the bottom of the bowl, creating a valley in the middle. If the sides of your valley don't budge, you're ready to add the vanilla and continue to beat until well mixed. Then fold in your choice of options, if desired. Spoon about 2 tablespoons of the meringue per cookie onto the cookie sheets, leaving about 1-inch space between each cookie.

Bake for at least 1 to 1½ hours, or until dry and crispy. You can even leave them in the oven overnight without the burner on if they need longer to dry. Store in airtight container.

Mexican Peach Pastries

NUTRITION FACTS			
Servings per Recipe 6			
Amount Per Serving			
Calories 275		Calories from Fat 17	
			% Daily Value*
Total Fat 2g			**3%**
Saturated Fat 1g			**6%**
Cholesterol 11mg			**4%**
Sodium 280mg			**12%**
Total Carbohydrates 55g			**18%**
Dietary Fiber 8g			**31%**
Sugars 31g			
Protein 12g			
Vitamin A 8%	•	Vitamin C	6%
Calcium 32%	•	Iron	2%

¾ teaspoon cinnamon
¾ cup sugar
6 small (6-inch) fat-free flour tortillas
1½ cups low-fat ricotta cheese
2 cups sliced fresh peaches
¼ cup orange marmalade

Preheat oven to 350°.

Mix the cinnamon and sugar in a bowl and set aside.

On each tortilla round, spread about ¼ cup of the ricotta cheese to about ½ inch of the edge . Evenly sprinkle the cinnamon and sugar over the ricotta cheese. Place on ungreased baking sheet. Arrange peach slices decoratively in concentric circles over the cheese. Bake for 20 minutes. Remove from oven and let cool thoroughly.

In a small saucepan, heat the orange marmalade to a liquid state. Lightly brush the peaches with the melted marmalade.

Moroccan Orange Slices

NUTRITION FACTS	
Servings per Recipe 6	
Amount Per Serving	
Calories 140	Calories from Fat 1
	% Daily Value*
Total Fat 0g	**0%**
Saturated Fat 0g	**0%**
Cholesterol 0mg	**0%**
Sodium 1mg	**0%**
Total Carbohydrates 38g	**13%**
Dietary Fiber 3g	**11%**
Sugars 35g	
Protein 1g	
Vitamin A 4% •	Vitamin C 88%
Calcium 5% •	Iron 2%

3 medium oranges
⅜ cup honey
1 teaspoon ground cinnamon

Peel oranges and cut into ¼-inch slices. Arrange in a shallow dish. Heat the honey slightly and pour over the orange slices. Sprinkle with the ground cinnamon. Refrigerate for 1–2 hours before serving.

Rocky Road Rice Pudding

1 package (3.4 ounces) instant chocolate pudding
2 cups nonfat milk
2 cups cooked white rice (cooled to room temperature)
½ cup miniature marshmallows
¼ cup chopped walnuts
2 tablespoons rum (optional)

NUTRITION FACTS
Servings per Recipe 6

Amount Per Serving	
Calories 230	Calories from Fat 29
	% Daily Value*
Total Fat 3g	**5%**
Saturated Fat 1g	**2%**
Cholesterol 1mg	**0%**
Sodium 300mg	**12%**
Total Carbohydrates 45g	**15%**
Dietary Fiber 1g	**3%**
Sugars 19g	
Protein 6g	
Vitamin A 10% •	Vitamin C 2%
Calcium 11% •	Iron 10%

Prepare the chocolate pudding with the nonfat milk according to package instructions.

In a deep bowl, mix all the ingredients together, including the pudding. Then serve.

APPENDIXES

Appendix A

Animal Protein Sources

Food	**Low-Fat** Up to 3 grams of fat per serving (On food labels: 5% or less DV)	**Medium-Fat** 4-13 grams of fat per serving (On food labels: 6-19% DV)	**High-Fat** 14+ grams of fat per serving (On food labels: ≥20% DV)
Beef		Ground beef (10% fat), round, top loin, tenderloin, sirloin	Corned beef, ground beef (17% fat), meatloaf, prime cuts of beef, short ribs
Fish	Cod, flounder, halibut, trout, snapper, shark, tuna (canned in water)	Herring, oysters, salmon, sardines, tuna (canned in oil)	Fried fish
Lamb		Leg, loin chop	Ground lamb, rib roast
Pork		Center and top loin chops, roast, tenderloin 🧂 Canadian bacon, ham	Ground pork, spareribs 🧂 Bacon, pork sausage
Poultry	Skinless breast of chicken or turkey	Dark meat, ground turkey, ground chicken	Fried chicken
Shellfish	Clams, crab, lobster, scallops, shrimp, surimi (imitation shellfish)		
Egg	Whites, egg substitute	Whole	
Processed Meat	🧂 Fat-free or low-fat sandwich meat or hot dogs		🧂 Bologna, frankfurter, salami, sausage
Dairy	Cottage cheese, fat-free cheese, grated Parmesan, skim milk, low-fat milk, low-fat yogurt	Feta, low-fat cream cheese, mozzarella, ricotta	American, Brie, Blue, Cheddar, cream cheese, Monterey Jack, Swiss

🧂 = High salt content

Appendix B

Vegetable Protein Sources

Food	**Low-Fat** Up to 3 grams of fat per serving (On food labels: 5% or less DV)	**Medium-Fat** 4-13 grams of fat per serving (On food labels: 6-19% DV)	**High-Fat** 14+ grams of fat per serving (On food labels: ≥20% DV)
Legumes	Dried beans, lentils, peas	Tofu, tempeh (processed tofu product)	
Nuts	Chinese chestnuts, European chestnuts		Almonds, Brazil nuts, cashews, hazelnuts, peanuts, pecans, walnuts
Seeds		Pumpkin	Sesame, sunflower
Meat Substitutes		Falafel, veggie burgers	

Appendix C

Carbohydrate Sources

Food	**Low-Fat** Up to 3 grams of fat per serving (On food labels: 5% or less DV)	**Medium-Fat** 4-13 grams of fat per serving (On food labels: 6-19% DV)	**High-Fat** 14+ grams of fat per serving (On food labels: ≥20% DV)
BREADS, CEREALS, CRACKERS, GRAINS AND PASTA			
Breads	Bagels, breads, English muffins, rolls, pita, tortilla, pancakes	Biscuits, fried tortilla, breakfast bars, French toast, toaster pastries, waffles	Stuffing
Cereals	Cooked cereals, ready-to-eat cereals	Granola bars, specialty ready-to-eat cereals	
Crackers	Saltines	Snack rounds	
Pasta	Spaghetti, macaroni, Oriental noodles	Fried Oriental noodles, pasta and sauce	Pasta and cheese sauce
Rice and Other Grains	Steamed rice, amaranth, barley, groats, bulgar, couscous, quinoa, unbuttered popcorn	Fried rice, rice dishes, grain dishes, buttered popcorn	
Desserts	Angel food cake, graham crackers, low-fat cookies	Cookies, dessert bars, brownies, unfrosted cake, puddings	Frosted cakes, doughnuts, pie

Appendix C Continued

Food	**Low-Fat** Up to 3 grams of fat per serving (On food labels: 5% or less DV)	**Medium-Fat** 4-13 grams of fat per serving (On food labels: 6-19% DV)	**High-Fat** 14+ grams of fat per serving (On food labels: ≥20% DV)
		VEGETABLES	
	Fresh, frozen, canned, dried, baked potato	Potatoes with toppings (other than cheese)	Cheese-topped potatoes, potato skins, French fries
		FRUITS	
	Fresh, canned, frozen, dried, sorbet		Fruit pie
		EXTRAS	
Candy	Hard candy	Candied coconut, plain chocolate	Specialty chocolate candy
Sugar	White, brown, raw; soft drinks	Cookies, dessert bars, brownies, unfrosted cakes, puddings	Frosted cakes, doughnuts, pie
Syrup	Corn, chocolate, maple		

Appendix D

Water-Soluble Vitamins

Vitamin	Major Functions	Food Sources
C	Helps to make collagen, hormones, neurotransmitters; protective for firm blood vessels, healthy gums, wound healing, immune system	Asparagus, broccoli, Brussels sprouts, cantaloupe, cranberry juice, dark green leafy vegetables, kiwi, papaya, oranges, red and green peppers, potatoes, spinach, strawberries, tomatoes
Cobalamin (B_{12})	Works with folate to make red blood cells; helps with nerve function	Animal products
Folate	Helps in making DNA and RNA (master blueprints for cells); works with B_{12} to make hemoglobin (blood)	Green leafy vegetables, orange juice, legumes, liver, enriched grains
Niacin	Helps in energy metabolism; skin health; vision	Poultry, fish, beef, peanut butter, legumes
Pyridoxine (B_6)	Helps to make some amino acids; helps to make red blood cells; involved in fat metabolism	Poultry, fish, pork, shellfish, legumes, enriched grains, green and leafy vegetables
Riboflavin (B_2)	Helps in energy metabolism; skin health; vision	Milk, dairy products, green leafy vegetables, beef, pork, enriched grains, nuts
Thiamin (B_1)	Helps produce energy from carbohydrates; functioning of nervous system	Liver, pork, whole and enriched grain products, legumes (dried beans), nuts, sunflower seeds

Appendix E

Fat-Soluble Vitamins

Vitamin	Major Functions	Food Sources
A and Beta-carotene	Night vision; growth; prevent skin and eyes from drying out; promote resistance to bacterial infections; antioxidant when in the form of carotenoids	Broccoli, cantaloupe, carrots, collard greens, fortified milk, kale, liver, mango, mustard greens, pumpkin, spinach, sweet potato, Swiss chard, winter squash
D	Helps in the absorption of calcium from the intestine; promotes optimal amount of calcium in bone and teeth	Fortified milk, tuna fish, eggs, liver, salmon
E	Powerful antioxidant to protect cells from oxidation and damage	Nuts, fortified cereals, sweet potato, sunflower seeds, vegetable oils, wheat germ
K	Helps in blood clotting	Leafy green vegetables, broccoli, liver, wheat bran and germ

Appendix F

Minerals

Mineral	Major Functions	Food Sources
Calcium	Major component of bone and teeth; transmission of nerve impulses; contraction of muscle	Dairy products, tofu processed with calcium, canned fish with bones, broccoli, collards, kale, leafy vegetables
Iodide	Part of the thyroid hormone involved in metabolism	Iodized salt, seafood, fish, dairy products
Iron	An essential part of hemoglobin (blood) for carrying around oxygen in the blood; involved in immune function	Meats, seafood, spinach, broccoli, enriched grains, liver, oysters, dried beans
Magnesium	Part of many enzymes that regulate body functions; part of bones	Legumes, nuts, whole grains, green vegetables
Phosphorus	Involved in strength of bones and teeth; helps generate energy in cells; part of DNA and RNA cells	Dairy products, meat, poultry, fish, eggs, legumes, nuts
Potassium	Helps regulate fluid and mineral balances inside and outside of cells; helps regulate blood pressure; involved in nerve impulses and muscle contractions	Bananas, oranges, potatoes, spinach, vegetables, meat, poultry, fish, dairy products

Appendix F Continued

Mineral	Major Functions	Food Sources
Selenium	Acts with vitamin E as antioxidant to reduce cell destruction	Meats, eggs, fish, whole grains
Sodium	Helps regulate movement of fluid between inside and outside of cells; helps transmit nerve impulses; helps regulate blood pressure	Processed foods, table salt, cured meats, soy sauce, canned soups
Zinc	Helps in cell reproduction; aids growth and repair of tissue; part of many enzymes; involved in immune function	Seafood, meats, some vegetables, whole grains, plain yogurt, chick peas

Appendix G

Body Mass Index Table

	BODY MASS INDEX (BMI)													
	19	20	21	22	23	24	25	26	27	28	29	30	35	40
HEIGHT	WEIGHT (pounds)													
4′10″	91	96	100	105	110	115	119	124	129	134	138	143	167	191
4′11″	94	99	104	109	114	119	124	128	133	138	143	148	173	198
5′0″	97	102	107	112	118	123	128	133	138	143	148	153	179	204
5′1″	100	106	111	116	122	127	132	137	143	148	153	158	185	211
5′2″	104	109	115	120	126	131	136	142	147	153	158	164	191	218
5′3″	107	113	118	124	130	135	141	146	152	158	163	169	197	225
5′4″	110	116	122	128	134	140	145	151	157	163	169	174	204	232
5′5″	114	120	126	132	138	144	150	156	162	168	174	180	210	240
5′6″	118	124	130	136	142	148	155	161	167	173	179	186	216	247
5′7″	121	127	134	140	146	153	159	166	172	178	185	191	223	255
5′8″	125	131	138	144	151	158	164	171	177	184	190	197	230	262
5′9″	128	135	142	149	155	162	169	176	182	189	196	203	236	270
5′10″	132	139	146	153	160	167	174	181	188	195	202	207	243	278
5′11″	136	143	150	157	165	172	179	186	193	200	208	215	250	286
6′0″	140	147	154	162	169	177	184	191	199	206	213	221	258	294
6′1″	144	151	159	166	174	182	189	197	204	212	219	227	265	302
6′2″	148	155	163	171	179	186	194	202	210	218	225	233	272	311
6′3″	152	160	168	176	184	192	200	208	216	224	232	240	279	319
6′4″	156	164	172	180	189	197	205	213	221	230	238	246	287	328
	NORMAL						OVERWEIGHT					OBESE		

Source: National Institutes of Health, 1998.

Appendix H

Metropolitan Height and Weight Table for Females*

FEMALES			
Height (inches)	**Small Frame**	**Medium Frame**	**Large Frame**
57″	99–108	106–118	115–128
58″	100–110	108–120	117–131
59″	101–112	110–123	119–134
60″	103–115	112–126	122–137
61″	105–118	115–129	125–140
62″	108–121	118–132	128–144
63″	111–124	121–135	131–148
64″	114–127	124–138	134–152
65″	117–130	127–141	137–156
66″	120–133	130–144	140–160
67″	123–136	133–147	143–164
68″	126–139	136–150	146–167
69″	129–142	139–153	149–170
70″	132–145	142–156	152–173
71″	135–148	145–159	155–176

*Adapted version—weights shown are in pounds and without shoes and clothes.

Appendix H (Continued)

Metropolitan Height and Weight Table for Males*

MALES			
Height (inches)	**Small Frame**	**Medium Frame**	**Large Frame**
61″	123–129	126–136	133–145
62″	125–131	128–138	135–148
63″	127–133	130–140	137–151
64″	129–135	132–143	139–155
65″	131–137	134–146	141–159
66″	133–140	137–149	144–163
67″	135–143	140–152	147–167
68″	137–146	143–155	150–171
69″	139–149	146–158	153–175
70″	141–152	149–161	156–179
71″	144–155	152–165	159–183
72″	147–159	155–169	163–187
73″	150–163	159–173	167–192
74″	153–167	162–177	171–197
75″	157–171	166–182	176–202

*Adapted version—weights shown are in pounds and without shoes and clothes.

Appendix I

*% Daily Value Converter**

% Daily Value Listed on the Label	CALORIES						
	1200	**1500**	**1800**	**2200**	**2500**	**2800**	**3000**
1%	2	1	1	1	1	1	1
2%	3	3	2	2	2	1	1
3%	5	4	3	3	2	2	2
4%	7	5	4	4	3	3	3
5%	8	7	6	5	4	4	3
6%	10	8	7	5	5	4	4
7%	12	9	8	6	6	5	5
8%	13	11	9	7	6	6	5
9%	15	12	10	8	7	6	6
10%	17	13	11	9	8	7	7

% Daily Value (DV) is the portion of your daily nutrient needs supplied by the food. The % DVs listed on the label are for a 2,000 calorie diet.

If you eat more or fewer than 2000 calories a day, this converter adjusts % DV to your calorie level.

% Daily Value Listed on the Label	Adjusted % Daily Value						
11%	18	15	12	10	9	8	7
12%	20	16	13	11	10	9	8
13%	22	17	14	12	10	9	9
14%	23	19	16	13	11	10	9
15%	25	20	17	14	12	11	10
16%	27	21	18	15	13	11	11
17%	28	23	19	15	14	12	11
18%	30	24	20	16	14	13	12
19%	32	25	21	17	15	13	13
20%	33	27	22	18	16	14	13
21%	35	28	23	19	17	15	14
22%	37	29	24	20	18	16	15
23%	38	31	26	21	18	16	15
24%	40	32	27	22	19	17	16
25%	42	33	28	23	20	18	17

To use:

1. In the first column, find the % DV listed on the label for any nutrient (except cholesterol and sodium, which have the same % DV as on the label for all calorie levels).
2. Run your finger across that row until you come to the column with your calorie needs.
3. The number you see there is your **Adjusted % Daily Value** for your calorie level.

Appendix I Continued

% Daily Value Listed on the Label	CALORIES						
	1200	**1500**	**1800**	**2200**	**2500**	**2800**	**3000**
26%	43	35	29	24	21	18	17
27%	45	36	30	25	22	19	18
28%	46	37	31	25	22	20	19
29%	48	39	32	26	23	21	19
30%	50	40	33	27	24	21	20
31%	51	41	34	28	25	22	21
32%	53	43	36	29	26	23	21
33%	55	44	37	30	26	23	22
34%	56	45	38	31	27	24	23
35%	58	47	39	32	28	25	23

Adjusted % Daily Value

*From *Beyond Food Labels* by Roberta Schwartz Wennik, MS, RD, Perigee, 1996.

References and Resources for Further Reading

Psychological Type

Duniho, Terence. *Wholeness Lies Within: Sixteen Natural Paths Toward Spirituality.* Gladwyne, Pa.: Type and Temperament, 1991.

Hirsh, Sandra, and Jean Kummerow. *Life Types: Understand Yourself and Make the Most of Who You Are.* New York: Warner, 1989.

Keirsey, David, and Marilyn Bates. *Please Understand Me: Character and Temperament Types.* Del Mar, Calif.: Prometheus Nemesis, 1984.

Kroeger, Otto, and Janet Thuesen. *Type Talk: The 16 Personality Types That Determine How We Live, Love and Work.* New York: Dell, 1988.

Lawrence, Gordon. *People Types and Tiger Stripes.* Gainesville, Fla.: Center for Applications of Psychological Type, 1995.

Murray, William. *Give Yourself the Unfair Advantage!* Gladwyne, Pa.: Type and Temperament, 1995.

Myers, Isabel Briggs, and Mary McCaulley. *Manual: Guide to the Development and Use of the Myers-Briggs Type Indicator.* Palo Alto, Calif.: Consulting Psychologists, 1985.

Myers, Isabel Briggs, and Peter B. Myers. *Gifts Differing: Understanding Personality Type.* Palo Alto, Calif.: Davies-Black, 1995.

Quenk, Naomi. *Beside Ourselves: Our Hidden Personality in Everyday Life.* Palo Alto, Calif.: Davies-Black, 1993.

Tieger, Paul D., and Barbara Barron-Tieger. *Do What You Are:*

Discover the Perfect Career for You Through the Secrets of Personality Type. Boston: Little, Brown, 1992.

Health

Hunt, Sara, and James Groff. *Advanced Nutrition and Human Metabolism.* St. Paul: West, 1990.

Logue, A.W. *The Psychology of Eating and Drinking.* New York: W.H. Freeman, 1986.

Mahan, L.K., and Marian Arlin. *Krause's Food, Nutrition and Diet Therapy.* Philadelphia: W.B. Saunders, 1992.

Marieb, Elaine. *Human Anatomy and Physiology,* 2nd Ed. Redwood City, Calif.: Benjamin/Cummings, 1992.

McGee, Harold. *On Food and Cooking: The Science and Lore of the Kitchen.* New York: Collier, 1984.

Pennington, Jean A. *Bowes and Church's Food Values of Portions Commonly Used,* 16th Ed. Philadelphia: J.B. Lippincott, 1994.

Rahamimoff, P. *Appetite and Lack of Appetite in Infancy and Early Childhood.* Alabama: Strode, 1979.

University of California at Berkeley. *The New Wellness Encyclopedia.* Boston: Houghton Mifflin, 1995.

Vander, Arthur, James Sherman, and Dorothy Luciano. *Human Physiology: The Mechanisms of Body Function,* 4th Ed. New York: McGraw-Hill, 1985.

Heart Disease

About High Blood Pressure. 50-052-D. American Heart Association, 1989.

How Stroke Affects Behavior. 50-1019. American Heart Association, 1989.

Cancer

Dietary Guidelines to Lower Cancer Risk. AIRC Information Series. American Institute for Cancer Research, 1984.

Facts You Should Know About Outdoor Cooking. AIRC Information Series. American Institute for Cancer Research, March 1986.

The Cancer Process. AIRC Information Series. American Institute for Cancer Research, March 1986.

Cancer Facts and Figures—1997. 97-300M-No.5008.97. American Cancer Society, 1997.

Cancer Prevention—Good News, Better News, Best News. U.S. Department of Health and Human Services.

Cigarette Smoking: The Facts About Your Lungs. American Lung Association, March 1987.

Facts About . . . Second-Hand Smoke. American Lung Association, June 1988.

Nutrition and Cancer Prevention: A Guide to Food Choices by Charles DiSogra. Department of Health and Social Services, 1981.

Diabetes

Diabetes Info: Diabetes Facts and Figures. American Diabetes Association, 1997.

Stress and Relaxation

Benson, Herbert, and Eileen M. Stuart. *The Wellness Book: The Comprehensive Guide to Maintaining Health and Treating Stress-Related Illness.* New York: Simon & Schuster, 1992.

Benson, Herbert. *The Relaxation Response.* New York: Avon, 1976.

Cousins, Norman. *Anatomy of an Illness as Perceived by the Patient.* New York: W.W. Norton, 1979.

Cousins, Norman. *Head First: The Biology of Hope.* New York: E.P. Dutton, 1989.

Curtis, John D., and Richard A. Detert. *How to Relax: A Holistic Approach to Stress Management.* Palo Alto, Calif.: Mayfield, 1981.

Davis, Martha, Elizabeth Robbins Eshelman, and Matthew McKay. *The Relaxation and Stress Workbook.* Oakland, Calif.: New Harbinger, 1988.

Metcalf, C.W., and Roma Felible. *Lighten Up: Survival Skills for People Under Pressure.* Menlo Park, Calif.: Addison-Wesley, 1992.

Make It Last

Fletcher, Anne M. *Thin For Life: 10 Keys to Success.* Shelburne,VT: Chapters, 1994.

Marlatt, G. Alan, and Judith R. Gordon. *Relapse Prevention.* New York: Guilford, 1985.

Prochaska, James, John Norcross, and Carlo Diclemente. *Changing for Good.* New York: Avon, 1994.

Robertson, Douglas L. *Self-Directed Growth.* Muncie, Ind.: Accelerated Development, 1988.

Surveys and Trends

1995 Final Mortality Statistics. Released. National Center for Health Statistics, 1997.

1997 Heart and Stroke Statistical Update. American Heart Association, 1998.

"Nutrition and Cancer Prevention Knowledge, Beliefs, Attitudes, and Practices" by Nancy Cotugna et al. 1987 National Health Interview Survey. *Journal of the American Dietetic Association.* August 1992. Vol. 92, No. 8.

"Nutrition Trends Survey 1997 (Executive Summary)." The American Dietetic Association. September 1997.

"More Americans Are Eating Meals Away from Home, Says USDA (Federal Update)." Journal of the American Dietetic Association. February 1997. Vol 7, No. 1., 128.

"How Americans Are Making Food Choices." International Food Information Council. 1989 Survey.

"Report Card on the American Diet." USDA NEWS, Release No. 0568.95.

Consumer-Friendly Newsletters, Magazines, and Miscellaneous

Cooking Light. 4929 Wilshire Blvd., Suite 690, Los Angeles, CA 90010.

Eating Well. Telemedia Communications. Ferry Road, P.O. Box 1001, Charlotte, VT 05445–1001.

Environmental Nutrition. Environmental Nutrition, Inc. 52 Riverside Drive, New York, NY 10024–6599.

Health and Nutrition Letter. Tufts University Health & Nutrition Letter. 53 Park Place, New York, NY 10007.

Nutrition Action Health Letter. Center for Science in the Public Interest. 1875 Connecticut Avenue, NW, Suite 300, Washington, DC 20009–5728.

In Closing . . .

I'd love to hear from you about your success changing your habits using your personality type. What were you able to change? What did you find the most valuable part of this book? What challenges did you face in the process of changing? What excuses had you used in the past to avoid changing?

If you have any questions, thoughts, or ideas you'd like to share, I'd welcome hearing from you. Drop me a line at:

HealthPro
P.O. Box 83
Lynnwood, WA 98046-0083
or
E-mail me at roberta@foxinternet.net

When you write me, please include your personality type and address. That way I can send you pertinent information updates or newsletters.

To obtain me as a speaker, call me at (425) 778-1340. You can also write or E-mail me at the above addresses.

The best to you,

Roberta Wesnik

Metric Conversion Chart

Temperature Conversion

Formulas for conversion

Fahrenheit to Celsius: subtract 32, multiply by 5, then divide by 9

for example:

212°F – 32 = 180

180 × 5 = 900

900 ÷ 9 = 100°C

Celsius to Fahrenheit: multiply by 9, the divide by 5, then add 32

for example:

100°C × 9 = 900

900 ÷ 5 = 180

180 + 32 = 212°F

Temperatures (Fahrenheit to Celsius)

–10°F =	–23°C	coldest part of freezer
0°F =	–17°C	freezer
32°F =	0°C	water freezes
68°F =	20°C	room temperature
85°F =	29°C	
100°F =	38°C	
115°F =	46°C	water simmers
135°F =	57°C	water scalds

Temperatures (Fahrenheit to Celsius) *cont.*

140°F = 60°C	
150°F = 66°C	
160°F = 71°C	
170°F = 77°C	
180°F = 82°C	water simmers
190°F = 88°C	
200°F = 95°C	
205°F = 96°C	water simmers
212°F = 100°C	water boils, at sea level
225°F = 110°C	
250°F = 120°C	very low (or slow) oven
275°F = 135°C	very low (or slow) oven
300°F = 150°C	low (or slow) oven
325°F = 165°C	low (or moderately slow) oven
350°F = 180°C	moderate oven
375°F = 190°C	moderate (or moderately hot) oven
400°F = 205°C	hot oven
425°F = 220°C	hot oven
450°F = 230°C	very hot oven
475°F = 245°C	very hot oven
500°F = 260°C	extremely hot oven/broiling
525°F = 275°C	extremely hot oven/broiling

LIQUID MEASURES CONVERSION

For foods such as yogurt, applesauce, or cottage cheese that are not quite liquid, but not quite solid, use fluid measures for conversion.

Both systems, the US Standard and Metric, use spoon measures. The sizes are slightly different, but the difference is not significant in general cooking (It may, however, be significant in baking.)

Tbs = tablespoon   teas = teaspoon

Spoons, cups, pints, quarts	**Fluid oz**	**Milliliters (ml), deciliters (dl) and liters (l); rounded off**
1 teaspoon (tsp)	1/6 oz	5 ml
3 tsp (1 Tbs)	½ oz	15 ml
1 Tbs	1 oz	¼ dl (or 1 Tbs)
4 Tbs (¼ c)	2 oz	½ dl (or 4 Tbs)
⅓ c	2⅔ oz	¾ dl
½ c	4 oz	1 dl
¾ c	6 oz	1¾ dl
1 c	8 oz	250 ml (or ¼ L)
2 c (1 pint)	16 oz	500 ml (or ½ L)
4 c (1 quart)	32 oz	1 L
4 qt (1 gallon)	128 oz	3¾ L

Solid Measures Conversion

Converting solid measures between US standard and metrics is not as straightforward as it might seem. The density of the substance being measured makes a big difference in the volume to weight conversion. For example, 1 tablespoon of flour is ¼ ounce and 8.75 grams whereas 1 tablespoon of butter or shortening is ½ ounce and 15 grams. The following chart is intended as a guide only, some experimentation may be necessary to achieve success.

Formulas for conversion

ounces to grams: multiply ounces by 28.35

grams to ounces: multiply grams figure by .035

ounces	pounds	grams	kilograms
1		30	
4	¼	115	
8	½	225	
9		250	¼
12	¾	430	
16	1	450	
18		500	½
	2¼	1000	1
	5		2¼
	10		4½

Linear Measures Conversion

Pan sizes are very different in countries that use metrics versus the US standard. This is more significant in baking than in general cooking.

Formulas for conversion

inches to centimeters: multiply the inch by 2.54

centimeters to inches: multiply the centimeter by 0.39

inches	cm	inches	cm
½	1½	9	23
1	2½	10	25
2	5	12 (1 ft.)	30
3	8	14	35
4	10	15	38½
5	13	16	40
6	15	18	45
7	18	20	50
8	20	24 (2 ft.)	60

Index